Geriatric Dermatology Update

Editor

NICOLE M. BURKEMPER

CLINICS IN GERIATRIC MEDICINE

www.geriatric.theclinics.com

Consulting Editor
G. MICHAEL HARPER

February 2024 • Volume 40 • Number 1

ELSEVIER

1600 John F. Kennedy Boulevard • Suite 1800 • Philadelphia, Pennsylvania, 19103-2899

http://www.theclinics.com

CLINICS IN GERIATRIC MEDICINE Volume 40, Number 1
February 2024 ISSN 0749–0690, ISBN-13: 978-0-443-12149-4

Editor: Taylor Hayes
Developmental Editor: Anita Chamoli

Clinics in Geriatric Medicine (ISSN 0749-0690) is published quarterly by Elsevier Inc., 360 Park Avenue South, New York, NY 10010-1710. Months of issue are February, May, August, and November. Business and Editorial Offices: 1600 John F. Kennedy Blvd., Suite 1800, Philadelphia, PA 191023-2899. Periodicals postage paid at New York, NY, and additional mailing offices. Subscription prices are $321.00 per year (US individuals), $100.00 per year (US & Canadian student/resident), $340.00 per year (Canadian individuals), $457.00 per year (international individuals), and $195.00 per year (international student/resident). For institutional access pricing please contact Customer Service via the contact information below. Foreign air speed delivery is included in all *Clinics* subscription prices. All prices are subject to change without notice. POSTMASTER: Send address changes to *Clinics in Geriatric Medicine*, Elsevier Health Sciences Division, Subscription Customer Service, 3251 Riverport Lane, Maryland Heights, MO 63043. **Telephone: 1-800-654-2452 (U.S. and Canada); 314-447-8871 (outside U.S. and Canada). Fax: 314-447-8029.** E-mail: journalscustomerservice-usa@elsevier.com **(for print support) or** journalsonlinesupport-usa@elsevier.com **(for online support).**

Reprints. For copies of 100 or more, of articles in this publication, please contact the Commercial Reprints Department, Elsevier Inc., 360 Park Avenue South, New York, New York 10010-1710. Tel.: 212-633-3874; Fax: 212-633-3820, E-mail: reprints@elsevier.com.

Clinics in Geriatric Medicine is covered in *MEDLINE/PubMed (Index Medicus), EMBASE/Excerpta Medica, Current Contents/Clinical Medicine (CC/CM)*, and the *Cumulative Index to Nursing & Allied Health Literature*.

Contributors

CONSULTING EDITOR

G. MICHAEL HARPER, MD
Professor of Medicine, Geriatrics Department of Medicine, University of California, San Francisco San Francisco, California

EDITOR

NICOLE M. BURKEMPER, MD
Professor of Dermatology and Pathology, SSM Health Saint Louis University School of Medicine, St. Louis, Missouri

AUTHORS

ASHLEY ALLEN, MD
Resident Physician, Department of Dermatology, Tulane University School of Medicine, New Orleans, Louisiana

ANYA ANOKHIN, MD
Resident Physician, University of Missouri, Columbia, Missouri

NICOLE M. BURKEMPER, MD
Professor of Dermatology and Pathology, SSM Health Saint Louis University School of Medicine, St. Louis, Missouri

SOFIA CHAUDHRY, MD
Associate Professor, Department of Dermatology, Saint Louis University School of Medicine, St. Louis, Missouri

MARTHA LAURIN COUNCIL, MD, MBA, FAAD, FACMS
Director of Dermatologic Surgery, Professor of Dermatology, Department of Medicine (Dermatology), Washington University School of Medicine in St. Louis, St. Louis, Missouri

KAVITA DARJI, MD
Research Physician, Department of Dermatology, Saint Louis University, St. Louis, Missouri

JENNIFER FEHLMAN, MD
Assistant Professor, Saint Louis University SLU Care Physician Group - SSM Health, St. Louis, Missouri

AIBING MARY GUO, MD, MS
Assistant Professor, Department of Dermatology, Saint Louis University School of Medicine, St. Louis, Missouri

MONICA HESSLER-WANING, MD
Dermatology Research Fellow, Department of Dermatology, Saint Louis University, St. Louis, Missouri

GILLIAN HEINECKE, MD
Assistant Professor, Department of Dermatology, Saint Louis University, St. Louis, Missouri

MARIA YADIRA HURLEY, MD
Professor, Department of Dermatology, Saint Louis University School of Medicine, St. Louis, Missouri

MICHAEL KREMER, MD
Resident Physician, Department of Dermatology, Saint Louis University, St. Louis, Missouri

KATHRYN LEE, BA
Saint Louis University School of Medicine, St. Louis, Missouri

EAMONN MAHER, MD
Assistant Professor, Department of Dermatology, University of Minnesota, Minneapolis

SINO MEHRMAL, DO
Resident Physician, Department of Dermatology, Saint Louis University School of Medicine, St. Louis, Missouri

SHAKIRA MELTAN, BS
Medical Student, School of Medicine, Texas Tech University Health Sciences Center, Lubbock, Texas

TRICIA A. MISSALL, MD, PhD
Clinical Associate Professor, Department of Dermatology, University of Florida College of Medicine, Gainesville, Florida

RAFAEL MOJICA, DO
Resident Physician, Department of Dermatology, University of Florida College of Medicine, Gainesville, Florida

ANDREA MURINA, MD
Professor, Department of Dermatology, Tulane University School of Medicine, New Orleans, Louisiana

ADITYA NELLORE, MD
Resident Physician, Department of Internal Medicine, St. Luke's Hospital, St. Louis, Missouri

AMANDA A. ONALAJA-UNDERWOOD, MD
Resident Physician, Department of Dermatology, Vanderbilt University Medical Center, Nashville, Tennessee

BHARAT PANUGANTI, MD
Assistant Professor, Department of Otolaryngology, The University of Alabama at Birmingham, School of Medicine, Birmingham, Alabama

MACKENZIE POOLE, MBA
Medical Student, Saint Louis University School of Medicine, St. Louis, Missouri

SANIYA SHAIKH, DO
Department of Dermatology, SSM Health SLU Care Physician Group Saint Louis
University School of Medicine, St. Louis, Missouri

SHEETAL K. SETHUPATHI, MD
Resident Physician, Department of Dermatology, Saint Louis University, St. Louis,
Missouri

DAVID M. SHEINBEIN, MD
Professor of Dermatology, Department of Medicine (Dermatology), Washington University
School of Medicine in St. Louis, St. Louis, Missouri

OLAYEMI SOKUMBI, MD
Associate Professor, Department of Dermatology, Department of Laboratory Medicine
and Pathology, Mayo Clinic, Jacksonville, Florida

MICHELLE TARBOX, MD
Associate Professor, Department of Dermatology, Texas Tech University Health Sciences
Center, Lubbock, Texas

Contents

categories of bullous disease: allergic, autoimmune, infectious, mechanical, and metabolic. These diseases affect individuals in all decades of life, but older adults, age 65 and older, are particularly susceptible to bullous diseases of all etiologies. The incidence of these disorders is expected to increase given the advancing age of the general population. In this comprehensive review, we will outline the common bullous diseases affecting older individuals and provide an approach to evaluation and management.

Venous insufficiency is a common medical condition that affects many individuals, especially those with advanced age. Chronic venous insufficiency can lead to secondary cutaneous changes that most commonly present as stasis dermatitis but can progress to more serious venous ulcers. Although venous ulcers are the most common cause of lower extremity ulcers, the differential diagnosis of leg ulcers is broad. This article will discuss clinical clues to help guide patient workup and will review basic clinical evaluation and management of common leg ulcers.

Pruritus is the most common dermatologic complaint in the geriatric population. Its growing prevalence coincides with the rapid growth of the elderly population (>65 years of age) in the United States. According to the US Census Bureau, 16.9% of the population, or more than 56 million adults 65 years and older, lived in the United States in 2022. Pruritus is a condition that accompanies a diverse array of underlying etiologic factors. The mechanism of normal itch impulse transmission has been recently elucidated. The itch sensation originates from epidermal/dermal receptors connected to unmyelinated, afferent C-fibers that transmit the impulse from the periphery.

This article focuses on bacterial infections that commonly affect geriatric patients. The elderly population is at a higher risk of contracting bacterial infections due to weakened immune systems and comorbidities. The article explores the cause, pathogenesis, clinical manifestations, and treatment options of these infections. Additionally, antibiotic resistance is a growing concern in the treatment of bacterial infections. The article highlights the importance of preventing these infections through proper hygiene and wound care. This article aims to provide an understanding of bacterial infections in geriatric patients and inform health-care providers on the most effective ways to manage and prevent these infections.

The population of older adults continues to increase in the United States, leading to a concomitant increase in cutaneous disease. Fungal disease, specifically, commonly affects this population but often goes undiagnosed for too long. It is therefore important that providers be aware of common fungal pathogens, recognizable symptoms of disease, and treatment options. This article discusses 3 groups of pathogens: dermatophytes, *Candida* species, and *Pityrosporum* species, all of which cause a host of conditions that can be debilitating for older adults.

Herpesviruses are medium-sized double-stranded DNA viruses. Of more than 80 herpesviruses identified, only 9 human herpesviruses have been found to cause infection in humans. These include herpes simplex viruses 1 and 2 (HSV-1 and HSV-2), varicella-zoster virus (VZV), human cyto-megalovirus (HCMV), Epstein–Barr virus (EBV), and human herpesvirus (HHV-6A, HHV-6B, HHV-7, HHV-8). HSV-1, HSV-2, and VZV can be problematic given their characteristic neurotropism which is the ability to invade via fusion of its plasma membrane and reside within neural tissue. HSV and VZV primarily infect mucocutaneous surfaces and remain latent in the dorsal root ganglia for a host's entire life. Reactivation causes either asymptomatic shedding of virus or clinical manifestation of vesicular lesions. The clinical presentation is influenced by the portal of entry, the immune status of the host, and whether the infection is primary or recurrent. Affecting 60% to 95% of adults, herpesvirus-associated infections include gingivostomatitis, orofacial and genital herpes, and primary varicella and herpes zoster. Symptomatology, treatment, and potential complications vary based on primary and recurrent infections as well as the patient's immune status.

Paraneoplastic syndromes include a variety of cutaneous presentations that have an associated internal malignancy. Some syndromes have a strong correlation to specific internal malignancies, whereas others are associated with a multitude of tumors. There are many cutaneous manifestations that suggest hematologic disorders, which will be reviewed in detail. Cutaneous metastases are commonly from breast and lung cancers and can present as nodules, vascular lesions, eczematous dermatitis, or inflammatory lesions. The most common histologic presentation of cutaneous metastasis is that of a dermal-based or subcutaneous-based nodule with sparing of the epidermis. Determination of origin of tumor requires immunohistochemistry and clinical correlation.

It is important to understand that each layer of facial tissue, from the underlying facial skeleton to the overlying skin, undergoes significant changes during the aging process. Bony support is lost along the mandible and maxilla and the orbital aperture widens. Superficial and deep fat pads undergo volume loss and migration and the overlying skin begins to reveal signs of both intrinsic aging with skin laxity and fine rhytids as well as extrinsic aging in the form of coarse, deeper rhytids and dyspigmentation.

CLINICS IN GERIATRIC MEDICINE

ISSUES OF RELATED INTEREST

Dermatologic Clinics
https://www.derm.theclinics.com/
Facial Plastic Surgery
https://www.facialplastic.theclinics.com/
Medical Clinics
https://www.medical.theclinics.com/

THE CLINICS ARE AVAILABLE ONLINE!
Access your subscription at:
www.theclinics.com

Foreword

Can You Please Take a Look at This Rash with Me?

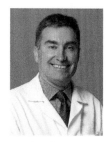

G. Michael Harper, MD
Consulting Editor

"Can you please take a look at this rash with me?" "Do you have a minute to eyeball a skin lesion?" These are two requests I often get from geriatrics fellows when I'm precepting in their primary care clinic. Sometimes they may be seeking conformation that a painful eruption of fluid-filled blisters distributed on the skin over a single unilateral dermatome is the rash from herpes zoster. Other times the lesion or rash is more mysterious, and it may require the opinion of a clinician with dermatologic expertise. Either way, the two questions serve as a stark reminder of the prevalence of skin diseases among older adults and the potential impacts on their health.

Anyone who has practiced in a primary care setting can attest to how common skin complaints and findings are among this population. In a Swedish study of adults aged 70 to 93 years, a whole-body skin examination performed by dermatologists found that 75% of these adults had at least one skin condition that required treatment or follow-up.[1] More than one in three of these subjects had three or more skin diseases simultaneously. While I don't find anything particularly surprising about the results of this study, a few questions come to mind. What skin conditions can I reassure my patient about, and which ones should I worry about? When is it okay to use surveillance, and when should I refer them to a dermatologist? Do I need to treat a basal cell cancer on the nose of a frail nursing home resident?

That brings me to this excellent issue of *Clinics in Geriatric Medicine* where our guest editor, Dr. Nicole Burkemper, and her team of experts help us answer many questions about the evaluation and treatment of skin diseases in older adults. This issue covers a broad range of topics, including the aging skin and wound healing, common skin cancers and inflammatory skin diseases, and venous stasis disease and leg ulcers. After

Clin Geriatr Med 40 (2024) xiii–xiv
https://doi.org/10.1016/j.cger.2023.10.001
0749-0690/24/© 2023 Published by Elsevier Inc.

reading it, I know that the next time I'm asked to look at a rash or a skin lesion, I'll do so with new knowledge and confidence.

G. Michael Harper, MD
Geriatrics Department of Medicine
University of California, San Francisco
4150 Clement Street, Rm 310B
San Francisco, CA 94121, USA

E-mail address:
Michael.harper@ucsf.edu

REFERENCES

1. Sinikumpu SP, Jokelainen J, Haarala AK, et al. The high prevalence of skin diseases in adults aged 70 and older. J Am Geriatr Soc 2020;68(11):2565–71.

Preface

Dermatology

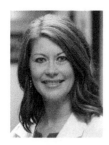

Nicole M. Burkemper, MD
Editor

The number of people in the United States older than 65 years is growing. By 2030, 20% of the US population will be older than 65 years, making the geriatric population the same size as the pediatric population. The number of people older than 85 years is the fastest growing segment of the American population, expected to double from 4.7 million in 2003 to 9.6 million in 2030, and will reach 20 million by 2060. Along with this population increase, the incidence of dermatologic conditions is also increasing, with more than 27 million visits to dermatologists and more than 5 million new skin cancers each year. The National Ambulatory Medical Care Survey of 2000 showed that 4.4% of all ambulatory visits for patients older than 65 years were to the dermatologist.[1] The idea that dermatology is focused on "antiaging" minimizes dermatology's impact on all patients, regardless of age. This dermatology issue of *Clinics in Geriatric Medicine* will hopefully provide a framework for providing dermatologic care to the older patient population. The field of geriatric dermatology relies on the appreciation of the multitude of factors that contribute to the skin health of older adults.

A review of the intrinsic age-related changes in barrier function and the systemic immune system is provided in this issue. In addition, the extrinsic elements that affect the skin, most importantly, sun exposure, are discussed. What follows are articles on both common dermatologic diseases and conditions as well as those more prevalent in older patients with an emphasis on evaluation and treatment, taking into account the nuances that are encountered in the aging population. The geriatrics principles are as follows: life expectancy are more than age; lag time to benefit; polypharmacy and medication adverse effects; cognition, function and mobility; caregivers and social

Clin Geriatr Med 40 (2024) xv–xvi
https://doi.org/10.1016/j.cger.2023.09.011
0749-0690/24/© 2023 Published by Elsevier Inc.

support; and patient preferences matter. These should all be taken into account when dealing with dermatologic conditions in older patients.[2]

Nicole M. Burkemper, MD
Department of Dermatology
SSM Health
Saint Louis University School of Medicine
1008 S Spring Avenue
St. Louis, MO 63104, USA

E-mail address:
nicole.burkemper@slucare.ssmhealth.com

REFERENCES

1. Rui P, Hing E, Okeyode T. National ambulatory medical care survey: 2014 state and national summary tables. National Center for Health Statistics; 2014.
2. Linos E, Chren MM, Covinsky K. Geriatric dermatology—a framework for caring for older patients with skin disease. JAMA Dermatol 2018;154(7):757–8.

Aging Skin and Wound Healing

Michael Kremer, MD[a], Nicole Burkemper, MD[a],*

KEYWORDS

- Aging • Photoaging • Wound healing • Skin structure • Skin function
- Chronic wounds

KEY POINTS

- Each of the many components of skin undergo changes with age that affect structure and function.
- Wound healing occurs in a highly regulated and evolutionarily conserved manner.
- Wound healing in the elderly is delayed but not defective.
- The higher prevalence of chronic wounds in aged populations is primarily due to comorbidities.

THE SKIN AND AGING

As the human body's largest organ, the skin is responsible for a myriad of essential functions, including immunologic surveillance, thermoregulation, sensation, excretion, and protection from external forces, such as UV radiation and foreign agents. Each of the 3 layers of the skin, the epidermis, the dermis, and the subcutaneous tissue, undergoes significant changes with aging.

The outermost layer of the skin is the epidermis, which gives rise to the cutaneous appendages, including sebaceous glands, sweat glands, hair follicles, and nails. The stratum corneum, the most superficial layer of the epidermis, gives the skin its waterproof barrier properties. The state of hydration of the stratum corneum is governed by 3 factors: water that reaches it from the epidermis, water lost from the skin's surface by evaporation, and the intrinsic ability of the stratum corneum to retain water. The ability of the stratum corneum to hold onto water relies on 2 mechanisms. The first mechanism involves the skin lipids, which consist of ceramides, cholesterol, and fatty acids. It is the ratio of each of these lipids, rather than one particular component, that is key to skin moisturization.[1] The second mechanism is the natural moisturizing factor, a mixture of amino acids, organic acids, urea, and inorganic ions that are extremely

[a] Department of Dermatology, SSM Saint Louis University Hospital, 1225 South Grand Boulevard 3L, St. Louis, MO 63104, USA
* Corresponding author.
E-mail address: nicole.burkemper@slucare.ssmhealth.com

Clin Geriatr Med 40 (2024) 1–10
https://doi.org/10.1016/j.cger.2023.06.001
0749-0690/24/© 2023 Elsevier Inc. All rights reserved.

water soluble and can absorb large amounts of water.[2–4] The elderly have a decreased amount of lipids and amino acids in the stratum corneum, thus contributing to the clinical presentation of dry skin (xerosis).[5–7]

Melanocytes are the pigment-producing cells of the epidermis. The density of melanocytes varies depending on the anatomic location, with more melanocytes concentrated on the face and fewer on the extremities. Aging takes its toll on melanocytes and their activity. Beginning at age 30 years, melanocyte density decreases by 6% to 8% with each decade of life.[8] In addition, melanocytes do not produce melanin pigment as efficiently with age, which explains why the elderly do not tan as easily as when they were young.[8]

Langerhans cells are the antigen-presenting cells within the epidermis. They act as immunologic sentinels by presenting foreign antigens to T lymphocytes. With aging and UV light exposure, the number and function of epidermal Langerhans cells decline, thereby decreasing the incidence of contact allergy in elderly patients.[9–11]

Sebaceous (oil) glands produce lipid-rich sebum, which prevents transepidermal water loss and has antimicrobial properties, inhibiting growth of certain fungi and bacteria. After peaking in adolescence, sebum production decreases about 23% per decade in men and 32% per decade in women.[12] Although sebaceous gland function diminishes with age, sebaceous gland size increases, which explains the yellow skin lesions of sebaceous gland hyperplasia that occur commonly in middle-aged and elderly adults.[13]

Eccrine sweat glands are responsible for thermoregulation, maintenance of electrolyte homeostasis, and excretion of metabolic byproducts. Certain heavy metals, organic molecules, and macromolecules may also be excreted in the sweat.[14] In elderly persons, the number and size of the sweat glands diminish, leading to the decreased sweating capacity of older adults.[14]

Hair follicles develop as downgrowths of the epidermis and function as a secondary sexual characteristic, as touch receptors, and as reservoirs for proliferating cells to help regenerate the epidermis after trauma. With age, the number, the growth rate, and the diameter of the hair shaft decline.[15] Gray hair results from decreased amounts of pigment within the hair shaft. Melanocytes are present in the hair follicles of people with gray hair, but melanin production is diminished in a comparable manner to the epidermis.[15]

Beneath the epidermis lies the dermis, which is composed of a fibrous connective tissue component and ground substance. Because the dermis is the main contributor to the thickness of skin, it is particularly important in the skin's cosmetic appearance. As a person ages, the dermis loses its thickness, elasticity, and water content.

Collagen gives the dermis its structural stability and resilience. Chronic UV light exposure upregulates the production of collagen-degrading enzymes called matrix metalloproteinases, such as collagenase and gelatinase. These degradative enzymes induce collagen damage, resulting in thinner, less-resilient skin with increased wrinkle formation.[16]

The skin's ability to return to its original shape after being stretched is due to the presence of elastic tissue in the dermis. Chronic sun exposure and aging cause a characteristic change in the elastic fibers of the skin, a finding called elastosis, in which elastic fibers appear thickened, coiled, and haphazardly arranged. It is controversial whether elastosis represents an increased breakdown of elastic fibers or an overproduction of abnormal elastic fibers.[17] Regardless of the mechanism, the elastic tissue in aging and photodamaged skin does not function normally, which leads to decreased skin recoil and a wrinkling effect.[18–20]

Collagen and elastin reside in the dermis within a gellike milieu called ground substance composed of glycoproteins and glycosaminoglycans. Glycoproteins are involved in cell migration, adhesion, and orientation, which allow for production of granulation tissue, re-epithelialization, and other aspects of wound healing. One of the primary roles of glycosaminoglycans is to bind water and give skin its supple appearance. In aging skin, the predominant glycosaminoglycan in the dermis, hyaluronic acid, is replaced by chondroitin sulfate, which has less effective water-binding capacity, leading to decreased skin suppleness.[21]

Aged skin has fewer dermal blood vessels, resulting in decreased blood flow, diminished nutrient exchange, impaired thermoregulation, lower skin surface temperature, and skin pallor. In addition, pericytes surrounding the cutaneous vessels decrease in number and synthetic activity with aging.[22] This loss of vascular stromal support explains the increased susceptibility to bruising in the elderly.

Beneath the dermis lies the subcutaneous fat, which serves as an energy reservoir, contributes to thermoregulation, and provides mechanical support. During the aging process, certain parts of the body, such as the face and the dorsal hands, lose subcutaneous fat, whereas other body parts, such as the abdomen in men and the thighs in women, gain subcutaneous fat.[23]

Significant structural and functional changes occur in the skin with aging. Two major forces contribute to this process: chronologic aging of the skin related to the intrinsic passage of time and photoaging resulting from cumulative UV light exposure. Many of the functions of skin that decline with age show an accelerated decline in photoaged skin. Photoaging likely causes a decrease in skin thickness in the upper dermis, but chronologic age is associated with an increase in thickness in the lower dermis. No general relationship between skin thickness and age has been observed.[24] Photoaging accounts for many of the cosmetic concerns associated with aging, such as dyspigmentation, yellow hues, enlargement of pores, wrinkling, laxity, telangiectasia, and leathery appearance.[25] Although the accumulation of actinic damage owing to solar injury seems to account for a major portion of observed skin change with aging, it is difficult to separate the degree of photoaging from chronologic aging in humans in vivo.

Delayed wound healing seen in elderly people can be explained by a 50% decrease in epidermal turnover rate between the third and eighth decades and the vascular changes mentioned above.[26] Vascular changes also increase the risk of bruising during activities of daily life and during medical procedures. As the skin becomes less elastic, configurational changes in the skin become irreversible and wrinkles develop. Loss and redistribution of the subcutaneous tissue produce further changes with folds and drooping skin. The impact of these changes on human wound healing is not clear. Reports have been complicated by lack of adjustment for environmental, solar, and comorbid factors as well as for specific skin sites.

NORMAL WOUND HEALING

Wound healing occurs in a carefully regulated and evolutionarily conserved fashion and relies on complex interactions of cells and extracellular matrix components. Acute wound healing progresses temporally through 3 distinct but overlapping phases: inflammatory, proliferative, and remodeling.

Within seconds after injury, the tissue repair process begins, as arriving platelets secrete proinflammatory cytokines and growth factors, including platelet-derived growth factor (PDGF), which facilitate the recruitment of inflammatory cells and fibroblasts into the nascent wound.[27] As the coagulation cascade proceeds, it releases anaphylatoxins C3a and C5a, which attract neutrophils, the predominant inflammatory cell type of the initial portion of the inflammatory phase.[28] Upon activation, neutrophils release additional proinflammatory cytokines, including interleukin-8 (IL-8) and tumor necrosis factor (TNF). This leads to the upregulation of cellular adhesion molecules, which are essential for leukocytes to migrate into the wound. Within 24 to 48 hours, macrophages replace neutrophils as the predominant cell type. In addition to cleaning the wound of foreign substances, macrophages synthesize and release growth factors important for the initiation of angiogenesis, such as vascular endothelial growth factor (VEGF), and for the stimulation of fibroblasts, including transforming growth factors (TGF-α, TGF-β), fibroblast growth factor (FGF), and IL-1.[29]

These growth factors usher in the second phase of wound healing, the proliferative phase. Characteristic changes include capillary growth, granulation tissue formation, fibroblast proliferation with collagen synthesis, and increased macrophage and mast cell activity. This stage is responsible for the development of wound tensile strength. Growth factors, especially PDGF and TGF-β, acting in concert with the extracellular matrix molecules, stimulate nearby fibroblasts to proliferate, express integrin receptors, and migrate into the wound space.[30–32] The expression of integrin receptors on epidermal cells allows them to interact with a variety of extracellular matrix proteins (eg, fibronectin and vitronectin) that interact with stromal type I collagen at the margin of the wound and in the fibrin clot in the wound space.[33–35] Plasminogen activator also stimulates collagenase (matrix metalloproteinase 1) and therefore facilitates the degradation of collagen and extracellular matrix proteins.[36] The process of neovascularization in this phase produces a granular appearance of the wound owing to formation of loops of capillaries and migration of macrophages, fibroblasts, and endothelial cells into the wound matrix. FGF sets the stage for angiogenesis during the first 3 days of wound repair, and VEGF is critical for angiogenesis during the formation of granulation tissue.[37] Re-epithelialization begins soon after injury and continues throughout the proliferative phase. In partial-thickness wounds, the stem cells originate from the hair follicles and sweat glands. In full-thickness wounds, epithelial cells migrate from the wound margin. The rate of migration of epithelial cells is dependent on tissue oxygen tension and moisture of the wound.[38,39] Migration is mediated in part by epidermal growth factor (EGF), TGF-α, FGF, heparin-binding EGF, PDGF, insulin-like growth factor 1, and IL-6.[40–47]

The third phase of wound healing is defined by maturation. This long phase of contraction, tissue remodeling, and increasing tensile strength lasts up to a year. Fibroblasts are responsible for the synthesis, deposition, and remodeling of the extracellular matrix. Fibroblast proliferation and collagen remodeling lead to contraction. This contracted tissue, or scar tissue, is functionally inferior to original skin and is a barrier to diffused oxygen and nutrients.[48] At maximum strength, a scar is only 80% as strong as normal skin.[49]

If the inflammatory response persists rather than resolves during the maturation phase, a disturbed healing response may result, leading to a chronic wound. Certain conditions can impair the process of wound healing, allowing an acute wound to progress to a chronic wound. The most common conditions that contribute to poor wound healing are diabetes, atherosclerosis, venous insufficiency, and pressure.[50,51] These conditions impede wound healing by reducing the supply of oxygen, nutrients, and mediators involved in the repair process.

WOUND HEALING IN OLDER ADULTS

Because most chronic wounds occur in aged populations, it has been concluded that aging itself may worsen wound healing. Indeed, many age-related morphologic and structural changes in skin have the potential to negatively influence wound healing.

Elderly skin demonstrates flattening of the dermal-epidermal junction, leading to increased vulnerability to shearing forces.[52] Older skin has a reduction in nerve endings that increases the risk of injury.[53] It has reduced and disorganized microcirculation, which may result in the development of ischemic ulcers.[54] It has fewer and less-effective Langerhans cells, leading to decreased recognition and elimination of foreign pathogens.[55] Older skin has decreased proliferation of keratinocytes and increased keratinocyte migration time, which may lead to delayed re-epithelialization.[56] In aged skin, fibroblasts decrease in number and produce less extracellular matrix material, which leads to delayed collagen deposition and remodeling.[57] Taking all of these contributing factors together, it seems intuitive that aged skin would demonstrate less efficient and effective wound healing compared with younger skin.

However, this concept has been challenged by recent research, which has shown that wound healing in healthy older people is delayed but not defective.[58–60] Impaired wound healing leading to chronic wounds in the elderly seems to be primarily due to higher prevalence of comorbidities rather than innate deficiencies in the wound healing process. It is important to consider that certain diseases that are associated with poor wound healing, including peripheral arterial disease, venous stasis, and diabetes mellitus, are much more prevalent in aged persons. Older patients are also more likely to receive treatments such as chemotherapy or corticosteroids, which may inhibit proper wound healing. In addition, as aged individuals more often undergo surgery and as their physical abilities and dexterity decline, they are at higher risk of developing more wounds overall.

The effect of age on wound tensile strength has been measured in several animal models, but in few human studies. The basis for the first reports on impaired healing in elderly persons came from a study in 1970 that showed increasing rates of dehiscence with age. Dehiscence occurred in 0.9% of surgical wounds in patients aged 30 to 39 years, in 2.5% in patients aged 50 to 59 years, and in 5.5% in patients over age 80 years.[61] However, adjustment for comorbidity or other potential confounders was not done. In 2015, a retrospective review of 25,967 plastic surgery patients showed that aging was not associated with an increased incidence of wound dehiscence.[62]

The visual quality of scarring and microscopic evaluation of scarring have been shown to be superior in older subjects.[63] A trial of experimental forearm wounding demonstrated that persons greater than 80 years of age had a nonsignificant decrease in tensile strength compared with persons less than 70 years of age.[64] Collagen deposition is similar in both young and elderly wounded subjects. No difference in hydroxyproline accumulation in polytetrafluoroethylene tubes was seen in young healthy volunteers compared with elderly healthy volunteers.[65] Age has no effect on collagen synthesis 2 weeks after wounding.[65] In fact, aging may be associated with increased amounts of fibrillin and elastin during acute wound healing and may lead to an improved quality of scarring, particularly in women. The messenger RNA (mRNA) expression of elastin was greatest in the wounds of older persons.[66]

The rate of epithelialization does seem to differ with age. Complete epithelialization of partial-thickness wounds occurs approximately 2 days faster in young healthy patients compared with elderly healthy patients.[65] A difference in in vitro growth of epidermal cells has been shown among newborns, young adults, and older adults. Although there was large interdonor variability, growth of keratinocytes obtained from upper arm biopsies of young adult (ages 22–27 years) and elderly adult (ages 60–82 years) donors significantly decreased with age. Cell yields at 7 days showed an 8-fold increase for young adults but only a 4-fold increase for elderly adults.[67]

Fibroblasts have a significant role in the synthesis and reorganization of the extracellular matrix during wound repair. An impaired functional response of these cells to stimulation by growth factors might contribute to the delayed wound healing reputed in aging. Cultures of dermal fibroblasts from young and elderly individuals exposed to TGF-β demonstrated a 1.6-fold to a 5.5-fold increase in the levels of secreted type I collagen and extracellular matrix proteins and exhibited a 2.0-fold to a 6.2-fold increase in the amounts of the corresponding mRNAs.[68] The dose-response to TGF-β was as vigorous in contractile properties in cells from aged donors as in cells from a young donor.[68] The response of cultured fibroblasts to cytokines does not seem to change with age. In fibroblast cell lines derived from persons aged 3 days to 84 years, synthesis of collagen in response to EGF, TNF-α, PDGF, and TGF-β did not vary with the age of the donor.[69]

Studies have suggested that microscopic structure of wounds in older persons is better than in younger persons and that the formation and quality of scarring may improve with age. This lack of inferior wound healing with aging is supported by clinical observation that there does not seem to be a significant difference in surgical wound healing in healthy older persons undergoing elective surgery. The rate of epithelialization does seem to be slower in older persons, but the magnitude of the delay may not be clinically important. The response to TGF-β and wound contractility does not seem to be different with aging.[69] Most age-related effects on the inflammatory process are modest.

Chronic wounds are defined as wounds that fail to proceed as expected in structural and functional integrity. Loss of subcutaneous tissue, failure of re-epithelization, necrosis, or infection can complicate wound healing. The use of growth factors found in acute wounds to accelerate healing in chronic wounds has received considerable attention in the field of wound healing.[70] Unfortunately, despite initial success in animal models, the only growth factor proven to improve wound healing in a double-blind randomized trial is PDGF, and those results were only modest.[71] Ultimately, it should not be too surprising that treatment with one growth factor is not likely to cure chronic wounds, considering that wound repair is the result of a complex set of interactions among cytokines, growth factors, extracellular matrix, and cells.

SUMMARY

Evidence for age-related effects on wound healing has been derived mostly from empirical observations without adjustment for confounders. Changes in the structure of the skin have been observed with aging, but the effects in skin unexposed to solar radiation appear modest. The clinical impact of these changes in acute wound healing seems to be small in comparison to other factors. Poor healing of chronic wounds, predominantly seen in older populations, is more often attributable to comorbid conditions rather than age alone.

CLINICS CARE POINTS

- When caring for older patients, it is important to keep in mind the physiologic changes of the skin associated with aging and how this can affect wound healing.

DISCLOSURE

The authors have nothing to disclose.

REFERENCES

1. Menon GK, Norlen L. Stratum corneum ceramides and their role in skin barrier function. New York: Marcel Dekker; 2002. p. 43.
2. Harding CR, Scott IR. Stratum corneum moisturizing factors. New York: Marcel Dekker; 2002. p. 76.
3. Lee SH, Jeong SK, Sung SK. An update of the defensive barrier function of skin. Yonsei Med J 2006;47:293–306.
4. Segre JA. Epidermal barrier function and recovery in skin disorders. Clin Invest 2006;116:1150–8.
5. Ghadially R. The aged epidermal permeability barrier: structural, functional, and lipid biochemical abnormalities in humans and a senescent murine model. J Clin Invest 1995;95:2281–90.
6. Horii I. Stratum corneum hydration and amino acid content in xerotic skin. Br J Dermatol 1989;121:587–92.
7. Holt DR, Kirk SJ, Regan MC, et al. Effect of age on wound healing in healthy human beings. Surgery 1992;112:293–8.
8. Gilchrest BA, Blog FB, Szabo G. Effects of aging and chronic sun exposure on melanocytes in human skin. J Invest Dermatol 1979;73:141–3.
9. Sunderkotter C, Kalden H, Luger TA. Aging and the skin immune system. Arch Dermatol 1997;133:1256–62.
10. Stigl G, Katz SI, Clement L. Immunologic functions of 1a-bearing epidermal Langerhans cells. Immunology 1978;121:2005.
11. Mizumoto N, Takashima A. CD1a and langerin: acting as more than Langerhans cell markers. Clin Invest 2004;113:658–60.
12. Jacobsen E, Billings J, Frantz R. Age-related changes in sebaceous wax ester secretion rates in men and women. J Invest Dermatol 1985;85:483.
13. Plewig G, Koigman AM. Proliferative activity of the sebaceous glands of the aged. J Invest Dermatol 1978;70:314.
14. Fenske NA, Lober CW. Structural and functional changes of normal aging skin. J Am Acad Dermatol 1986;15:571–85.
15. Van Neste D, Tobin DF. Hair cycle and hair pigmentation: dynamic interactions and changes associated with aging. Micron 2004;35:193–200.
16. Fisher GF, Wang ZQ, Datta SC. Pathophysiology of premature skin aging induced by ultraviolet light. N Engl J Med 1997;337:1419.
17. Fernandez-Flores A, Saeb-Lima M. Histopathology of cutaneous aging. Am J Dermatopathol 2019;41(7):469–79.
18. Braverman IM, Fonferko E. Studies in cutaneous aging. The elastic fiber network. J Invest Dermatol 1982;28:434.
19. Muto J. Accumulation of elafin in actinic elastosis of sun-damaged skin: elafin bids to elastin and prevents elastolytic degradation. J Invest Dermatol 2007;127:1358–66.
20. Schalkwijk J. Cross-linking of elafin/SKALP to elastic fibers in photodamaged skin: too much of a good thing? J Invest Dermatol 2007;127:1286–7.
21. Waller JM, Maibach HI. Age and skin structure and function, a quantitative approach (II): protein, glycosaminoglycan, water, and lipid content and structure. Skin Res Technol 2006;12:145–54.
22. Waller JM, Maibach HI. Age and skin structure and function, a quantitative approach (I): blood flow, pH, thickness, and ultrasound echogenicity. Skin Res Technol 2005;11:221–35.

23. Kanehisa H, Miyatani M, Azuma K, et al. Influences of age and sex on abdominal muscle and subcutaneous fat thickness. Eur J Appl Physiol 2004;91(5–6):534–7.
24. Gniadecka M, Jemec GB. Quantitative evaluation of chronological ageing and photoaging in vivo: studies on skin echogenicity and thickness. Br J Dermatol 1998;139(5):815–21.
25. Rabe JH, Mamelak AJ. Photoaging: mechanisms and repair. J Am Acad Dermatol 2006;55:1–19.
26. Grove GL, Kligman AM. Age-associated changes in human epidermal cell renewal. J Gerontol 1983;38(2):137–42.
27. Martin P, Leibovich SJ. Inflammatory cells during wound repair: the good, the bad and the ugly. Trends Cell Biol 2005;15(11):599–607.
28. Eming SA, Martin P, Tomic-Canic M. Wound repair and regeneration: mechanisms, signaling, and translation. Sci Transl Med 2014;6(265):265.
29. Lucas T, Waisman A, Ranjan R, et al. Differential roles of macrophages in diverse phases of skin repair. J Immunol 2010;184(7):3964–77.
30. Roberts AB, Sporn MB. Transforming growth factor-(beta). In: Clark RAF, editor. The molecular and cellular biology of wound repair. 2nd edition. New York: Plenum Press; 1996. p. 275–308.
31. Gray AJ, Bishop JE, Reeves JT, et al. A(alpha) and B(beta) chains of fibrinogen stimulate proliferation of human fibroblasts. J Cell Sci 1993;104:409–13.
32. Xu J, Clark RAF. Extracellular matrix alters PDGF regulation of fibroblast integrins. J Cell Biol 1996;132:239–49.
33. Clark RAF. Fibronectin matrix deposition and fibronectin receptor expression in healing and normal skin. J Invest Dermatol 1990;94:128S–34S.
34. Larjava H, Salo T, Haapasalmi K, et al. Expression of integrins and basement membrane components by wound keratinoctyes. J Clin Invest 1993;92:1425–35.
35. Clark RAF, Ashcroft GS, Spencer MJ, et al. Re-epithelialization of normal human excisional wounds is associated with a switch from (alpha)v(beta)5 to (alpha)v(beta)6 integrins. Br J Dermatol 1996;135:46–51.
36. Mignatti P, Rifkin DB, Welgus HG, et al. Proteinases and tissue remodeling. In: Clark RAF, editor. The molecular and cellular biology of wound repair. 2nd edition. New York: Plenum Press; 1996. p. 427–74.
37. Nissen NN, Polverini PJ, Koch AE, et al. Vascular endothelial growth factor mediates angiogenic activity during the proliferative phase of wound healing. Am J Pathol 1998;152:1445–52.
38. Kanzler MH, Gorsulowsky DC, Swanson NA. Basic mechanisms in the healing cutaneous wound. J Dermatol Surg Oncol 1986;12:1156–64.
39. Kirsner RS, Eaglstein WH. The wound healing process. Dermatol Clin 1993;11:629–40.
40. Dawson RA, Goberdhan NJ, Freedlander E, et al. Influence of extracellular matrix proteins on human keratinocyte attachment, proliferation and transfer to a dermal wound model. Burns 1996;22:93–100.
41. Barrandon Y, Green H. Cell migration is essential for sustained growth of keratinocyte colonies: the roles of transforming growth factor alpha and epidermal growth factor. Cell 1987;50:1131–7.
42. Werner S, Peters KG, Longaker MT, et al. Large induction of keratinocyte growth factor in the dermis during wound healing. Proc Natl Acad Sci USA 1992;89:6896–900.
43. Higashiyama S, Abraham JA, Miller J, et al. A heparin-binding growth factor secreted by macrophage-like cells that is related to EGF. Science 1991;251:936–9.

44. Meddahi A, Caruelle JP, Gold L, et al. New concepts in tissue repair: skin as an example. Diabetes Metab 1996;22:274–8.
45. Antoniades HN, Galanopuulos T, Neville-Golden J, et al. Injury induces in vivo expression PDGF and PDGF receptor mRNAs in skin epithelial cells and PDGF mRNA in connective tissue fibroblasts. Proc Natl Acad Sci U S A 1991;88:565–9.
46. Krane JF, Murphy DP, Carter DM, et al. Synergistic effects of epidermal growth factor and insulin-like growth factor 1/somatemedin C on keratinocyte proliferation may be medicated by IGF 1 transmodulation of the EGF receptor. J Invest Dermatol 1991;96:419–24.
47. Grossman RM, Krueger J, Yourish D, et al. Interleukin 6 is expressed in high levels in psoriatic skin and stimulates proliferation of cultured human keratinocytes. Proc Natl Acad Sci U S A 1989;86:6367–71.
48. Chvapil M, Koopman CF. Scar formation: physiology and pathological states. Otolaryngol Clin North Am 1984;17:265–72.
49. Schilling JA. Wound healing. Surg Clin North Am 1976;56:859.
50. Baltzis D, Eleftheriadou I, Veves A. Pathogenesis and treatment of impaired wound healing in diabetes mellitus: new insights. Adv Ther 2014;31(8):817–36.
51. Natarelli L, Schober A. MicroRNAs and the response to injury in atherosclerosis. Hämostaseologie 2015;35(02):142–50.
52. Broderick VV, Cowan LJ. Pressure injury related to friction and shearing forces in older adults. J Dermatol Skin Sci 2021;3(2):9–12.
53. Chang YC, Lin WM, Hsieh ST. Effects of aging on human skin innervation. Neuroreport 2004;15(1):149–53.
54. Jin K. A microcirculatory theory of aging. Aging Dis 2019;10(3):676.
55. Pilkington SM, Ogden S, Eaton LH, et al. Lower levels of interleukin-1β gene expression are associated with impaired Langerhans' cell migration in aged human skin. Immunology 2018;153:60–70.
56. Keyes BE, Liu S, Asare A, et al. Impaired epidermal to dendritic T cell signaling slows wound repair in aged skin. Cell 2016;167(5):1323–38.
57. Salzer MC, Lafzi A, Berenguer-Llergo A, et al. Identity noise and adipogenic traits characterize dermal fibroblast aging. Cell 2018;175(6):1575–90.
58. Gould L, Abadir P, Brem H, et al. Chronic wound repair and healing in older adults: current status and future research. Wound Repair Regen 2015;23(1):1–13.
59. Gosain A, DiPietro LA. Aging and wound healing. World J Surg 2004;28(3):321–6.
60. Engeland CG. Mucosal wound healing. Arch Surg 2006;141(12):1193.
61. Mendoza CB Jr, Postlethwait RW, Johnson WD. Incidence of wound disruption following operation. Arch Surg 1970;101:396–8.
62. Karamanos E, Osgood G, Siddiqui A, et al. Wound healing in plastic surgery. Plast Reconstr Surg 2015;135(3):876–81.
63. Horan MA, Ashcroft GS. Ageing, defence mechanisms and the immune system. Aging 1997;26:15S–9S.
64. Lindstedt E, Sandblom P. Wound healing in man: tensile strength of healing wounds in some patient groups. Ann Surg 1975;181:842–6.
65. Kurban R, Bhawan J. Histological changes in skin associated with aging. J Dermatol Surg Oncol 1990;16:908–14.
66. Pienta KJ, Coppey DS. Characterization of the subtypes of cell motility in ageing human skin fibroblasts. Mech Ageing Dev 1990;56:99–105.
67. Stanulis-Praeger BM, Gilchrest BA. Growth factor responsiveness declines during adulthood for human skin-derived cells. Mech Ageing Dev 1986;35:185–98.

68. Reed MJ, Vernon RB, Abrass IB, et al. TGF-beta 1 induces the expression of type I collagen and SPARC, and enhances contraction of collagen gels, by fibroblasts from young and aged donors. J Cell Physiol 1994;158:169–79.

69. Freedland M, Karmiol S, Rodriguez J, et al. Fibroblast responses to cytokines are maintained during aging. Ann Plast Surg 1995;35:290–6.

70. Emmerson E, Campbell L, Davies FC, et al. Insulin-like growth factor-1 promotes wound healing in estrogen-deprived mice: new insights into cutaneous IGF-1R/ERalpha cross talk. J Invest Dermatol 2012;132(12):2838–48.

71. Smiell JM, Wieman TJ, Steed DL, et al. Efficacy and safety of becaplermin (recombinant human platelet-derived growth factor-BB) in patients with nonhealing, lower extremity diabetic ulcers: a combined analysis of four randomized studies. Wound Repair Regen 1999;7(5):335–46.

Diagnosis and Management of Common Inflammatory Skin Diseases in Older Adults

Monica Hessler-Waning, MD, Gillian Heinecke, MD*

KEYWORDS

- Inflammatory • Dermatitis • Psoriasis • Elderly • Geriatric • Skin

KEY POINTS

- Many common dermatoses begin or continue in elderly patients.
- Management considerations in this population need to account for increased likelihood of difficulty with mobility and dexterity, of concurrent medical conditions, and of polypharmacy.
- The primary complaint of inflammatory dermatoses can be pruritus, so a careful history must be obtained to discern the correct diagnosis.

INTRODUCTION

Inflammatory skin conditions affect people of all ages, genders, and races and are frequent causes of visits to the dermatologist. The geriatric population is often afflicted by these conditions because many are chronic and relapsing diseases. Examples include but are not limited to psoriasis, atopic dermatitis (AD), contact dermatitis, rosacea, seborrheic dermatitis, and Grover disease. Chronic inflammatory skin conditions place a large burden on the health care system in the United States and have many associated comorbidities.[1] Herein, we discuss the common inflammatory dermatoses that affect the geriatric population.

RELEVANT CLINICAL QUESTIONS

- When was the onset of the eruption?
- What underlying diseases are present and could be contributing to the eruption?
- Is there an association between the eruption and a certain trigger?
- What type of management is required for this condition based on the associated risks of the condition versus the risks of the treatment options taking into account the patient's comorbidities and current medications?

Department of Dermatology, Saint Louis University, 1225 South Grand Avenue, St. Louis, MO 63110, USA
* Corresponding author.
E-mail address: gillian.heinecke@health.slu.edu

Clin Geriatr Med 40 (2024) 11–23
https://doi.org/10.1016/j.cger.2023.09.007
0749-0690/24/© 2023 Elsevier Inc. All rights reserved.

- How long is treatment required for the condition?

PSORIASIS

Psoriasis is a chronic inflammatory condition with several subtypes including plaque, guttate, pustular, inverse, and erythrodermic. According to a recent study in 2021, the prevalence of psoriasis of US adults age 20 and older is 3%.[2] Although psoriasis can occur at any age, it most commonly presents before the age of 35 years old.[3] Several studies have shown that psoriasis has a bimodal age of onset with the first peak occurring in the 30s and the second in the early 60s.[4] Kwon and colleagues[5] describes elderly onset psoriasis as those who first develop clinical manifestations of psoriasis at greater than 60 years old. Given the chronicity of the condition, this disease still has a prevalence of 1.23% in the older population from the US Medicare beneficiary database.[2] Associated psoriatic arthritis is debilitating and often hinders ambulation and dexterity for elderly patients. In a study from France, 19.4% of psoriasis patients greater than 70 years old also had psoriatic arthritis.[6]

Clinical Presentation

- Plaque psoriasis is the most common form of psoriasis seen in the elderly population and presents as well-demarcated, thick plaques with silvery scale (**Fig. 1**) most often affecting the extensor surfaces and scalp.
- Plaques can also be seen in the intertriginous regions with maceration and fissuring more often than scaling because of occlusion in these areas.
- Psoriasis also has several associated serious medical comorbidities: psoriatic arthritis, cardiovascular disease, and the metabolic syndrome.

Differential and Diagnosis

- Differentials: Seborrheic dermatitis, AD, nummular eczema, fungal infections, crusted scabies, and secondary syphilis.
- Diagnosis: Often clinical, but skin biopsy is useful in ruling out other conditions.

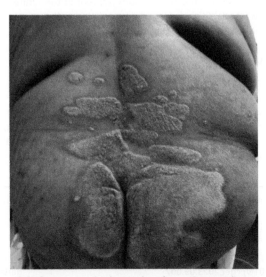

Fig. 1. Well-demarcated plaques on the buttocks of a patient with severe plaque psoriasis.

Pathogenesis

- The cause of psoriasis involves interleukin (IL)-17 and IL-23 and crosstalking between the innate and adaptive immune systems in a feed-forward amplification that leads to the inflammatory cascade occurring in psoriasis.

Treatment

Treatment of psoriasis is individualized to meet the severity of the case and the willingness of the patient to use different therapeutic regimens with the primary goal being to improve quality of life in conjunction with interval improvement in disease status. First-line treatments for limited plaque psoriasis in the elderly are topical agents, such as topical steroids; however, special attention should be given to monitoring of the cutaneous side effects including purpura (**Fig. 2**), telangiectasia, atrophy, and secondary skin infections. Vitamin D analogues are other topical treatment options (calcipotriene/calcipotriol) that are used alone or in combination with topical steroids. It is also important to assess for any risk factors for hypercalcemia when using vitamin D_3 analogues. Topical retinoids, such as tazarotene, are another option for treatment, but use is often limited by skin irritation. Topical calcineurin inhibitors are beneficial in intertriginous areas. Phototherapy is an effective option that circumvents any drug interactions or side effects but is often cumbersome in the elderly because frequent visits several times weekly are needed and caregivers may need to provide transportation.

Systemic agents are widely effective and convenient options for those with a larger body surface area involved. Methotrexate is a folic acid antagonist that is a traditional first-line medication used in moderate to severe psoriasis.[7] However, extra care should be given to monitoring renal function and hepatic function because the medication is renally excreted and is hepatotoxic and older patients are more likely to have renal insufficiency. Because of this, smaller doses may be required in the geriatric population when compared with younger populations.[8] Dosing is done orally;

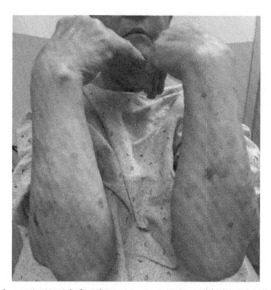

Fig. 2. Patient with psoriasis with focal concurrent purpura, likely partially caused by recent topical steroid use.

however, the intramuscular injection is better tolerated in the geriatric population with difficulty swallowing. A newer systemic agent is apremilast, a phosphodiesterase-4 inhibitor. This is an oral option that is also approved for psoriatic arthritis. It has a known side effect of causing diarrhea and often causes modest weight loss, which is beneficial in the right patient.[9] Apremilast is less immunosuppressive than conventional immunosuppressants or biologic agents and therefore is useful in patients with a history of malignancy or chronic infection. Acitretin is another option that is considered in a patient with a history of malignancy or chronic infection, but it can cause significant xerosis and dyslipidemia and hepatotoxicity, which may be of particular concern in older patients.

The next systemic agents are the biologic medications. In terms of safety profile, biologics typically cause less organ dysfunction as compared with the conventional immunosuppressants, which is beneficial in the geriatric population, but overall, these drugs have been less studied in the elderly population. The biologics are broadly classified by targeted elements of the immune system and are broken down into the tumor necrosis factor (TNF)-α inhibitors, IL-17 inhibitors, IL-23 inhibitors, and IL-12/23 inhibitors.

TNF-α inhibitors were the first biologics to be approved for psoriasis and typically have an onset of action at 12 to 16 weeks.[10] These include etanercept, adalimumab, certolizumab, and infliximab, with the first three being offered as subcutaneous (SQ) injections and the last given intravenously.[11] This class of medications are approved for psoriasis and psoriatic arthritis, but are contraindicated in patients with comorbidities, such as congestive heart failure class III and IV and multiple sclerosis.[12] Although chronic infection is a contraindication, in some circumstances, they are used in patients with HIV, hepatitis B, and hepatitis C infections if the patient is actively treated with concurrent antiviral therapy and if they are being followed by infectious disease specialists.[10,12] IL-12/23 inhibitors include ustekinumab, which is available in an SQ formulation. Full effect of therapy is usually seen after 12 weeks. This class of drugs can also be used in combination with other systemic agents to increase efficacy and the only absolute contraindication to use is history of allergic reaction to the therapeutic agent. Of note, ustekinumab is less effective than the TNF-α inhibitors in treating psoriatic arthritis.

IL-17 inhibitors include secukinumab, ixekizumab, and brodalumab, which are all available in SQ formulations. As a class, the response to therapy is best appreciated after 12 weeks. Efficacy is comparable among the agents in this class.[10] The IL-17 inhibitors are associated with increased mucocutaneous *Candida* infection, and this class should be avoided in patients with a history of irritable bowel disease. Injection site reactions are seen in up to 20% of patients with pruritis at the injection site as the primary complaint.[10] Brodalumab stands alone in that rare cases of suicidal ideation have resulted in a black box warning and brodalumab should not be used in patients with a history of or current suicidal ideation.

IL-23 inhibitors are the last class of biologics that include guselkumab, Risankizumab, and tildrakizumab. Response to the IL-23 class is seen after 12 weeks of therapy and increasing the dose is considered in patients who partially respond. Rare cases of increased liver transaminases have been seen with this class of medications. Temporary discontinuation of the drug is recommended if the patient has a febrile illness, particularly if they are receiving systemic antibiotics.[10] The drug is restarted after symptom resolution.

Newer classes of medications called tyrosine kinase and janus kinase (JAK) inhibitors are emerging as treatment options for psoriasis and psoriatic arthritis. Deucravacitinib, an oral tyrosine kinase-2 inhibitor, is currently the one medication approved for psoriasis in this class.[13] Because this is a newer medication just approved in Fall of 2022, not all side effects are known. It is known that deucravacitinib may increase the risk of infections with the most common being mild to moderate including upper respiratory infections, herpes simplex infections, and folliculitis.[13,14] Other JAK inhibitors are approved for psoriatic arthritis, but are not yet approved for psoriasis alone. Tofacitinib and upadacitinib are Food and Drug Administration (FDA)-approved for psoriatic arthritis and may be approved for psoriasis in the future. Side effects of JAK inhibitors include increased risk of infections and increased risk of thromboembolic events, which must be considered if using in the geriatric population.[15]

For all biologics and immunomodulators, baseline laboratory studies should include a complete metabolic panel, complete blood count with differential, tuberculosis test (purified protein derivative, Quantiferon Gold, or T-spot), serologic tests for hepatitis B and C, and possible HIV testing depending on physician discretion and risk factors of the patient.[10]

ATOPIC DERMATITIS

AD is another chronic, inflammatory disease that can impact the elderly. Because many older adults see their physicians for dry, flaky skin, diagnosing and treating AD correctly is paramount in this population. There is a degree of age-related skin barrier breakdown and a switch to primarily type 2 helper T cellular responses with age, but this should not exclude proper diagnosis and treatment of AD in the geriatric population. It has been estimated that 2% to 7% of adults have AD.[16,17]

Clinical Presentation

- Adult type AD: Lichenified plaques involving the flexural areas of the extremities, the head, and the neck.
- Elderly type AD: Lichenified plaques more commonly seen affecting the buttocks or genitals. Lesions are less likely to be located within the flexural regions, but may involve the areas surrounding the skinfolds.[18]

Differential and Diagnosis

- Differential diagnosis: Asteatotic dermatitis, nummular eczema, contact dermatitis, cutaneous T-cell lymphoma, and adverse drug eruptions.
- Diagnosis:
  - Often based on the clinical findings of eczematous dermatitis with lichenification that involves flexural regions of the extremities (**Fig. 3**) or chronic eczematous patches involving the face and neck.
  - Positive family history of atopic conditions (asthma, seasonal allergies, AD) or personal elevated total IgE and allergen-specific IgE is supportive of the diagnosis.
  - Skin biopsy is recommended for older patients without a history of prior AD to rule out cutaneous T-cell lymphoma.

Pathogenesis

- The pathophysiology of AD is multifactorial including cellular barrier dysfunction, environmental factors, IgE hypersensitivity, in addition to changes in cell-mediated immune responses.[19]
- Loss of function mutations in filaggrin are implicated in classic AD, but a down-regulation of filaggrin occurs with age adding to pathophysiology of AD in the geriatric population.[17,19]
- Cytokine imbalances that lead to increased expression of IL-4 and IL-13.

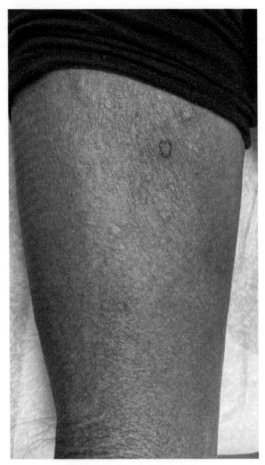

Fig. 3. Thin lichenified papules in xerotic plaques on forearm of patient with atopic dermatitis. Biopsy performed to rule out mycosis fungoides.

Treatment

Initial therapy for AD in the geriatric population should be targeted toward education about the chronicity of the disease, treatments to maintain the skin barrier, avoidance of possible triggers, and anti-inflammatory medications. All patients should be counseled to avoid harsh topical products and to use products that are free of dyes and perfumes. Emollients should be used liberally and frequently to prevent general xerosis of the skin. Topical corticosteroids are first line in AD and should be applied once or twice daily with decreasing steroid potency as the disease status improves.[18] Topical calcineurin inhibitors (tacrolimus and pimecrolimus) are steroid-sparing agents that can be applied to sensitive areas, such as the face, neck, and groin.[20] However, use of these topical steroids or other topical medications may be limited if the patient has a lower self-care ability. Light therapy is viable option for treatment of AD, but logistical complications of transportation can become burdensome in the geriatric population.

Common systemic agents that are recommended for geriatric populations include dupilumab and methotrexate.[18,21] Because randomized controlled trials often exclude geriatric subjects and those with many complex medical comorbidities the full safety profiles of systemic and biologic agents in older patients are not known.[21,22] Dupilumab is the most commonly recommended first-line systemic agent for geriatric patients with AD and blocks IL-4 and IL-13 signaling.[21,22] It is dosed every 2 weeks and often results in rapid improvement in skin lesions with minimal adverse events. Methotrexate is a treatment option that is available in once-weekly dosing as either oral tablets or SQ injections. This treatment is often referred to as a second-line systemic therapy in geriatric adults after dupilumab and should be started at lower doses with close monitoring.[22]

Newer treatment options include JAK inhibitors, which are available as oral abrocitinib and upadacitinib and topical ruxolitinib.[15,23] The oral options are approved for moderate to severe AD in adults. Risks of the oral JAK inhibitors are still being investigated; however, there is a known increased risk of infection and a potential increase in venous thromboembolism.[15,23] Topical ruxolitinib offers similar efficacy to triamcinolone with less risk of skin atrophy and striae formation, which could be favorable for the geriatric population.[23]

CONTACT DERMATITIS

Contact dermatitis is inflammation of the skin that is a direct result of an interaction of the skin with a chemical substance. Contact dermatitis has two forms, irritant contact dermatitis (ICD) and allergic contact dermatitis (ACD), which are dichotomized by their pathogenesis. Eighty percent of all contact dermatitis is irritant and 20% is allergic.[24] Asteatotic and perineal irritant dermatitis are important common variants of ICD in older patients.[25] For ACD, older literature has found nickel, balsam of Peru, rubber accelerators, topical antibacterials, fragrance mix, and potassium dichromate common allergens in the elderly.[26] More recent data from 2023 have shown fragrance mix, nickel sulfate, and preservatives, such as methylchloroisothiazolinone/methylisothiazolinone, to be among the most commonly encountered allergens in the geriatric population.[27] The same study also found that the frequency of patch test positives was lower in the aging population.[27] Patients with leg ulcers, which occur in more than 1.7% of patients aged 65 and older, have a higher risk of ACD with their sensitization rate increasing with duration of the ulceration.[26]

Clinical Presentation

- Despite different pathogenesis, ACD and ICD are difficult to differentiate clinically.
- Acute phase: Erythematous papules and vesicles, often weeping.
- Subacute phase: Erythematous patches, scaling, serous exudate.
- Chronic phase: Fissures, lichenified plaques, and hyperkeratosis.

Pathogenesis

- ACD: The allergic process requires sensitization to a specific allergen, which is determined by a genetic predisposition. On reexposure to the allergen, the host mounts an immune response.
- ICD: An irritant reaction does not require prior sensitization and can occur at any time. The properties of the substance, such as pH, vehicle, humidity, occlusion, and duration of exposure, all contribute to the reaction.

Differential and Diagnosis

- Differentials vary based on phases

Acute: Impetigo, drug eruptions, herpetic infections, viral exanthems, and urticaria.
- Subacute: Dermatophyte infections, psoriasis, AD, early cutaneous T-cell lymphoma, and squamous cell carcinoma in situ.
- Chronic: Lichen simplex chronicus, psoriasis, nummular eczema, and crusted scabies.

- Diagnosis
  - Diagnosis is usually made on the pattern of distribution and history of the eruptions.
  - Well-defined eczematous plaques that align with belt buckles, zippers, or watches are clinical indicators of ACD, but often distinguishing the ACD from ICD depends on a careful history of exposures and timing of eruptions.
  - Patch testing is useful for ACD and can test for specific allergies.

Treatment

The mainstay of treatment of ACD and ICD is avoidance of the allergen or irritant. For ACD, identification of the allergen is critical and is commonly done through patch testing. In addition to avoidance of triggers, the acute dermatitis is treated with emollients; topical corticosteroids; and other steroid-sparing agents, such as topical calcineurin inhibitors. When using topical steroids in the geriatric population, it is especially important to consider the potency used and to be aware of side effects, such as striae, skin thinning, and telangiectasia. Physicians must also be mindful of which topical corticosteroid is prescribed because they may contain allergens.[28] Above all, avoidance of the allergen or irritant must be at the forefront and patients should be counseled on avoidance practices, such as wearing gloves, minimizing exposure, and using alternative products.

SEBORRHEIC DERMATITIS

Seborrheic dermatitis is a chronic inflammatory condition characterized by pruritic erythematous scaly patches or plaques seen in infancy and adulthood.[29] Although this condition is usually mild, it is often chronic and can reoccur frequently if not kept under control. The prevalence of the condition is estimated to be between 2.35% and 11.3%, with increased frequency in immunocompromised individuals and patients with neurologic conditions.[29]

Clinical Presentation

- Erythematous patches, papules, or plaques with fine or greasy-appearing scaling most often seen in regions with high numbers of sebaceous glands.
- Commonly affected areas: Scalp, face, flexural regions, and chest.

Pathogenesis

- Proposed pathogenesis involves disruption of the skin microbiome and an abnormal immune response to the fungus *Malassezia* sp on the skin.[30]
- It is thought that there is abnormal keratinocyte shedding and increased amount of unsaturated fatty acids in the skin.[31]

Differential and Diagnosis

- Differentials: AD, psoriasis, contact dermatitis, dermatophyte infection, lupus erythematosus, rosacea, pityriasis rosea, Grover disease, and Darier disease.
- Diagnosis

- ○ Seborrheic dermatitis is usually a clinical diagnosis that does not require biopsy.
- ○ Clinically, distribution of lesions is in regions with high number of sebaceous glands, particularly the scalp and face. The pink patches often have greasy scale.
- ○ If considering other differentials, a KOH examination, bacterial swab, serum antinuclear antibodies/extractable nuclear antigen/erythrocyte sedimentation rate, and histology with or without direct immunofluorescence can help rule out other etiologies.[31]

Treatment

Treatment of seborrheic dermatitis depends on the extent and severity of the condition and the desire of the patient to treat this chronic relapsing condition. Treatment rotation is helpful to maintain effectiveness and minimize adverse events. Typical first-line therapies are topical antifungals, such as ketoconazole, miconazole, clotrimazole, ciclopirox olamine, selenium sulfide, or zinc pyrithione. These work to decrease the *Malassezia* burden and reduce inflammation and show similar remission rates to topical corticosteroids but with lower risk of adverse events.[32] The vehicle for the agent selected depends on the area of the body to which it is being applied. Shampoo formulation should be applied to the scalp or body and left on the skin for 5 to 10 minutes before rinsing. Topical corticosteroids of low to mid potencies help mitigate the inflammatory component of seborrheic dermatitis but should be used intermittently to minimize the risk of skin thinning, atrophy, and telangiectasia. The use of steroid-sparing agents, such as calcineurin inhibitors (tacrolimus and pimecrolimus), can also be considered.

Oral systemic agents should only be used in refractory and severe cases. Oral systemic antifungals include itraconazole, fluconazole, and terbinafine.[32] Oral fluconazole is a systemic option that is well tolerated and is used in the elderly, with attention to the risk of the QT prolongation.

ROSACEA

Rosacea is another chronic inflammatory condition that affects 16 million American adults and is estimated to affect 10% of fair-skinned people.[33] Rosacea is typically diagnosed after the age of 30 and is more common in females except for phymatous rosacea, which is more common in men younger than 60 years old.[34] Although more common in Fitzpatrick type I-II, rosacea also affects skin of color.[33]

Clinical Presentation

- • Four clinical subtypes of rosacea: Erythematotelangiectatic, papulopustular, phymatous, and ocular.
  - ○ Erythematotelangiectatic: Persistent central facial erythema, with or without telangiectasia and flushing.
  - ○ Papulopustular: Persistent central facial erythema, facial papules, and/or pustules in the central face.
  - ○ Phymatous: Thickening of the skin with resultant surface nodularities and enlargement. Often affects nose, chin, forehead, cheeks, or ears and is most commonly seen in older men.[33]
  - ○ Ocular: Gritty sensation, burning/stinging, dryness and itching of the eye. Often with blurred vision and telangiectasia of the sclera. Can have periorbital edema.

- Variant: Granulomatous rosacea presents with firm, indurated, yellow, brown, or red papules and nodules.

Pathogenesis

- Rosacea is a multifactorial disease that is comprised of genetic predispositions that cause neurovascular dysregulation and immune dysregulation in combination with aberrant responses to environmental triggers.
- Those with genetic predisposition have exaggerated responses to temperature changes, emotional stress, ultraviolet light, and microbial antigens.[33]

Differential and Diagnosis

- Differentials: Adult acne vulgaris, seborrheic dermatitis, contact dermatitis, photodermatitis, actinic damage, and systemic lupus erythematosus.
- Diagnosis
  - Rosacea is diagnosed clinically and can present in a variety of ways. According to the National Rosacea Society, it is defined by one or more of the following primary features: flushing, papules, pustules, or persistent erythema.[33,35]
  - Secondary features include burning, stinging, itching, edema, dryness, erythematous plaques, ocular manifestations, and phymatous changes.[33,35]

Treatment

Treatment depends on the severity of the disease presentation and clinical phenotype of the condition. Topical therapies should be chosen based on the signs and symptoms, tolerability, and past treatments used. The FDA-approved topical therapy options include azelaic acid (15%) gel, metronidazole (1% cream and gel; 0.75% gel, cream, and lotion), sodium sulfacetamide/sulfur (gel, cleanser, lotion, suspension, and cream), brimonidine tartrate (0.33%) gel, oxymetazoline hydrochloride (1%) cream, and ivermectin (1% cream). Azelaic acid or metronidazole treat mild-moderate rosacea and reduce erythema and inflammatory lesions through decreasing reactive oxygen species activity.[35] Sodium sulfacetamide/sulfur wash is also anti-inflammatory, but should be avoided in those with renal disease and known sulfa allergy.[35] Also, the odor is off-putting for patients.[35,36] Topical medications brimonidine tartrate and oxymetazoline hydrochloride are approved for treatment of persistent erythema associated with rosacea, with fast onset of action.[35] Ivermectin cream is thought to have anti-inflammatory actions because it upregulates anti-inflammatory cytokine IL-10; decreases phagocytosis of neutrophils; and targets demodex mites, which are thought to play a role in rosacea activity. It is thought to have less itching and burning compared with azelaic acid and once-daily use of ivermectin 1% cream was more effective than 0.75% metronidazole cream applied twice daily.[37] Topical calcineurin inhibitors are a treatment option for steroid-induced rosacea and lead to improvement in erythema.

Oral therapy for rosacea includes tetracyclines, macrolides, metronidazole, and isotretinoin. Doxycycline (100–200 mg/day) and minocycline (100–200 mg/day) are most used because of tolerability and can be combined with topical agents, such as azelaic acid or metronidazole to achieve control of papulopustular rosacea. Low-dose doxycycline (40 mg) has also recently become available and is another systemic treatment. Ocular rosacea tends to respond to lower doses of doxycycline for long-term treatment.[35] Macrolide antibiotics (azithromycin and clarithromycin) and metronidazole are used in patients with papulopustular rosacea who are intolerant to tetracyclines or have an allergy. Oral isotretinoin is used in erythematotelangiectatic and papulopustular rosacea that have been refractory to other treatments. Although antibiotics have a faster onset of action when compared with oral isotretinoin, oral isotretinoin is an alternative treatment option with doses of 0.3 mg/kg/day being best tolerated and most effective.[35] Additionally, oral ivermectin has been used off-label because it is not approved by the FDA for rosacea at this time.[35] Laser therapy is used to treat telangiectasia including pulsed dye laser, intense pulsed light, and Nd:YAG laser.

GROVER DISEASE

Grover disease, also known as transient and persistent acantholytic dermatosis, is an inflammatory condition that most commonly affects older White men with a history of extensive photodamage.[38] Some patients report flaring in the winter, whereas others report flares in the summer. The lesions themselves usually last 2 to 4 weeks, but relapses and reoccurrences are common.

Clinical Presentation

- Skin-colored to pink papules and papulovesicles, often excoriated, on the trunk and proximal extremities.
- Lesions can also have crusting or hyperkeratosis and associated pruritis.

Pathogenesis

- Direct pathogenesis is unknown, but exacerbating factors include heat, sweating, low humidity, cold, friction, and radiation (ultraviolet and ionizing).

Differential and Diagnosis

- Differentials: Folliculitis, multiple lichenoid keratoses, arthropod bites, pemphigus foliaceous (early), and Darier disease.
- Diagnosis:
  - Although often diagnosed clinically, biopsy is sometimes needed to differentiate from other dermatoses (discussed previously). Direct and indirect immunofluorescence are negative.

Treatment

There is no cure to Grover disease, but avoidance of triggers and providing symptomatic treatments is standard practice. In mild cases, xerosis should be treated with emollients. Topical corticosteroids (triamcinolone) are recommended to decrease inflammation and reduce pruritis. Other topical treatments include vitamin D analogues and calcineurin inhibitors. Oral antihistamines, such as fexofenadine and hydroxyzine hydrochloride, is added to help ease pruritis, but do not prevent new lesions from forming. Second-line therapy includes oral retinoids, such as isotretinoin. Careful monitoring of liver function and lipids is important, particularly in this geriatric population. For severe cases of Grover disease in which systemic therapies are not tolerated, another treatment option includes phototherapy.

DISCLOSURE

The authors have nothing to disclose.

REFERENCES

1. Pezzolo E, Naldi L. Epidemiology of major chronic inflammatory immune-related skin diseases in 2019. Expert Rev Clin Immunol 2020;16(2):155–66.
2. Armstrong AW, Mehta MD, Schupp CW, et al. Psoriasis prevalence in adults in the United States. JAMA Dermatol 2021;157(8):940–6.

3. Parisi R, Iskandar IYK, Kontopantelis E, et al, Global Psoriasis Atlas. National, regional, and worldwide epidemiology of psoriasis: systematic analysis and modelling study. BMJ 2020;369:m1590.
4. Tseng IL, Yang CC, Lai EC, et al. Psoriasis in the geriatric population: a retrospective study in Asians. J Dermatol 2021;48(6):818–24.
5. Kwon HH, Kwon IH, Youn JI. Clinical study of psoriasis occurring over the age of 60 years: is elderly-onset psoriasis a distinct subtype? Int J Dermatol 2012; 51(1):53–8.
6. Galezowski A, Maccari F, Hadj-Rabia S, et al. Psoriatic arthritis in France, from infants to the elderly: findings from two cross-sectional, multicenter studies. Ann Dermatol Venereol 2018;145(1):13–20.
7. Reid C, Griffiths CEM. Psoriasis and treatment: past, present and future aspects. Acta Derm Venereol 2020;100(3):adv00032.
8. Yosipovitch G, Tang MB. Practical management of psoriasis in the elderly: epidemiology, clinical aspects, quality of life, patient education and treatment options. Drugs Aging 2002;19(11):847–63.
9. Kaushik SB, Lebwohl MG. Psoriasis: which therapy for which patient: psoriasis comorbidities and preferred systemic agents. J Am Acad Dermatol 2019;80(1): 27–40.
10. Menter A, Strober BE, Kaplan DH, et al. Joint AAD-NPF guidelines of care for the management and treatment of psoriasis with biologics. J Am Acad Dermatol 2019;80(4):1029–72.
11. Xu Q, Adabi S, Clayton A, et al. Swept-source optical coherence tomography-supervised biopsy. Dermatol Surg 2018;44(6):768–75.
12. Dave R, Alkeswani A. An overview of biologics for psoriasis. J Drugs Dermatol 2021;20(11):1246–7.
13. Hoy SM. Deucravacitinib: first approval. Drugs 2022;82(17):1671–9.
14. Sotyku (deucravacitinib) [package insert]. Princetown, NJ: Bristol-Myers Squibb Pharmaceutical Company; 2022.
15. Shalabi MMK, Garcia B, Coleman K, et al. Janus kinase and tyrosine kinase inhibitors in dermatology: a review of their utilization, safety profile and future applications. Skin Therapy Lett 2022;27(1):4–9.
16. Chello C, Carnicelli G, Sernicola A, et al. Atopic dermatitis in the elderly caucasian population: diagnostic clinical criteria and review of the literature. Int J Dermatol 2020;59(6):716–21.
17. Bocheva GS, Slominski RM, Slominski AT. Immunological Aspects of Skin Aging in Atopic Dermatitis. Int J Mol Sci 2021;22(11):5729.
18. Tanei R. Atopic dermatitis in older adults: a review of treatment options. Drugs Aging 2020;37(3):149–60.
19. David Boothe W, Tarbox JA, Tarbox MB. Atopic dermatitis: pathophysiology. Adv Exp Med Biol 2017;1027:21–37.
20. Tanei R. Atopic dermatitis in the elderly. Inflamm Allergy - Drug Targets 2009;8(5): 398–404.
21. Adam DN, Gooderham MJ, Beecker JR, et al. Expert consensus on the systemic treatment of atopic dermatitis in special populations. J Eur Acad Dermatol Venereol 2023;37(6):1135–48.
22. Drucker AM, Lam M, Flohr C, et al. Systemic therapy for atopic dermatitis in older adults and adults with comorbidities: a scoping review and international eczema council survey. Dermatitis 2022;33(3):200–6.
23. Tampa M, Mitran CI, Mitran MI, Georgescu SR. A New Horizon for Atopic Dermatitis Treatments: JAK Inhibitors. J Pers Med 2023;13(3):384.

24. Schalock PC, Dunnick CA, Nedorost S, et al. American Contact Dermatitis Society core allergen series: 2020 update. Dermatitis 2020;31(5):279–82.
25. Seyfarth F, Schliemann S, Antonov D, et al. Dry skin, barrier function, and irritant contact dermatitis in the elderly. Clin Dermatol 2011;29(1):31–6.
26. Balato A, Balato N, Di Costanzo L, et al. Contact sensitization in the elderly. Clin Dermatol 2011;29(1):24–30.
27. Slodownik D, Mousa M, Bar J. Allergic contact dermatitis in the older adults: a comparative cross-sectional study. Dermatitis 2023;34(4):329–33.
28. Prakash AV, Davis MD. Contact dermatitis in older adults: a review of the literature. Am J Clin Dermatol 2010;11(6):373–81.
29. Gupta AK, Richardson M, Paquet M. Systematic review of oral treatments for seborrheic dermatitis. J Eur Acad Dermatol Venereol 2014;28(1):16–26.
30. Leachman SA, Carucci J, Kohlmann W, et al. Selection criteria for genetic assessment of patients with familial melanoma. J Am Acad Dermatol 2009;61(4):e671–7.
31. Tucker D, Masood S. Seborrheic dermatitis. In: StatPearls. Treasure island (FL): StatPearls Publishing Copyright © 2022, StatPearls Publishing LLC.; 2022.
32. Borda LJ, Perper M, Keri JE. Treatment of seborrheic dermatitis: a comprehensive review. J Dermatolog Treat 2019;30(2):158–69.
33. Cices A, Alexis AF. Patient-focused solutions in rosacea management: treatment challenges in special patient groups. J Drugs Dermatol 2019;18(7):608–12.
34. Rainer BM, Kang S, Chien AL. Rosacea: epidemiology, pathogenesis, and treatment. Dermatoendocrinol 2017;9(1):e1361574.
35. Sharma A, Kroumpouzos G, Kassir M, et al. Rosacea management: a comprehensive review. J Cosmet Dermatol 2022;21(5):1895–904.
36. Oge LK, Muncie HL, Phillips-Savoy AR. Rosacea: diagnosis and treatment. Am Fam Physician 2015;92(3):187–96.
37. Cardwell LA, Alinia H, Moradi Tuchayi S, et al. New developments in the treatment of rosacea: role of once-daily ivermectin cream. Clin Cosmet Investig Dermatol 2016;9:71–7.
38. Weaver J, Bergfeld WF. Grover disease (transient acantholytic dermatosis). Arch Pathol Lab Med 2009;133(9):1490–4.

Common Skin Cancers in Older Adults Approach to Diagnosis and Management

Martha Laurin Council, MD, MBA*, David M. Sheinbein, MD

KEYWORDS

- Skin cancer • Melanoma • Lentigo maligna • Basal cell carcinoma
- Squamous cell carcinoma • Mohs micrographic surgery

KEY POINTS

- Malignant melanoma accounts for the greatest number of skin cancer-related deaths in the elderly.
- Basal cell carcinoma is the most common type of skin cancer, with over 2 million diagnosed each year.
- Squamous cell carcinoma is the 2nd most common type of skin cancer. Although typically curable when treated early, melanoma has the potential to metastasize.
- Surgery remains the gold standard for treatment of most skin cancers. Systemic therapies such as immunotherapy are used in advanced and metastatic disease.

INTRODUCTION

Skin cancer affects an estimated 4.4 million Americans each year.[1–5] Although predominantly a disease of the elderly white population, skin cancer can affect individuals of all ages and races. The most common type of skin cancer is basal cell carcinoma, followed in incidence by squamous cell carcinoma.[6] A third type of skin cancer, melanoma, is less common than basal and squamous cell carcinomas but accounts for the greatest skin cancer-related morbidity and mortality.[5] The purpose of this article is to review the epidemiology, diagnosis, staging, histologic subtyping, and treatment of melanoma and nonmelanoma skin cancers.

MELANOMA

Epidemiology

In 2023, it is estimated that 97,610 new cases of invasive and 89,070 cases of in situ melanoma will be diagnosed in the United States.[7] Risk factors include a personal history of melanoma, exposure to ultraviolet radiation (natural sunlight or indoor tanning

Department of Medicine (Dermatology), Washington University School of Medicine in St. Louis, 969 North Mason Road, Suite 200, St Louis, MO 63141, USA
* Corresponding author.
E-mail address: mcouncil@wustl.edu

Clin Geriatr Med 40 (2024) 25–36
https://doi.org/10.1016/j.cger.2023.09.001
0749-0690/24/© 2023 Elsevier Inc. All rights reserved.

device), and white skin, with exposure to ultraviolet radiation being the single most important modifiable risk.[7]

Clinical Diagnosis

When diagnosed in early stages, melanoma has great potential for cure.[7] Skin self-examinations and screening examinations by a primary care physician or dermatologist are important for identification of worrisome lesions. Patients should be educated with regard to the ABCDEs of melanoma (**Fig. 1**). Any existing lesions that fall into this category should be evaluated. Additionally, new pigmented lesions arising after the age of 40 should be evaluated.

One technique that can aid in the evaluation of a new or changing pigmented lesion is dermoscopy. Dermoscopy is the use of magnification and polarized light to examine a patient's lesion for findings characteristic of a benign or malignant process. Although helpful in assessing whether or not further evaluation is warranted, dermoscopy is not a substitute for histopathological examination and, therefore, does not replace the skin biopsy as the gold standard for the diagnosis of melanoma.

Various biopsy techniques are available to further evaluate a pigmented lesion. A shave biopsy uses a surgical blade to remove a thin piece of tissue. Shave biopsies

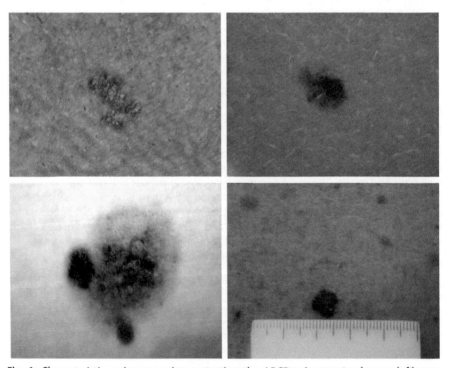

Fig. 1. Characteristic melanomas demonstrating the ABCDs: *Asymmetry* (*upper left*): one-half of the lesion does not mirror the other; *Border irregularity* (*upper right*): edge of the lesion is indistinct or variegated; *Color change* (*lower left*): multiple colors exist within the lesion or lesion changes color/darkens; *Diameter* (*lower right*): lesion is ≥ 6 mm in diameter. A final letter, *E* for *Evolution* is added to the acronym (ABCDE) to indicate that lesions that are evolving in size, shape, or color should also be evaluated. (*From* Council ML. Common skin cancers in older adults: approach to diagnosis and management. Clin Geriatr Med. 2013 May;29(2):361-72.)

can be used to evaluate thin lesions, such as melanoma in situ, but are less helpful in assessing invasive melanomas because the biopsy typically expends no deeper than the papillary or superficial reticular dermis. A shave biopsy of an invasive melanoma risks transection of the lesion and an inadequate measurement of Breslow thickness (important for staging the lesion). A deeper biopsy can be accomplished with either a punch biopsy or a complete excision. A punch biopsy uses a punch tool of a certain diameter (typically 2 mm – 1 cm) to remove a circular piece of tissue to the level of subcutaneous fat. This allows for evaluation of the deep margin, but can only assess a piece of tissue the size of the corresponding punch tool. For complete assessment of larger or irregularly shaped lesions, an excisional biopsy of the entire lesion, extending to the subcutaneous fat, could be performed.

Once a diagnosis of melanoma has been made, patients may question whether further studies are indicated. This is largely dependent upon the stage of the disease at diagnosis and the need for further treatment.

Staging

Melanoma staging guidelines were most recently updated with the 8th Edition of the American Joint Commission on Cancer.[8] Melanoma uses a staging system for tumors, lymph nodes, and distant metastases (TNM) (**Table 1**). Prognosis is directly related to cancer stage, with a 5-year survival rate greater than 99% for stage I disease, and 32% for distant metastatic disease.[7]

Histologic Subtype

Histologically, melanomas can be categorized into 4 main subtypes. Superficial spreading is the most common type of melanoma and is characterized by irregular nests of atypical melanocytes in the epidermis and dermis.[9] Nodular melanomas tend to be more invasive and have a deeper nodular component. Lentigo maligna is a subtype of melanoma typically found on the head and neck of elderly individuals. These tend to be broad and not deep lesions. Acral lentiginous melanoma is typically found on acral sites—palms and soles. Although rare, it accounts for the most common subtype among Black individuals.[10] Extracutaneous locations, including the

Table 1
American Joint Committee on Cancer melanoma staging guidelines

Stage	T	N	M
Stage 0	Tis	N0	M0
Stage I	T1a, T1b, T2a	N0	M0
Stage II	T2b, T3, T4	N0	M0
Stage III	T any	N1	M0
Stage IV	T any	N any	M1

Tis, in situ disease; T1a, tumor less than 0.8 mm thick and nonulcerated; T1b, tumor less than 0.8 mm thick and ulcerated or tumor between 0.8 mm and 1 mm in thickness; T2a, tumor greater than 1 but less than or equal to 2 mm thick, nonulcerated; T2b, tumor greater than 1 but less than or equal to 2 mm thick, ulcerated; T3, tumor greater than 2 and less than or equal to 4 mm thick; T4, tumor greater than 4 mm thick; N0, no nodal metastases; N1, involvement of a single node or in-transit metastases; N2, involvement of 2 to 3 nodes or involvement of a node and in-transit metastases; N3, involvement of more than or equal to 4 nodes or matted nodes, or in-transit metastases with 2 metastatic node(s); M0, no distant metastases; M1, distant metastases.
From Council ML. Common skin cancers in older adults: approach to diagnosis and management. Clin Geriatr Med. 2013 May;29(2):361-72.

eye, mucosal membranes, and lymphatic system, account for a small subset of melanomas.

Treatment

Treatment of melanoma varies depending on the stage of the primary tumor. The Breslow thickness is 1 of the most important prognostic indicators of the primary lesion.[11] The thickness is defined as the histologic depth of the tumor when measured from the top of the granular cell layer of the epidermis to the depth of the bulk of the tumor. This measurement is used to categorize a lesion as thin (≤1 mm), intermediate (1.1–4 mm), or thick (>4 mm). In addition to the Breslow thickness, additional histologic factors (see **Table 1**) are used to further stage the tumor and guide treatment.

After a diagnosis of melanoma is made histologically, a patient should undergo wide local excision of the primary tumor. Margins vary based on Breslow thickness. In situ lesions (Breslow 0 mm) are excised with 5 to 10 mm margins. Invasive melanomas less than or equal to 1 mm in thickness are excised with a 1 cm margin. Melanomas between 1 mm and 2 mm in thickness are excised with a 1 or 2 cm margin. Melanomas greater than 2 mm in thickness are excised with 2 cm margins.

In addition to wide local excision, patients stage T1b or greater are advised to consider sentinel lymph node biopsy. This is typically performed at the time of wide local excision by a surgical oncologist. If a sentinel lymph node is positive, active observation or completion lymphadenectomy are discussed.

Sentinel lymph node status also guides adjuvant therapy. A patient with high-risk disease is subsequently imaged for metastatic disease. Additionally, patients with stage IIB and higher disease may be offered immunotherapy or other systemic treatment. Various treatment modalities exist, including checkpoint inhibitors (ie, ipilimumab, nivolumab, pembrolizumab), cytokines (interferon, interleukins), BRAF inhibitors (vemurafenib, dabrafenib, encorafenib), oncolytic viruses (talimogene laherparepvec), MEK inhibitors (trametinib, cobimetinib, binimetinib), chemotherapeutic agents (dacarbazine), vaccines (bacillus Calmette-Guerin vaccine), and immune stimulators (imiquimod).[12] Radiation therapy is sometimes used for locoregional control of inoperable disease. See **Fig. 2** for the standard treatment algorithm of local disease. Finally, ongoing clinical trials may be available to interested patients. A searchable list may be found at http://clinicaltrials.gov.

Prevention

Because individuals with a history of melanoma have 12 times the likelihood of developing a second primary lesion compared to patients without melanoma,[13] continued monitoring by a dermatologist is crucial. Patients should be reminded to wear sun-protective clothing and to apply and re-apply a broad-spectrum sunscreen of sun protection factor 30 or greater to exposed areas. Patients should be advised to avoid tanning, either outdoors or in a tanning bed, because this is the single most modifiable risk factor for the development of melanoma.[14] Finally, immediate family members of those with melanoma should also be screened as they may have a similar phenotype, genetic risk, or exposure practice.[15]

NONMELANOMA SKIN CANCER

Nonmelanoma skin cancers are the most commonly diagnosed malignancies in humans. Additionally, the incidence is rising along with the aging population. As with melanoma, early recognition and treatment is an important component of preventing advanced disease. Although rare, cases of metastatic basal cell carcinoma

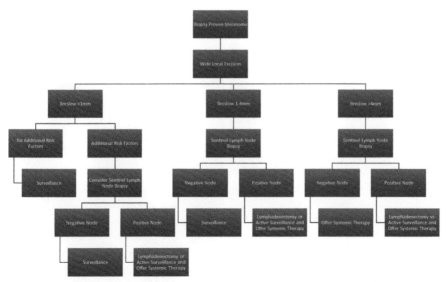

Fig. 2. Treatment algorithm for melanoma. After a diagnosis of melanoma, patients should undergo a wide local excision with or without sentinel lymph node biopsy. Sentinel lymph node status gives important prognostic information and can guide further work-up and treatment.

have been reported.[16,17] Squamous cell carcinoma has a greater tendency toward local recurrence, nodal, or distant metastasis.[18]

Epidemiology

As with melanoma, the greatest modifiable risk factor for nonmelanoma skin cancer is sun exposure. Unlike melanoma, however, chronic sun exposure is believed to play a greater role in the formation of nonmelanoma skin cancers than intermittent sun exposure.[19] Photoprotective measures, such as avoiding the sun during the peak midday hours, wearing sunscreen and sun-protective clothing, and avoiding tanning bed use, are believed to decrease the incidence of nonmelanoma skin cancers.[20]

Clinical Diagnosis

Basal cell carcinoma typically appears as a nonhealing sore or a pearly pink papule (**Fig. 3**). Although most commonly located on sun-exposed areas, basal cell carcinoma may develop in areas of minimal or no exposure as well. Four main subtypes of basal cell carcinoma exist: superficial multifocal, nodular, morpheaform/infiltrative, and basosquamous (metatypical). Superficial multifocal tumors are limited to the outermost layer of skin, the epidermis. These tumors may be found overlying a deeper subtype of basal cell carcinoma, and an adequate biopsy is needed to ascertain whether or not this is the case.[21] In addition, these tumors may be broad and ill-defined, often appearing as a faint scaly pink patch. Nodular basal cell carcinoma is the most common subtype. These lesions typically appear with the classic features of a pink or skin-colored, dome-shaped papule with overlying prominent vasculature. Another histologic variant, the micronodular tumor, clinically appears similarly but may behave more aggressively. Morpheaform or infiltrative tumors can have a sclerotic or scar-like appearance. Basosquamous or metatypical tumors have features of both

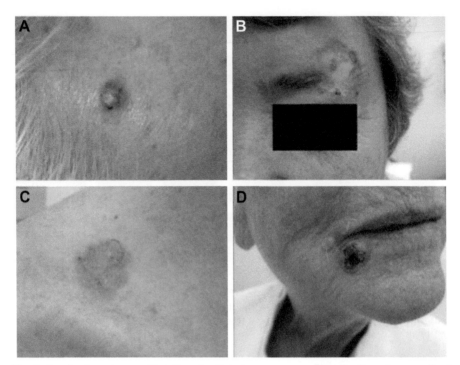

Fig. 3. Basal cell carcinoma. Variations in clinical appearance of basal cell carcinoma reflect histologic variants. Shown here are pigmented (*A*), morpheaform (*B*), superficial multifocal (*C*), and nodular (*D*) subtypes. (*From* Council ML. Common skin cancers in older adults: approach to diagnosis and management. Clin Geriatr Med. 2013 May;29(2):361-72.)

basal and squamous cell carcinomas.[22] Although metastatic basal cell carcinoma is rare, tumors may be locally destructive (**Fig. 4**).

Squamous cell carcinoma likewise may be categorized into several subtypes (**Fig. 5**). A precursor to squamous cell carcinoma formation is the actinic keratosis. It is estimated that up to 16% of actinic keratoses become invasive if untreated.[23] These lesions clinically appear as scaly pink papules, most commonly, on the head, face, and dorsal hands/forearms. If untreated, actinic keratoses may progress to squamous cell carcinoma in situ, squamous cell carcinoma that involves only the outermost layer of skin, the epidermis. Like superficial basal cell carcinoma, squamous cell carcinoma in situ is typically a broad, scaly pink plaque on a sun-exposed area. Squamous cell carcinoma in situ is also known as Bowen disease. Invasive squamous cell carcinoma clinically appears as a nonhealing sore or wart-like growth. More aggressive tumors are classically larger in size, invade more deeply into tissue, have perineural invasion, and are less well differentiated (**Fig. 6**).

Other rare nonmelanoma skin cancers include Merkel cell carcinoma, sebaceous carcinoma, extramammary Paget's disease, dermatofibrosarcoma protuberans, endocrine mucin-producing sweat gland carcinoma, atypical fibroxanthoma, mucinous carcinoma, microcystic adnexal carcinoma, and angiosarcoma, among others. As with other types of skin cancer, diagnosis is based on histopathological evaluation. Treatment is typically surgical removal, followed by adjuvant therapies when indicated.

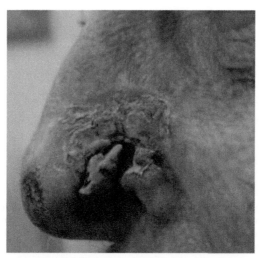

Fig. 4. Locally advanced basal cell carcinoma. Although metastasis is extraordinarily rare, basal cell carcinoma can be locally destructive. The lesion shown here has eroded the alar rim. (*From* Council ML. Common skin cancers in older adults: approach to diagnosis and management. Clin Geriatr Med. 2013 May;29(2):361-72.)

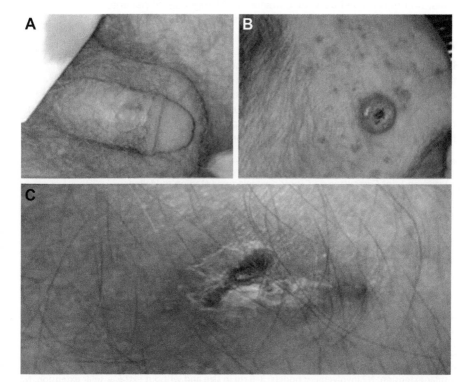

Fig. 5. Squamous cell carcinoma. Clinical appearance of squamous cell carcinoma is also varied. Shown here are the human papillomavirus associated (*A*), keratoacanthoma (*B*), and in situ subtypes (*C*). (*From* Council ML. Common skin cancers in older adults: approach to diagnosis and management. Clin Geriatr Med. 2013 May;29(2):361-72.)

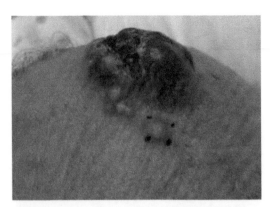

Fig. 6. Locally advanced squamous cell carcinoma. Left untreated, squamous cell carcinoma carries significant morbidity and mortality. This longstanding lesion demonstrates a locally aggressive tumor and in-transit metastasis. (*From* Council ML. Common skin cancers in older adults: approach to diagnosis and management. Clin Geriatr Med. 2013 May;29(2):361-72.)

Staging

Nonmelanoma skin cancer uses the TNM staging system. See **Table 2** for the American Joint Committee on Cancer staging guidelines for the staging of basal, squamous, and non-Merkel adnexal carcinomas.[8] Prognosis of patients with early stage basal and squamous cell carcinoma is excellent.

Treatment

Surgical removal of nonmelanoma skin cancer is the mainstay of treatment. Primary tumors on the trunk or extremity less than 2 cm in diameter are typically excised with 4 mm margins. This results in a cure rate of approximately 95% for basal cell carcinoma.[24]

In certain circumstances, such as with tumors located on the head/neck, large tumors, or recurrent tumors, Mohs micrographic surgery may be used. Developed by the late Frederick Mohs, MD, the Mohs technique allows for the preservation of normal

Table 2
American Joint Committee on Cancer nonmelanoma staging guidelines

Stage	T	N	M
Stage 0	Tis	N0	M0
Stage I	T1	N0	M0
Stage II	T2	N0	M0
Stage III	T3	N0	M0
	T any	N1	M0
Stage IV	T any	N 2–3	M0
	T any	N Any	M1

Tis, in situ disease; T1 tumor up to 2 cm in greatest dimension; T2 tumor more than 2 cm but less than 4 cm; T3 tumor more than or equal to 4 cm or minimal bone erosion or perineural invasion or invasion beyond fat; T4 extensive bone involvement or invasion through foramen; N0 no nodal involvement; N1 involvement of 1 ipsilateral node less than or equal to 3 cm and without extracapsular extension; N2 involvement node(s) 3–6 cm in size and without extracapsular extension; N3 involvement of a node more than 6 cm in size or with extracapsular extension; M0, no distant metastasis; M1, distant metastasis.
From Council ML. Common skin cancers in older adults: approach to diagnosis and management. Clin Geriatr Med. 2013 May;29(2):361-72.

tissue and complete resection of the tumor. During the procedure, a curette or scalpel is used to debulk the clinical lesion. A narrow (approximately 2 mm) margin is then taken for frozen section analysis. The specimen is inked for precise orientation and embedded so that the entire deep and peripheral margin can be evaluated. If residual tumor is noted on histopathological review, additional resection is performed only in the precise area of involvement. This tissue is likewise inked and processed for review. Repetition of these steps occurs until the entire margin is clear of tumor, at which time reconstruction may commence. The American Academy of Dermatology, the American Society for Dermatologic Surgery Association, the American College of Mohs Surgery, and the American Society for Mohs Surgery published Appropriate Use Criteria for Mohs Micrographic Surgery.[25] The Mohs procedure is typically performed under local anesthesia in the office setting, an ideal situation for elderly patients who may not tolerate greater sedation.

In certain circumstances, local destruction may be appropriate management of nonmelanoma skin cancers. One method is electrodesiccation and curettage. In this procedure, a metal curette is used to mechanically debulk the tumor. Curettage relies on malignant tissue being more friable than its surrounding skin. After curettage, electrodesiccation is performed for further destruction. This cycle is typically repeated 2 additional times. Advantages of electrodesiccation and curettage include the short duration and low cost of the procedure. Disadvantages include the absence of tissue confirmation of clear margins and potential for hypertrophic scarring.

Cryotherapy, alone or in combination with curettage, is another method of nonmelanoma skin cancer destruction. In order for substantial tumor damage to occur, tissue must be treated to a temperature of $-60^{\circ}C$.[26] This is typically accomplished with liquid nitrogen. Although not commonly the sole modality in the treatment of invasive skin cancer, cryotherapy is commonly used to treat actinic keratoses.

Imiquimod and 5-fluorouracil are 2 topical therapies that have United States Food and Drug Administration approval for superficial basal cell carcinoma. Application of imiquimod should occur 5 times weekly for 6 weeks. Topical 5-fluoroutacil should be applied twice daily for 6 to 12 weeks. Both medications typically cause erythema and inflammation of the treated area, and patients must be monitored for adequate response. Although not approved by the United States Food and Drug Administration for this purpose, imiquimod and 5-fluorouracil have been used to treat other superficial skin cancers, including melanoma in situ/lentigo maligna[27] and squamous cell carcinoma in situ (Bowen disease).[28] Both are indicated for the treatment of precancerous actinic keratoses.

Intralesional treatment of nonmelanoma skin cancers has been reported in select cases. Agents include 5-fluorouracil, methotrexate, interferon, and bleomycin. These treatments are believed to work via local tissue destruction. Tissue necrosis, pain, and systemic side effects may occur.[29]

Radiation is used for treatment of advanced, inoperable basal and squamous cell carcinomas. In addition, radiation can be adjuvant therapy for nodal disease or high-risk lesions.[30]

Several systemic agents have been approved for advanced and metastatic nonmelanoma skin cancers. Vismodegib and sonidegib, oral hedgehog pathway inhibitors, have been approved for the treatment of advanced and metastatic basal cell carcinoma. Cemiplimab and pembrolizumab, programmed cell death 1 receptor inhibotors, have been approved for advanced and metastatic cutaneous squamous cell carcinoma. Additionally, cemiplimab has been approved for advanced and metastatic basal cell carcinoma in patients who fail or cannot tolerate treatment with a hedgehog inhibitor.

SUMMARY

Melanoma and nonmelanoma skin cancers are a growing concern among elderly individuals. Prompt diagnosis and management are keys in minimizing disease morbidity and mortality. Patients with a history of disease should be followed regularly by a dermatologist to monitor for recurrence and/or development of new lesions. In advanced disease, a multidisciplinary approach with primary care physicians, dermatologists, surgical oncologists, medical oncologists, and radiation oncologists assures optimal management. Current therapies for advanced disease are promising, but prevention of melanoma and nonmelanoma skin cancers remains of paramount importance.

CLINICS CARE POINTS

- Skin cancer is the most common malignancy in adults.
- The diagnosis of skin cancer is confirmed with a tissue biopsy.
- Treatment of localized disease is typically surgical. Systemic and radiation therapy are used for advanced disease.

DISCLOSURE

M.L. Council has served as a consultant for Castle Biosciences, Abbvie, and Regeneron, and a researcher for Castle Biosciences.

REFERENCES

1. Aggarwal P, Knabel P, Fleischer AB. United States burden of melanoma and nonmelanoma skin cancer from 1990 to 2019. J Am Acad Dermatol 2021;85(2): 388–95.
2. Rogers H, Beveridge M, Puente J, et al. Incidence of nonmelanoma skin cancer in the United States population aged 65 years and older, 2014. J Am Acad Dermatol 2021;85(3):741–3.
3. Cameron MC, Lee E, Hibler BP, et al. Basal cell carcinoma: Epidemiology; pathophysiology; clinical and histological subtypes; and disease associations. J Am Acad Dermatol 2019;80(2):303–17.
4. Rogers HW, Weinstock MA, Feldman SR, et al. Incidence estimate of nonmelanoma skin cancer (keratinocyte carcinomas) in the U.S. population, 2012. JAMA Dermatol 2015;151(10):1081–6.
5. Perez M, Abisaad JA, Rojas KD, et al. Skin cancer: primary, secondary, and tertiary prevention. Part I. J Am Acad Dermatol 2022;87(2):255–68.
6. Skin Cancer Facts and Statistics. Skin Cancer Foundation. Available at: https://www.skincancer.org/skin-cancer-information/skin-cancer-facts/. Accessed March 26, 2023.
7. Cancer Facts and Figures. American Cancer Society. Available at: https://www.cancer.org/content/dam/cancer-org/research/cancer-facts-and-statistics/annual-cancer-facts-and-figures/2023/2023-cancer-facts-and-figures.pdf. Accessed March 27, 2023.
8. American Joint Committee on Cancer. Melanoma of the Skin. In: AJCC cancer staging Manual. 8th edition. New York, NY: Springer; 2017. p. 563–85.

9. Elston DM, Ferringer T. Requisite in dermatology: dermatopathology. New York: Saunders Elsevier; 2008.

10. Fernandez JM, Poling KL, Desai AD, Koblinski JE, Borgstrom M, Abraham I, Behbahani S. Primary cutaneous melanoma in Black patients: An analysis of 2464 cases from the National Cancer Database 2004-2018.

11. White RL, Ayers GD, Stell VH, et al. Sentinel Lymph Node Working Group. Factors predictive of the status of sentinel lymph nodes in melanoma patients from a large multicenter database. Ann Surg Oncol 2011;18(13):3593-600.

12. Drugs Approved for Melanoma. National Cancer Institute. Available at: https://www.cancer.gov/about-cancer/treatment/drugs/melanoma. Accessed April 16, 2023.

13. Van der Leest RJ, Liu L, Coebergh JW, et al. Risk of second primary in situ and invasive melanoma in Durch population-based cohort: 1989-2008. Br J Dermatol 2012;167(6):1321-30.

14. Zhang M, Qureshi AA, Geller AC, et al. Use of tanning beds and incidence of skin cancer. J Clin Oncol 2012;30(14):1588-93.

15. Ghiorzo P, Bonelli L, Pastorino L, et al. MC1R variation and melanoma risk in relation to host/clinical and environmental factors in CDKN2A positive and negative melanoma patients. Exp Dermatol 2012;21(9):718-20.

16. Nigro O, Chini C, Marcon IGA, et al. Metastatic basal cell carcinoma to the bone: A case of bone metastasis in uncommon sites. Dermatol Reports 2022;14(3):9267.

17. Fordham SA, Shao EX, Banney L, et al. Management of basal cell carcinoma with pulmonary metastasis. BMJ Case Rep 2023;16(1):e251700.

18. Soleymani T, Brodland DG, Arzeno J, et al. Clinical outcomes of high-risk cutaneous squamous cell carcinomas treated with Mohs surgery alone: An analysis of local recurrence, regional nodal metastases, progression-free survival, and disease-specific death. J Am Acad Dermatol 2023;88(1):109-17.

19. Samarasinghe V, Madan V. Nonmelanoma skin cancer. J Cutan Aesthet Surg 2012;5(1):3-10.

20. Raymond-Lezman JR, Riskin S. Attitudes, behaviors, and risks of sun protection to prevent skin cancer amongst children, adolescents, and adults. Cureus 2023; 15(2):e34934.

21. Wolberink EA, Pasch MC, Zeiler M, et al. High discordance between biopsy and excision in establishing basal cell carcinoma subtype: analysis of 500 cases. J Eur Acad Dermatol Benereol 2013;27(8):985-9.

22. Sgouros D, Apalla Z, Theofili M, et al. How to spot a basosquamous carcinoma: a study on demographics, clinical-dermatoscopic features and histopathological correlations. Eur J Dermatol 2021;31(6):779-84.

23. Ratushny V, Gober MD, Hick R, et al. From keratinocyte to cancer: the pathogenesis and modeling of cutaneous squamous cell carcinoma. J Clin Invest 2012; 122(2):464-72.

24. Gulleth Y, Goldberg N, Silverman RP, et al. What is the best surgical margin for a basal cell carcinoma: a meta-analysis of the literature. Plast Reconstr Surg 2010; 126(4):1222-31.

25. Hoc Task Force Ad, Connolly SM, Baker DR, et al. AAD/ACMS/ASDSA/ASMS 2012 Appropriate use criteria for Mohs micrographic surgery: a report of the American Academy of Dermatology, American College of Mohs Surgery, American Society for Dermatologic Surgery Association, and the American Society for Mohs Surgery. J Am Acad Dermatol 2012;67(4):531-50.

26. Kuflik EG. Cryosurgery. In: Bolognia JL, editor. Dermatology. 2nd edition. Spain: Mosby Elsevier; 2008. p. 2124.

27. Ellis LZ, Cohen JL, High W, et al. Melanoma in situ treated successfully using imiquimod after nonclearance with surgery: a review of the literature. Dermatol Surg 2012;38(6):937–46.
28. Nemer KM, Council ML. Topical and systemic modalities for chemoprevention of nonmelanoma skin cancer. Dermatol Clin 2019;37(3):287–95.
29. Kirby JS, Miller CJ. Intralesional chemotherapy for nonmelanoma skin cancer: a practical review. J Am Acad Dermatol 2010;63(4):689–702.
30. Hulyalkar R, Rakkhit T, Garcia-Zuazaga J. The role of radiation therapy in the management of skin cancers. Dermatol Clin 2011;29(2):287–96.

Diagnosis and Management of Bullous Disease

Amanda A. Onalaja-Underwood, MD[a], Maria Yadira Hurley, MD[b],
Olayemi Sokumbi, MD[c,d,]*

KEYWORDS

- Bullous diseases • Dermatoses • General population • Anatomic level

KEY POINTS

- Bullous diseases are a group of dermatoses primarily characterized by the presence of vesicles (0.1–0.9 cm) or bullae (>1 cm).
- The complex process of aging, which involves cumulative environmental, genetic, and cellular interplay, is evident in the skin.
- The clinical approach to reaching a diagnosis includes a thorough history and physical examination.

INTRODUCTION

Bullous diseases are a group of dermatoses primarily characterized by the presence of vesicles (0.1–0.9 cm) or bullae (>1 cm). There are various categories of bullous disease: allergic, autoimmune, infectious, mechanical, and metabolic. These diseases affect individuals in all decades of life, but older adults, age 65 and older, are particularly susceptible to bullous diseases of all etiologies. The incidence of these disorders is expected to increase given the advancing age of the general population.

The complex process of aging, which involves cumulative environmental, genetic, and cellular interplay, is evident in the skin. Vasculature atrophies, the dermis deteriorates, and the extracellular matrix and its components become more disorganized. The dermal papillae flatten causing attenuation in the surface area of dermal and epidermal adhesion that contributes to an increased risk of blister formation.[1] Simultaneously, the process of immune system dysregulation that accompanies normal aging contributes greatly to autoimmune bullous diseases.[2]

a Department of Dermatology, Vanderbilt University Medical Center, 719 Thompson Lane, Suite 26300, Nashville, TN 37204, USA; b Department of Dermatology, Saint Louis University, School of Medicine, 1225 South Grand Boulevard, St. Louis, MO 63104, USA; c Department of Dermatology, Mayo Clinic, 4500 San Pablo Road S, Jacksonville, FL 32224, USA; d Department of Laboratory Medicine & Pathology, Mayo Clinic, 4500 San Pablo Road S, Jacksonville, FL 32224, USA
* Corresponding author. Mayo Clinic, 4500 San Pablo Road S, Jacksonville, FL 32224.
E-mail address: Sokumbi.olayemi@mayo.edu

Clin Geriatr Med 40 (2024) 37–74
https://doi.org/10.1016/j.cger.2023.09.002
0749-0690/24/© 2023 Elsevier Inc. All rights reserved.

geriatric.theclinics.com

In this comprehensive review, the bullous dermatoses will focus on those applicable to adults and will be categorized primarily by the anatomic level of the split. Additionally, this article includes clinical and epidemiologic data concerning the disease, pathophysiology, diagnostic methods, and therapies. Recognition and diagnosis of a bullous disease are crucial for timely intervention and limitation of complications.

RELEVANT CLINICAL QUESTIONS

The clinical approach to reaching a diagnosis includes a thorough history and physical examination. The following are focused points to consider while narrowing the differential diagnosis.

- Did the eruption coincide with a change in medication or general health status?
- Are the blisters flaccid or tense?
- Are the blisters pruritic, painful, or asymptomatic?
- Is there surrounding erythema/induration or noninflamed/normal skin?
- Are the blisters cutaneous, mucosal, or mucocutaneous?
- Are the blisters localized (acral, sun-exposed, extensor surfaces) or generalized?
- Does the morphology of the eruption have a particular pattern (annular, linear, clusters)?

INITIAL WORKUP CONSIDERATIONS

When a blistering disorder is suspected, but a diagnosis cannot be established, a skin biopsy is indicated. An early, intact lesion with adjacent skin should be biopsied to ensure that an accurate histopathological diagnosis is made. This sample is submitted in formalin for routine hematoxylin and eosin staining. If autoimmune blistering dermatoses are being considered, an additional biopsy for direct immunofluorescence (DIF) should be performed. To properly submit a specimen for immunobullous DIF testing, the ideal sample is taken from immediately adjacent unaffected, healthy-appearing skin surrounding the bulla and submitted in Michel media. Other special studies such as salt-split skin immunofluorescence, serum indirect immunofluorescence (IIF), and electron microscopy may be useful adjuncts. Serologic tests, specifically enzyme-linked immunosorbent assays (ELISAs), are available for bullous pemphigoid and pemphigus and can be used when the diagnosis is in doubt (**Box 1**).

Box 1
Diseases with an intracorneal/subcorneal split

Pemphigus foliaceus

Pemphigus erythematosus

Fogo selvagem

Subcorneal pustular dermatosis

IgA pemphigus

Acute generalized exanthematous pustulosis

Impetigo

Staphylococcal/Streptococcal scalded-skin syndrome

Dermatophytosis

Miliaria crystallina

Pemphigus Foliaceus

Pemphigus foliaceus (PF) represents 10% to 20% of all pemphigus cases. PF is the second most common form of pemphigus and considered milder compared to pemphigus vulgaris. Like pemphigus vulgaris, it can be associated with myasthenia gravis, thymoma, and autoimmune thyroiditis. The antibodies are directed toward desmoglein 1 which is why oral lesions are rare. Adult mucosal surfaces contain enough desmoglein-3 to compensate for the disruption of the desmoglein-1 attachments and are therefore not usually involved. A similar compensation is believed to protect the growing fetus from maternal autoantibodies against desmoglein-1. **Table 1** lists characteristics of variants of pemphigus foliaceus: Fogo selvagem and pemphigus erythematosus. Drug-induced PF is most caused by thiol-containing drugs, such as D-penicillamine and captopril. Other implicated drugs are listed in **Box 2**

Pathogenesis

- The pathogenesis is secondary to antibodies (immunoglobulin [Ig]G4 subclass) against desmoglein 1, which is a transmembrane glycoprotein of desmosomes in the epidermis.

Clinical features

- Superficial vesicles of the scalp, face, and trunk break open and lead to crusted erosions that heal without scarring. **Fig. 1**.
- "Cornflake" scale is common **Fig. 2**.
- Mucosal involvement is rarely seen.
- Nikolsky sign is positive (light rubbing of unaffected skin adjacent to a blister or erosion will cause separation of the skin).
- Adults are most affected, usually during midlife.

Differential diagnosis

- Seborrheic dermatitis
- Impetigo (especially the bullous form)
- Dermatitis herpetiformis

Table 1 Variants of pemphigus foliaceus		
Disease		**Clinical presentation**
Fogo selvagem	• Endemic form of pemphigus foliaceus mainly found in rural areas of Brazil, Columbia, El Salvador, Paraguay, and Peru • Transmitted by *Simulium* species (black fly) • Increasing frequencies in families with HLA-DRB1 mutations	Identical clinical and histologic features to pemphigus foliaceus
Pemphigus erythematosus (Senear – Usher syndrome)	• Represents 10% of all cases of pemphigus foliaceus, with features of lupus erythematosus • Sunlight may worsen the disease • Clinical course is generally chronic	Localized to malar region of face and other seborrheic areas

Box 2
Medications associated with pemphigus

Captopril

Cephalosporins

Enalapril

Gold

Interferon-alpha

Interleukin-2

Levodopa

Oxyphenylbutazone

Penicillamine

Peniclillin's

Phenobarbital

Phenylbutazone

Piroxicam

Propranolol

Pyritinol

Rifampin

- Subacute cutaneous lupus erythematosus
- Drug reaction
- Allergic contact dermatitis
- Darier disease

Diagnostic testing

- Lesional biopsy for histopathology.
- Perilesional biopsy for DIF.
- IIF on guinea pig esophagus.
- ELISA for desmogleins 1 and 3.

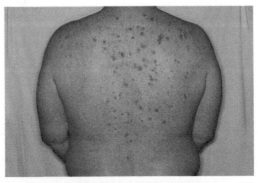

Fig. 1. Widespread erythematous plaques on the back of a patient with pemphigus erythematosus. (*Courtesy of* O Sokumbi, MD)

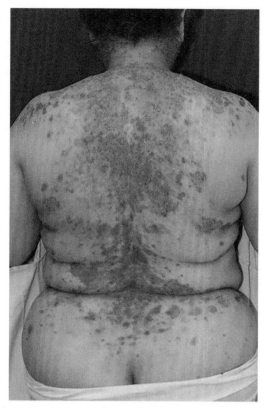

Fig. 2. Widespread erosions, crusts, and thin, erythematous, scaly plaques on the back of a patient with pemphigus foliaceous. (*Courtesy* of O Sokumbi, MD)

Treatment

- Localized disease can typically be managed by potent topical steroids.
- For more widespread disease, the mainstay is prednisone followed by steroid-sparing immunosuppressants such as azathioprine, mycophenolate mofetil, rituximab, or dapsone.

Subcorneal Pustular Dermatosis

Subcorneal pustular dermatosis (SPD), also known as Sneddon–Wilkinson disease, is a chronic, waxing-waning neutrophilic dermatosis characterized by sterile pustules that erupt into polycyclic patterns. Like the subcorneal pustular subtype of IgA pemphigus, the pustular lesions found in Sneddon–Wilkinson disease coalesce in an annular pattern and eventually evolve into crusted plaques. Diagnosis is made based on physical examination findings, histologic findings of a subcorneal neutrophilic vesicle, and by ruling out other potential and related diagnoses with laboratory evaluation. Associated conditions include hematologic disorders (polycythemia rubra vera, Ig A monoclonal gammopathy, and multiple myeloma), pyoderma gangrenosum, Raynaud's phenomenon, Sjogren's syndrome, systemic lupus erythematosus, and inflammatory bowel disease.

Pathogenesis

- The pathogenesis of SPD is poorly understood.

- SPD with associated autoantibodies to desmocollin 1 is best classified as SPD-like IgA pemphigus.
- Desmocollins function in cell adhesion with other structural proteins within the cadherin family; when these proteins are affected, the underlying scaffolding of a skin cell is compromised, leading to the formation of subcorneal bullae and vesicles.

Clinical features

- Flaccid, sterile pustules with yellowish fluid in the dependent half with clearer fluid in the top half of the lesion
- A predilection for the groin, trunk, axillae; avoids the mucosal surfaces
- It is mostly seen in women over 40 years old
- Chronic, relapsing clinical course

Differential diagnosis

- IgA pemphigus
- Acute generalized exanthematous pustulosis
- Amicrobial pustulosis associated with autoimmune disease
- Bacterial folliculitis
- Impetigo
- Pustular psoriasis
- Pustular vasculitis

Diagnostic testing

- Lesional biopsy for histopathology.
- Perilesional biopsy for DIF is negative.
- IIF is negative.
- Serum protein electrophoresis and DIF may be repeated every few years.

Treatment

- The typical first-line treatment for patients with SPD is oral dapsone 50 to 200 mg once daily.
- Second-line and salvage therapies include sulfapyridine, sulfasalazine (prodrug to sulfapyridine), immunosuppressants, colchicine, systemic retinoids, phototherapy (broad and narrowband *ultraviolet* [UV]A or psoralen plus UVA); they are reserved for those unable to take dapsone or who failed to respond to therapy.
- Evaluation for associated cutaneous and systemic diseases should be undertaken when clinically indicated.

IgA Pemphigus

IgA pemphigus is a poorly understood bullous disease defined by the presence of IgA anti-keratinocyte cell surface autoantibodies. It may have some clinical overlap with SPD, and the SPD type of IgA pemphigus presents with similar annular, crusted vesicles and pustules in the axilla and groin. The intraepidermal neutrophilic dermatosis (IEN) type of IgA pemphigus may preferentially involve the trunk, rather than the intertriginous areas.

Pathogenesis

- Target antigen in SPD type is desmocollin 1.
- Target antigens in IEN type are desmoglein-1 or 3.

Clinical features

- Presents in the axillae and groin in the middle-aged to elderly with pruritic and flaccid vesicles and pustules in annular configurations and central crusting.
- Oral involvement is rarely seen.
- Can be associated with IgA paraproteinemia and multiple myeloma.[3]
- Two subtypes are known:
  - Subcorneal pustular dermatosis type (SPD) is clinically indistinguishable from Sneddon–Wilkinson disease; DIF/IIF is needed to distinguish.
  - Intraepidermal neutrophilic type (IEN) presents with a "sunflower" arrangement of vesicles and pustules and may preferentially involve the trunk rather than the intertriginous areas.

Differential diagnosis

- Dermatitis herpetiformis
- Eosinophilic pustular folliculitis
- Pemphigus foliaceus
- Subcorneal pustular dermatosis

Diagnostic testing

- Lesional biopsy for histopathology.
- Perilesional biopsy for DIF shows intercellular staining with IgA in 100% of cases:
  - SPD type: intercellular IgA deposition in the upper epidermis
  - IEN type: intercellular IgA in the lower epidermis or throughout
- IIF is unreliable as only 50% have detectable circulating IgA.

Treatment

- Treatment is directed against neutrophils with dapsone 25 to 100 mg daily, being a medication in which dramatic responses are seen within 48 hours.
- Alternatively, if dapsone-intolerant: start sulfapyridine 500 mg twice a day and increase slowly.
- Some case reports include colchicine or retinoids as effective.

Acute Generalized Exanthematous Pustulosis

Acute generalized exanthematous pustulosis (AGEP) is a pustular, generalized drug eruption. Beta-lactam antibiotics, anticonvulsants, and calcium channel blockers are the most frequent culprits. Intravenous contrast and infections can also trigger the condition. Unlike other drug eruptions, such as drug rash with eosinophilia and systemic symptoms (DRESS) and Stevens–Johnson Syndrome/toxic epidermal necrolysis (SJS/TEN), AGEP can occur within 4 days of initial exposure. Hypocalcemia is a key laboratory finding in AGEP and is thought to occur due to hypoalbuminemia. Fever, neutrophilia, and eosinophilia are often found. The cutaneous eruption usually resolves in a few days, but hepatic and kidney involvement is possible.

Pathogenesis

- AGEP is thought to be T-cell mediated: drug-specific CD4+ T cells, cytotoxic CD8+ T cells, and inflammatory cytokines and chemokines are thought to be involved in tissue accumulation of neutrophils.
- 90% of reported cases of AGEP are drug induced with an onset of hours (antibiotics) to 3 weeks (other drugs).
- A minority of cases are linked to viral infections.

Clinical features

- The eruption begins as acute, erythematous edema on the face or intertriginous areas and is quickly followed by numerous pinpoint nonfollicular pustules.
- Most patients have a fever and a history of a recently added medication.
- Mucous membrane involvement is atypical but when present is limited to erosions of the lips.

Differential diagnosis

- Acute pustular psoriasis
- Bacterial folliculitis
- DRESS
- Cutaneous candidiasis

Diagnostic testing

- Lesional biopsy for histopathology.
- Perilesional biopsy for DIF will be negative.

Treatment

- Remove offending drug
- Antipyretics as needed
- Supportive care

Bullous Impetigo

Bullous impetigo is a superficial staphylococcal skin infection. The condition is primarily seen in children but can occur in adults. Infection is spread by direct contact with colonized or infected individuals. Undiagnosed human immunodeficienc virus (HIV) infection should be considered in an adult with bullous impetigo and appropriate risk factors.

Pathogenesis

- Superficial skin infection caused primarily by phage group II staphylococci.
- Staphylococcus . aureus produces exotoxin-mediated cleavage of desmoglein-1 causing bullae formation.[4]

Clinical features

- Vesicles which enlarge and lead to flaccid, serous superficial bullae.
- Eroded and crusted plaques may appear at the site of denuded bullae.

Differential diagnosis

- Bullous arthropod assault
- Bullous drug eruption
- Bullous tinea
- Herpes simplex virus
- Contact dermatitis
- Autoimmune blistering disorders

Diagnostic testing

- Gram stain of blister fluid may show gram-positive cocci.
- Bacterial culture with sensitivities.
- Biopsy is usually not necessary.

- Lesional biopsy for histopathology.
- DIF is negative.

Treatment

- Topical antibiotic ointments such as mupirocin or retapamulin ointment can be used twice daily for 5 days in limited disease.
- For widespread infections, systemic antibiotics can be used; dicloxacillin or cephalexin for methicillin-sensitive *Staphylococcus aureus* (MSSA) or doxycycline, clindamycin, or sulfamethoxazole-trimethoprim if methicillin-resistant *Staphylococcus* aureus (MRSA) is suspected (**Box 3**).

Trauma Bullae

Trauma bullae are blisters that are typically found on acral surfaces due to repeated physical forces. Occupations or recreational activities that require prolonged running or walking are at the highest risk. Moist skin can produce higher frictional forces than wet or dry skin and increase the risk of bullae formation.[5]

Pathogenesis

- Development is linked to the magnitude of frictional force and the number of cycles across the skin.
- Shearing forces cause the disassociation of keratinocytes which leads to epidermal splitting and fluid filling.

Clinical features

- Noninflamed blister on the palms and soles.
- The most affected sites include the tips of the toes, the balls of the feet, and the posterior heel.
- Occurs in vigorously active populations.

Differential diagnosis

- Epidermolysis bullosa simplex
- Epidermolysis bullosa acquisita
- Bullous arthropod assault
- Bullosis diabeticorum
- Bullous fixed drug eruption
- Bullous tinea

Diagnostic Testing

- History and location
- Biopsy is usually not necessary

Box 3
Diseases with an intraepidermal split

Amicrobial pustulosis associated with autoimmune diseases

Trauma bullae

Spongiotic diseases

Palmoplantar pustulosis

Viral blistering

- Lesional biopsy for histopathology
- DIF is negative

Treatment

- Maintain blister roof intact to speed healing time; larger lesions may need to be drained.
- Prevention can be achieved by avoiding friction using acrylic socks, closed-cell neoprene insoles, and thin polyester socks combined with thick wool or propylene socks.

Herpes Zoster

Herpes zoster, also known as shingles, is caused by the reactivation of the varicella-zoster virus (VZV). This occurs in about 20% of immunocompetent individuals and is more commonly seen in immunocompromised individuals or the elderly. Clinically, they have grouped vesicles, and/or erosions on an erythematous base. Herpes zoster can be triggered by a condition such as immunosuppression, radiation, UV exposure, trauma, stress, or be idiopathic.

Clinical features

- Painful grouped vesicles with scalloped borders on an erythematous base in a dermatomal pattern. **Fig. 3**.
- Disseminated disease will have a dermatomal pattern and 20 or more lesions outside of the primary dermatome.
- The thorax is the most common location, followed by the face, lumbar, and sacrum.

Pathogenesis

- VZV is dormant in the dorsal root ganglia for life after primary infection (varicella).
- Reactivation of the latent varicella-zoster virus.

Differential diagnosis

- Herpes simplex virus infection
- Allergic contact dermatitis
- Bullous arthropod assault
- Other poxviruses

Diagnostic testing

- Polymerase chain reaction (PCR)-based testing from base of a blister is the test of choice as it is sensitive and can have a relatively fast turnaround time.
- Tzanck smear from base of blister
- Viral culture from base of blister
- Histology will show an intraepidermal vesicle with epithelial necrosis, ground-glass-appearing ballooned nuclei within keratinocytes and multinucleated cells.

Treatment

- Antiviral therapy with acyclovir and pro-drug forms; skin lesions remain contagious until all lesions are crusted over (**Box 4**).

Pemphigus Vulgaris

Pemphigus vulgaris is the most common type of pemphigus, representing 70% or more of all subtypes. Characteristic flaccid bullae rupture and leave denuded areas.

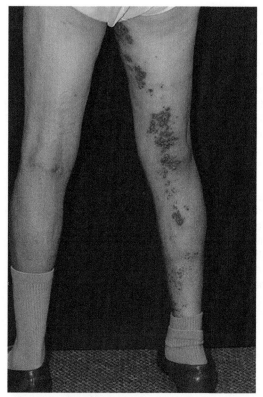

Fig. 3. Multiple grouped and confluent vesicles and bullae on a background of erythema in the S2 dermatome. (*Courtesy* of O Sokumbi, MD)

Pemphigus vulgaris is the classic disease associated with the Nikolsky sign, in which light friction on perilesional skin induces a blister. The Asboe-Hansen sign, in which pressure on the surface of a bulla causes the blister to spread laterally, is also positive. Mucosal, in particular oral involvement is often the initial manifestation in PV.

This disease process can be associated with myasthenia gravis, thymoma, and autoimmune thyroiditis. The hair follicles are extensively involved. Many different drugs have precipitated this disease, especially those with thiol groups, although pemphigus foliaceus rather than pemphigus vulgaris is more commonly induced.

Box 4
Diseases with a suprabasilar split
Pemphigus vulgaris
Pemphigus vegetans
Paraneoplastic pemphigus
Grover disease
Hailey–Hailey disease
Darier disease

Pathogenesis

- Both humoral and cell-mediated mechanisms contribute.
- Autoantibodies of the predominantly IgG4 subclass target desmoglein-3 early and later cross-react with desmoglein-1.
- In the adult, desmoglein-3 is concentrated in the basal and suprabasilar layers of the epidermis and mucosal surfaces.
- Desmoglein 1 is expressed in all levels of the epidermis and can compensate for desmoglein 3 loss in the upper layers of the skin; desmoglein 3 cannot compensate for the loss of desmoglein 1 in mucosa which leads to the oral manifestation seen in PV.

Clinical features

- Flaccid bullae break to form painful erosions **Fig. 4**.
- Oral involvement occurs first in 60% of cases, followed by the skin **Fig. 5**.
- Other mucosal surfaces may be involved
- Commonly involves the trunk, groin, axillae, scalp, and face
- Positive Nikolsky sign
- The average age at presentation is in the fifth or sixth decade
- More common in Jewish/Mediterranean populations
- Associations: other autoimmune disorders (myasthenia gravis and thymoma)

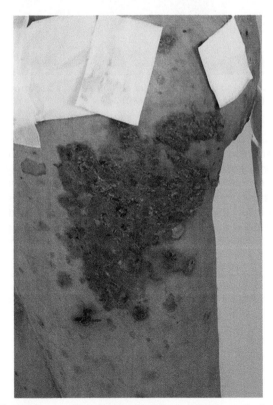

Fig. 4. Flaccid bullae with secondary erosion, crusting, and scale on the lower extremity of a patient with pemphigus vulgaris. (*Courtesy* of O Sokumbi, MD)

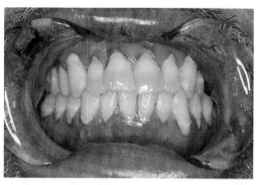

Fig. 5. Erosions along the gum line giving rise to marginal gingivitis in a patient with pemphigus vulgaris. (*Courtesy* of O Sokumbi, MD)

Differential diagnosis

- Pemphigus foliaceus
- Drug-induced pemphigus
- Erythema multiforme
- Stevens–Johnson syndrome
- Bullous pemphigoid

Diagnostic testing

- Lesional biopsy for histopathology.
- Perilesional biopsy for DIF.
- IIF on monkey esophagus can be used to assess patient's sera for circulating IgG antibodies and as a proxy for disease state and treatment status.
- ELISA for desmogleins 1 and 3.

Treatment

- Rituximab has been Food and Drug Administration (FDA) approved for moderate to severe PV since June 2018.
- Short-term systemic corticosteroids (1 mg/kg/day) combined with adjuvant immunosuppressants (ie, azathioprine, mycophenolate mofetil, or rituximab) can also be used.[6]
- Other steroid-sparing immunosuppressive agents to consider include cyclophosphamide, intravenous immunoglobulin (IVIG), methotrexate, and plasmapheresis.
- Treatment response can be monitored clinically or with IIF and ELISA levels.

Pemphigus Vegetans

Pemphigus vegetans is the rarest clinical variant in the pemphigus group of vesiculobullous autoimmune diseases and represents less than 2% of all pemphigus.[7] Vegetative plaques in intertriginous areas and the oral mucosa help to distinguish it from pemphigus vulgaris. Pemphigus vegetans has traditionally been classified into Neumann and Hallopeau types.

- Neumann type: Lesions typically begin as typical flaccid blisters of pemphigus vulgaris, become eroded, and form vegetating plaques. Plaques are often studded with pustules. Tends to have a chronic course.
- Hallopeau type: Pustular lesions evolve into vegetating plaques. The Hallopeau type may be more benign and remit spontaneously.

Pathogenesis

- Autoantibodies against desmoglein-3 are pathogenic; often desmoglein-1 is also involved as in PF.
- IgG and IgA antibodies against desmocollins have also been reported[8].

Clinical features

- Vesicles or pustules that become vegetating plaques often on the axillae/groin (flexural), trunk, and extremities. **Fig. 6**.
- Most patients present with stomatitis.
- Mean age of onset is in the fifth decade.

Differential diagnosis

- Hailey–Hailey disease
- Iododerma/bromoderma
- Syphilitic condyloma
- Granuloma inguinale
- Leishmaniasis
- Condyloma acuminata
- Deep fungal infection

Diagnostic testing

- Lesional biopsy for histopathology.

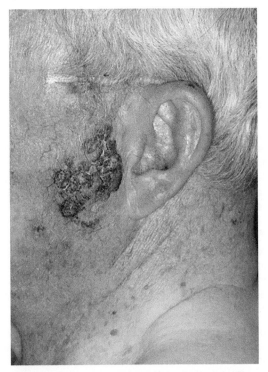

Fig. 6. Verrucous and vegetative plaque on the left cheek in pemphigus vegetans. (*Courtesy* of O Sokumbi, MD)

- DIF of perilesional skin.
- ELISA can identify desmoglein 3 autoantibodies in sera with a specificity and sensitivity of 98% to 100%, respectively.[9]

Treatment

- As with pemphigus vulgaris, the goal is to decrease or eliminate circulating anti-desmoglein antibodies and then the bound antibodies in the skin.
- The gold standard of therapy is systemic corticosteroids which are thought to up-regulate desmoglein expression.
- Transition to steroid-sparing immunosuppressive agents such as azathioprine, dapsone, methotrexate, rituximab, or mycophenolate mofetil.

Paraneoplastic Pemphigus

Paraneoplastic pemphigus (PNP) is alternatively referred to as paraneoplastic auto-immune multiorgan syndrome. PNP is often fatal and pulmonary involvement in the form of bronchiolitis obliterans is significantly associated with decreased survival. Some cases have been described following treatment with interferon or radiation.[10] A variety of internal malignancies are associated with paraneoplastic pemphigus, with non-Hodgkin lymphoma being the most common. Other associations include chronic lymphocytic leukemia, Castleman disease (especially in children), thymoma, poorly differentiated sarcoma, Waldenström macroglobulinemia, inflammatory fibrosarcoma, Hodgkin disease, T-cell lymphoma, and treatment with fludarabine.

Pathogenesis

- Autoantibodies to envoplakin and periplakin, desmoplakin-1 and desmoplakin-3, desmoglein-1 and desmoglein-3, bullous pemphigoid antigen (BPAg1), and plectin.[11]
- Epitope spreading may be responsible for the diverse clinicopathologic findings and many antibodies.

Clinical features

- The presentation usually starts with severe, intractable stomatitis with character-istic lip involvement. **Fig. 7.**
- Mucositis can involve the conjunctiva, esophagus, anogenital, and nasopharynx.

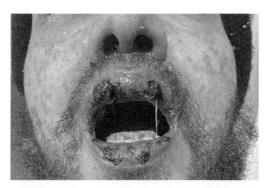

Fig. 7. Diffuse hemorrhagic crusting of the lips in a patient with paraneoplastic pemphigus. (*Courtesy* of O Sokumbi, MD)

- Polymorphic skin lesions with features of bullous pemphigoid (tense and friable bullae and erosions), toxic epidermal necrolysis, erythema multiforme (targetoid plaques), pemphigus, lichen planus, or linear IgA disease.

Differential diagnosis

- Erythema multiforme
- Bullous pemphigoid
- Pemphigus vulgaris
- SJS/TEN
- Linear IgA bullous dermatosis
- Lichen planus
- Mucous membrane pemphigoid
- Bullous lupus erythematosus

Diagnostic testing

- Lesional biopsy for histopathology.
- Perilesional biopsy for DIF.
- IIF shows intercellular IgG staining on rat bladder epithelium.

Treatment

- Includes treatment of the underlying neoplasms and initiation of immunosuppression.
- Systemic corticosteroids are the mainstay of therapy at 1 to 2 mg/kg per day.
- Adjunctive immunosuppressive drugs as needed (rituximab, IVIG, cyclophosphamide, azathioprine, mycophenolate mofetil).
- Plasmapheresis may be initiated.

Transient Acantholytic Dermatosis

Transient acantholytic dermatosis, also known as Grover disease, is a relatively common disorder that presents with excoriated papules and papulovesicles on the trunk. It tends to affect Caucasian middle-aged men with a significant history of sun damage. The disease is benign and, in some cases, self-limited.

Pathogenesis

- The exact pathogenesis is unknown but is linked to heat, sweating, and dysfunction of the sweat glands.

Clinical features

- Excoriated papules and vesicles on the central chest, abdomen, and back
- Middle-aged to older adults

Differential diagnosis

- Pityrosporum folliculitis
- Bacterial folliculitis
- Acne
- Miliaria rubra
- Pemphigus
- Darier disease
- Hailey–Hailey disease
- Galli–Galli disease

- Allergic contact dermatitis
- Drug eruption

Diagnostic testing

- Biopsy is usually not necessary.
- Lesional biopsy for histopathology.
- DIF is negative.
- Five histologic patterns can be seen: Darier-like, Hailey-Hailey–like, pemphigus vulgaris–like, pemphigus foliaceus–like, and spongiotic.

Treatment

- The goal of therapy is supportive care: avoidance of ultraviolet (UV) exposure, sweating, heat, and friction followed by emollient application.
- If conservative measures fail, mid to high-potency topical steroids twice daily and/or topical vitamin D-analogs can be utilized.

- Refractory cases can be treated with isotretinoin 0.5 to 1 mg/kg/day for 2 to 12 weeks, psoralen with ultraviolet A (PUVA), methotrexate, and dapsone (**Box 5**).

Bullous Allergic Contact Dermatitis

Allergic contact dermatitis is a type IV (cell-mediated) hypersensitivity reaction to allergen contact in a sensitized individual. An erythematous eruption develops within

Box 5
Diseases with a subepidermal split
Bullous pemphigoid
Cicatricial pemphigoid
Lichen planus pemphigoides
Pemphigoid gestationis
Epidermolysis bullosa acquisita
Dermatitis herpetiformis
Linear IgA bullous dermatosis
Bullous systemic lupus erythematosus
Arthropod bite
Cryotherapy blister
Burn blister
Suction blister
Drug overdose bullae
Bullous lesions in diabetes mellitus
Epidermolysis bullosa
Porphyria cutanea tarda
Toxic epidermal necrolysis
Bullous drug reaction
Erythema multiforme
Bullous fixed drug reaction

days, with the formation of plaques, papules, and rarely vesicles and bullae. A robust response can lead to bullae and systemic symptoms such as fatigue, fever, and diffuse myalgia.

Pathogenesis

- Sensitization occurs when Langerhans or dendritic cells present allergens to naïve T-helper lymphocytes causing clonal expansion of sensitized lymphocytes.
- Cell-mediated, delayed-type hypersensitivity occurs on subsequent exposure.

Clinical features

- The acute presentation is an erythematous eruption with vesicles or bullae.
- Chronic presentation commonly manifests as hyperkeratosis, fissuring, and lichenification.
- Symptoms occur 24 to 48 hours following exposure to an allergen for the acute presentation.
- On physical examination, rash distribution corresponds to contact exposure.

Differential diagnosis

- Phytophotodermatitis
- Bullous pemphigoid
- Bullous tinea

Diagnostic testing

- Historical correlation is essential to determine the clinical relevance of potential allergens.
- Lesional biopsy for histopathology.
- DIF is appropriately negative.
- Patch testing is the gold standard for identifying specific allergens.

Treatment

- Known allergens should be avoided.
- High or moderately potent topical steroids are usually effective in resolving symptoms.
- Systemic steroids are indicated for severe symptoms or if widespread areas are involved.
- Can consider oral antihistamines for pruritus.

Bullous Lymphedema

Bullous lymphedema blisters are non-infectious lesions that develop in the setting of poorly controlled edema. Concurrent medical conditions contributing to volume overload may include heart failure, renal failure, cirrhosis lymph node dissection, hypoalbuminemia, and venous thrombo-embolus.

Pathogenesis

- The rapid accumulation of interstitial fluid in patients with localized acute edema or anasarca causes these blisters to appear.

Clinical features

- Thin roofed bullae on dependent areas, typically the lower extremities, with associated acute edema.

- Bullae can drain sterile liquid although hemorrhagic or serous fluid can appear.
- Lesions are fragile and rupture easily.
- Bullae may increase in size and number over time.

Differential diagnosis

- Bullous arthropod assault
- Coma blister
- Bullosis diabeticorum
- Contact dermatitis
- Trauma blister
- Bullous pemphigoid

Diagnostic testing

- History of tense bullae that develop in temporal association with acute edema.
- Lesional biopsy for histopathology.
- DIF will be negative.

Treatment

- Supportive management with leg elevation, compression, a low-salt diet, diuretics.
- Optimize underlying medical conditions contributing to edema.

Bullous Pemphigoid

Bullous pemphigoid (BP) is the most common subepidermal bullous disease and it most commonly affects older adults (mean age 68–82 years). There is often a pro-drome that lasts weeks to months, in which patients present with urticarial or eczem-atous lesions. Blisters are tense and heal without scarring. Milia are rarely present in areas of resolving erosions. Patients tend to have a chronic course with remission after about 6 years. Morbidity and mortality are low with treatment. Medications implicated in the cause of BP include furosemide, sulfasalazine, penicillins, penicilla-mine, and captopril. **Box 6** lists other medications that induce bullous pemphigoid. BP has also been described after treatment with ultraviolet light, PUVA, and radiation.

Pathogenesis

- BP180 (BPAG2) and BP230 (BPAG1) are vital components of the hemidesmo-somes which adhere to the epidermis and dermis.
- Both antigens are targets of autoantibodies in pemphigoid; however, it is the NC16 A domain of BPAG2 that is thought to be pathogenic in bullous pemphigoid.
- This is the primary location for antibody binding in bullous pemphigoid and can be detected with the use of an ELISA assay in 85% of affected patients.[12]

Clinical features

- Tense bullae on normal or erythematous skin, urticarial/eczematous lesions **Fig. 8**.
- Early disease may be nonbullous as urticarial patches, plaques, and erythema.
- Bilateral, symmetric, often involving the lower abdomen and shins.
- Mucosal involvement in up to 20%.
- Onset usually in adults older than 65, but young adult and pediatric cases occur.

Box 6
Medications implicated in inducing bullous pemphigoid

Anti-influenza vaccine

Arsenic

Captopril

Clonidine

Dactinomycin

Enalapril

Furosemide

Gold

Ibuprofen

Interleukin-2

Methyldopa

Nadolol

Omeprazole

Penicillamine

Penicillins

Phenacetin

Poatassium iodide

Practolol

Psoralens (PUVA)

Risperidone

Sulfapyridine

Sulfasalazine

Sulfonamide

Terbinafine

Tolbutamide

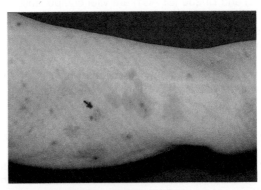

Fig. 8. Tense blisters and erythematous plaques on the upper extremity of a patient with bullous pemphigoid. (*Courtesy* of O Sokumbi, MD)

Differential diagnosis

- Cicatricial pemphigoid
- Lichen planus pemphigoides
- Epidermolysis bullosa acquisita
- Dermatitis herpetiformis
- Linear IgA bullous dermatosis
- Drug eruption
- Arthropod bite
- Urticaria

Diagnostic testing

- Lesional biopsy for histopathology.
- Perilesional biopsy for DIF will show linear complement component 3 (C3) (in an n-serrated pattern) and/or IgG at the basement membrane zone; sometimes IgA and IgM are also present.
- IIF on salt-split skin shows immunoreactants bound to the blister roof.
- Tissue-bound and circulating autoantibodies detected by ELISA; ELISAs are more sensitive than IIF for bullous pemphigoid.

Treatment

- Many patients can be successfully managed with the topical use of class I steroids, such as clobetasol.
- Tetracycline and nicotinamide are thought to help via their anti-inflammatory effects.
- Systemic corticosteroids with a transition to steroid-sparing immunosuppressants can be utilized; these include methotrexate, cyclosporine, mycophenolate mofetil, azathioprine, leflunomide, and rarely cyclophosphamide or chlorambucil.
- In recent years, off-label use of dupilumab and rituximab has been beneficial in moderate-to-severe cases.

Cicatricial/Mucous Membrane Pemphigoid

Mucous membrane pemphigoid encompasses a heterogeneous group of disorders characterized by autoantibodies against various proteins in the anchoring filament zone. There are many different target antigens found in patients with mucous membrane pemphigoid; it may be that this disorder represents a disease phenotype rather than a single entity. Limited cutaneous involvement may also be seen in about 25% of patients. Skin lesions resemble those seen in bullous pemphigoid and may be on the head, neck, or extremities. Patients may develop generalized bullae. There is a 2-to-1 female predominance, and the disease seems to affect older patients (sixth or seventh decade of life).

Significant morbidity may occur due to tissue destruction as the result of chronic mucosal inflammation, pain, and scarring. Oral lesions are the most common manifestation of this condition. Patients present with desquamative gingivitis, erythema, ulcers, and vesicles. The gingival and buccal mucosa, tongue, palate, and tonsillar pillars may be involved. Ocular involvement can also occur and begins with bilateral erythema and rare vesicles that develop into xerosis, fibrosis, and scarring. A localized variant of cicatricial pemphigoid referred to as Brunsting–Perry disease, consists of recurrent blisters on the head and neck that heal with scarring. These patients generally have no mucosal involvement.

Pathogenesis

- Suspected that molecular mimicry results in the development of autoantibodies that target different autoantigens (BPAg1 and 2, laminin 5 and 6, integrin subunit beta 4).

Clinical features

- Lesions tend to recur in the same area.
- Oral and ocular mucosal membrane erosions and painful ulcers that scar **Fig. 9**.
- Anogenital blisters and erosions that result in phimosis or vaginal scarring.
- Scarring may result in adhesions and strictures.
- Rare, tense bullae on erythematous plaques on the scalp, head, neck, and upper trunk.
- Scarring alopecia may develop.

Differential diagnosis

- Bullous pemphigoid
- Bechet disease
- Linear IgA bullous dermatosis
- Lichen planus
- Lichen sclerosus
- Epidermolysis bullosa acquisita

Diagnostic testing

- Lesional biopsy for histopathology:
  - Mucosal: subepidermal bullae with mixed infiltrate
  - Skin: subepidermal bullae with mostly neutrophils and eosinophils; dermal scarring
- Perilesional biopsy for DIF.
- 20% of IIF studies will show linear basement membrane zone with IgG and IgA.
- Anti-laminin 332 (Anti-epiligrin) positive cicatricial pemphigoid has an increased risk for solid organ cancers; therefore, malignancy screening is indicated.

Treatment

- Refer to an ophthalmologist and/or otolaryngologist.
- Minimize loss of gingival tissue and teeth through good oral hygiene.

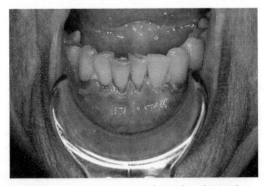

Fig. 9. Gingiva with several erosions. (*Courtesy* of O Sokumbi, MD)

- Mild disease limited to the mouth may respond to high-potency topical cortico-steroids (clobetasol or dexamethasone) or topical tacrolimus.
- Treatment of chronic lesions may include intralesional triamcinolone acetonide.
- If ocular, laryngeal, or urogenital epithelia are scarred, then aggressive treatment with a short course of glucocorticoids 1 mg/kg per day with a transition to steroid-sparing immunosuppressants is warranted.
- Alternatives include IVIG, rituximab, azathioprine, cyclophosphamide, methotrexate, and plasmapheresis.

Ocular Cicatricial Pemphigoid

Ocular cicatricial pemphigoid is also known as ocular mucous membrane pemphigoid. It is a subcategory of mucous membrane pemphigoid. The disease is characterized by chronic conjunctivitis, conjunctival injection, and conjunctival and corneal scar formation. Squamous metaplasia with keratinization of the ocular surface epithelium results in blindness.

Pathogenesis

- IgA antibodies to the intraepidermal portion of the b4 subunit of the $\alpha6$-$\beta4$ integrin.

Clinical features

- Erosions, ulcers with subsequent conjunctival and corneal scarring; blisters are rare. **Fig. 10**.
- Scarring is predominant with fornix obliteration and symblepharon (adhesion of the palpebral and bulbar conjunctiva) formation that leads to ankyloblepharon (fusion of eyelids).
- Entropion, trichiasis, and corneal neovascularization can occur.
- Uncontrolled disease may cause blindness.

Differential diagnosis

- Paraneoplastic pemphigus
- Mucous membrane pemphigoid
- Postinfectious conjunctivitis

Diagnostic testing

- Perilesional biopsy for DIF from conjunctiva will show linear basement membrane zone IgG and/or IgA in conjunctival biopsies.

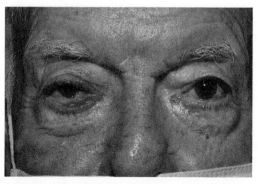

Fig. 10. Conjunctival injection and fibrosis in a patient with ocular cicatricial pemphigoid. (*Courtesy* of O Sokumbi, MD)

Treatment

- Referral to an ophthalmologist
- Dapsone 100 to 150 mg/day
- Oral low-dose weekly methotrexate or mycophenolate mofetil
- Systemic cyclophosphamide with short-term adjunctive high-dose prednisolone is the preferred treatment for severe and/or rapidly progressing ocular cicatricial pemphigoid.

Lichen Planus Pemphigoides

Lichen planus pemphigoides (LPP) is a rare autoimmune skin disorder that involves the simultaneous presence of 2 distinct skin conditions: lichen planus and bullous pemphigoid. In LPP, patients typically experience a combination of the skin lesions associated with lichen planus and the blisters associated with bullous pemphigoid. The skin lesions of lichen planus can occur before, after, or at the same time as the blisters of bullous pemphigoid.

Pathogenesis

- The exact pathogenesis of LPP is not fully understood. It is thought that autoantibodies against specific basement membrane proteins, such as BP180 and BP230, are produced and contribute to the development of bullous pemphigoid.
- Additionally, the T cells that are involved in the development of lichen planus may play a role in the activation of the immune response in LPP.

Clinical features

- Small, flat-topped, purplish, pruritic papules on the flexor arms, legs, and trunk.
- Bullae on skin uninvolved by lesions of lichen planus. **Fig. 11.**
- Erosions, blisters, and lichenoid striae can occur on mucosal surfaces.

Differential diagnosis

- Bullous pemphigoid (without lichen planus lesions)
- Bullous lichen planus
- Pemphigus vulgaris
- Epidermolysis bullosa acquisita
- Linear IgA bullous dermatosis
- Dermatitis herpetiformis
- Erythema multiforme
- Stevens–Johnson syndrome
- Drug-induced bullous eruptions

Diagnostic testing

- Lesional biopsy for histopathology.
- Perilesional biopsy for DIF.

Treatment

- Topical and systemic corticosteroids
- Immunosuppressive medications such as azathioprine, mycophenolate mofetil, methotrexate, or cyclophosphamide.
- In some cases, dupilumab, phototherapy, or plasmapheresis may also be used.

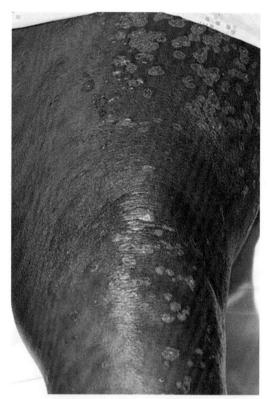

Fig. 11. Lower extremity with small, flat-topped, purple papules and bullae. (*Courtesy* of O Sokumbi, MD)

Epidermolysis Bullosa Acquisita

Epidermolysis bullosa acquisita (EBA) is a chronic, immunobullous disease seen in association with inflammatory bowel disease, hematologic malignancy, and other autoimmune diseases. It is characterized by autoantibodies against collagen VII. EBA usually develops in adulthood but can present at any age.

Pathogenesis

- Type VII collagen is the targeted autoantigen in EBA and the primary constituent of the hemidesmosomal dermal anchoring fibers.[13]

Clinical features

- EBA has 1 non-inflammatory presentation and 4 inflammatory presentations:
  - Classical (non-inflammatory) type: Formation of non-inflammatory tense vesicles and bullae that rupture; locations most susceptible to minor trauma like the hands and feet are most affected with subsequent scarring and milia formation. Patients may also develop scarring alopecia, loss of nails, and esophageal stenosis.
  - Inflammatory:
- Bullous pemphigoid-like type: characterized by a general eruption of blisters that have features of bullous pemphigoid surrounded by inflamed skin or urticaria.

- Mucous membrane type: erosions and scars on mucosal surfaces including buccal, conjunctival, gingival, nasopharyngeal, esophageal, rectal, and genital.
- Brunsting–Perry-type: bullous eruption localized to the head and neck with scarring, minimal mucosal involvement. **Fig. 12**.
- IgA type: presents with linear IgA deposits in the basement membrane (BMZ) that can be observed by DIF.
- Onset usually in adulthood but can occur at any age, no predilection for older adults.
- Trauma often precedes the formation of lesions.

Differential diagnosis

- Bullous pemphigoid
- Cicatricial pemphigoid
- Linear IgA dermatosis
- Porphyria cutanea tarda
- Bullous systemic lupus erythematosus

Diagnostic testing

- Lesional biopsy for histopathology.
- Perilesional biopsy for DIF.

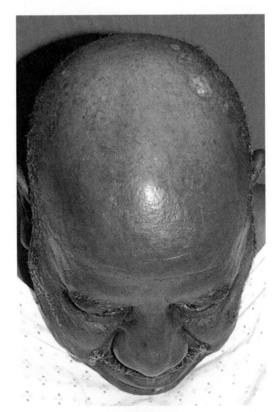

Fig. 12. Patient with Brunsting–Perry pemphigoid with erosions, and surrounding scarring on the parietal aspect of the left side of the scalp. (*Courtesy* of O Sokumbi, MD)

- IIF: linear basement membrane IgG in 50% of cases.
- Salt-split skin DIF demonstrates dermal pattern linear IgG, on the "floor" of the blister.
- ELISA will have autoantibody against non-collagenous (NC)1 domain of type VII collagen.

Treatment

- Minimize trauma to the skin and, if mucous membranes are involved, encourage good oral hygiene and a soft diet with little acid content.
- Oral corticosteroids and antineutrophilic agents or immunosuppressive agents are standard.
- Dapsone started at 50 mg daily and increase by 50 mg weekly, up to 300 mg once a day, until remission occurs. Maintain at remission dose for several months, then decrease slowly until the drug can be discontinued.
- Cyclosporine at 3 to 5 mg/kg per day divided into 2 doses, usually produces a rapid response.
- The noninflammatory variant is more resistant to treatment and may require intravenous immunoglobulin or extracorporeal photopheresis.

Dermatitis Herpetiformis

Dermatitis herpetiformis is a gluten-sensitive blistering dermatitis characterized by anti-transglutaminase 3 IgA antibodies. It is an extremely pruritic disorder that presents with clustered vesicles that are quickly excoriated. Vesicles arise in crops and are distributed symmetrically on the scalp, sacrum, and extensor extremities. Some patients, especially children, may have palmar involvement. The disease course is usually lifelong; spontaneous remissions occur in up to 10% of patients. Patients with dermatitis herpetiformis commonly have gluten-sensitive enteropathy or "celiac sprue." Thyroid disease, small bowel lymphoma, non-Hodgkin lymphoma are also associated. Of note, there is a strong association with *human leukocyte antigen* (HLA)-DQ2 and HLA-DQ8. Other alloantigens that have been reported are HLA-B8, HLA-DR3, and HLA-A1.

Pathogenesis

- The pathogenesis is uncertain but involves extrinsic and intrinsic factors.
- Granular deposition of IgA in the dermal papillae, activation of the complement system, chemotaxis of neutrophils followed by the release of enzymes that alter or destroy laminin and type IV collagen all contribute to the formation of blisters.

Clinical features

- The onset is usually young adulthood to middle age.
- Small, pruritic, and often excoriated, papules and vesicles with a predilection for extensor surfaces.
- Symmetric distribution, especially on elbows, knees, buttocks. **Fig. 13** and **14**
- Mucous membranes are rarely involved.

Differential diagnosis

- Linear IgA bullous dermatitis
- Bullous pemphigoid
- Scabies
- Contact dermatitis
- Bullous arthropod assault

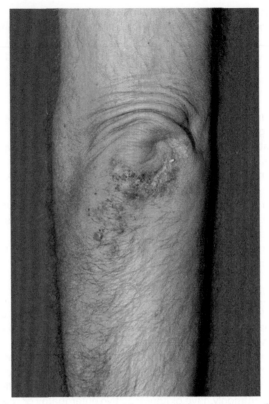

Fig. 13. Elbow with several excoriated papules and vesicles. (*Courtesy* of O Sokumbi, MD)

Diagnostic testing

- Lesional biopsy on an intact vesicle or pink papule (not an excoriated lesion) for histopathology.
- Perilesional biopsy for DIF.
- Serum antibodies include antiendomysial IgA, antireticulin, thyroid microsomal, antinuclear, and tissue transglutaminase.

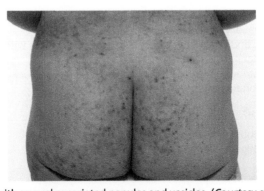

Fig. 14. Buttocks with several excoriated papules and vesicles. (*Courtesy* of O sokumbi, MD).

- Total IgA level is useful as IgA deficiency appears to be less common in dermatitis herpetiformis.[14]

Treatment

- A gluten-free diet is the preferred treatment for both cutaneous and gastrointestinal disease; long-term adherence decreases the risk of lymphoma.
- The skin often responds rapidly to dapsone:
  - Adult initial dose 25 to 50 mg daily
  - Average adult maintenance dose of 100 mg daily
  - Lesions return abruptly on discontinuation
  - Gastrointestinal disease is typically not adequately controlled with dapsone
- Alternative if dapsone-unresponsive or allergic: sulfapyridine 500 mg 3 times daily up to 2 g 3 times daily.
- Occasional application of topical steroids to control lesions.
- Lifelong treatment is needed.

Linear IgA Bullous Dermatosis

Linear IgA bullous dermatosis (LABD) is a rare, autoimmune subepidermal bullous disease that can affect the skin and/or mucous membranes. It has a bimodal age distribution with 2 forms of the disease: LABD occurs in older adults and chronic bullous disease of childhood occurs in children. LABD is marked by linear deposition of IgA along the basement membrane. It can present like other blistering cutaneous disorders, such as dermatitis herpetiformis or bullous pemphigoid. While it is often idiopathic, LABD can be drug induced, and vancomycin has historically been the most commonly associated drug. However, a strong causal relationship between vancomycin and LABD has not yet been established.

Pathogenesis

- Linear IgA bullous dermatosis-1 (LAD-1: 120 kDa) antigen and linear IgA bullous dermatosis (LABD: 97 kDa) antigen are breakdown products of the transmembrane protein BPAg2 (BP180).
- Rare cases in which the antigen is collagen VII of the anchoring fibril.
- The most common drug reported to be associated with LABD is vancomycin, but the pathophysiology remains unknown.[15]
- Other implicated medications include amiodarone, diclofenac, captopril, penicillins, ceftriaxone, metronidazole, interleukin-2, naproxen, and phenytoin.

Clinical features

- Discrete bullae that often are annular and occur in clusters: "cluster of jewels" or "string of pearls." **Fig. 15.**
- The lesions can be extremely pruritic.
- Adults generally present with rapid onset of tense vesicles and confluent erythematous plaques and papules that affect the trunk, face, buttocks, and extensor extremities.
- Typically, children present with bullae or vesicles on the trunk, face, genitalia, and extremities.

Differential diagnosis

- Bullous pemphigoid
- Cicatricial pemphigoid

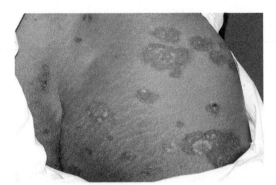

Fig. 15. Hyperpigmented plaques with peripheral "cluster of jewels" or "string of pearls" vesicles. (*Courtesy* of O Sokumbi, MD)

- Herpes simplex and zoster
- Dermatitis herpetiformis
- Pemphigus vulgaris
- Bullous impetigo

Diagnostic testing

- Lesional biopsy for histopathology.
- Perilesional biopsy for DIF.
- IIF on salt-split human skin may show linear IgA antibodies in 33% to 50% of adult patients.

Treatment

- First-line treatment is dapsone; screening for glucose-6-phosphate dehydrogenase deficiency should be performed and if positive, dapsone should be avoided for increased risk of hemolytic anemia. It is important to note that patients who are sulfa allergic can still be treated with dapsone, a sulfone.
- In patients who cannot tolerate dapsone, consider sulfapyridine or sulfamethoxypyridazine, sulfonamide agents that share structural similarities with dapsone.
- If these methods fail to control the disease, corticosteroids and/or other immunosuppressive agents can be used.
- Penicillin and macrolides have also been found to be highly effective.[15]

Bullous Systemic Lupus Erythematosus

Bullous systemic lupus erythematosus (BSLE) is seen in patients who meet the criteria for SLE and is characterized by autoantibodies to collagen VII. BSLE is a rare presentation of systemic lupus erythematosus. Bullae arise on sun-exposed skin on a noninflammatory or inflammatory base. The prognosis is usually excellent with treatment.

Pathogenesis

- Autoantibodies to type VII collagen (290-kDa protein) in the anchoring fibrils, similar to epidermolysis bullosa acquisita.

Clinical features

- Herpetiform vesicles or more often large, tense, fluid-filled to hemorrhagic bullae **Fig. 16**.
- Acute onset, usually on sun-exposed skin

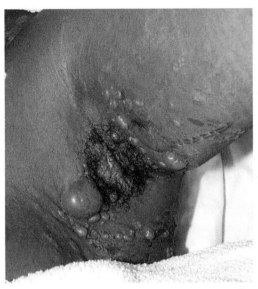

Fig. 16. The left axilla of a patient with bullous systemic lupus erythematosus with large, tense bulla. (*Courtesy* of O Sokumbi, MD)

Differential diagnosis

- Epidermolysis bullosa acquisita
- Dermatitis herpetiformis
- Linear IgA bullous dermatosis
- Bullous pemphigoid
- Bullous impetigo
- Bullous drug eruption
- Erythema multiforme

Diagnostic testing

- Lesional biopsy for histopathology.
- DIF demonstrates granular to linear basement membrane zone staining with IgG, IgA and/or IgM, and C3 ('lupus band').
- IIF is negative.

Treatment

- Dapsone (25–100 mg per day in an adult) is considered the treatment of choice for BSLE; new bullae formation usually ceases within days of starting therapy.
- Other treatments include hydroxychloroquine (200–400 mg per day), colchicine, corticosteroids, rituximab, anakinra, methotrexate, and mycophenolate mofetil.

Cryotherapy Blister

A cryotherapy blister is a blister that forms because of cryotherapy, which involves the use of extreme cold to treat various skin conditions, such as warts, skin tags, and precancerous lesions. Cryotherapy works by applying liquid nitrogen, which has a temperature of around −196°C, to the affected area, causing the cells to freeze and die.

Pathogenesis

- The disruption of the normal structure and function of the skin occurs due to the application of extreme cold, leading to damage to the skin cells and the accumulation of fluid and inflammatory cells, which can cause a blister to form.
- The blister is a natural part of the healing process and is important for tissue repair and regeneration.

Clinical features

- Tense blister at the site of prior cryotherapy.
- Usually, blisters form within 24 to 48 hours after the procedure and can range in size from small to large, depending on the extent of the treatment.

Differential diagnosis

- Herpes simplex virus
- Varicella-zoster virus
- Bullous pemphigoid
- Pemphigus vulgaris
- Epidermolysis bullosa
- Contact dermatitis
- Burn blister
- Arthropod assault

Diagnostic testing

- The clinical history of a recent cryotherapy procedure is the key.

Treatment

- Cryotherapy blisters are a normal part of the healing process after cryotherapy and usually resolve on their own within a few days to a week. However, if the blister is particularly large or causing discomfort, it may be drained using a sterile needle or scalpel.

Burn Blister

A burn blister forms on the skin because of exposure to heat or chemicals. Burn blisters occur when the skin is damaged by a burn, which causes the skin cells and tissues to separate and fluid to accumulate between the layers of the skin. The formation of a burn blister serves as a protective mechanism, as it helps to protect the underlying tissue from further damage and provides a moist environment for the healing process to occur. However, it is important to be cautious when dealing with burn blisters, as they can be fragile and easily ruptured, which can increase the risk of infection or slow down the healing process.

Pathogenesis

- The pathogenesis of a burn blister involves the disruption of the normal structure and function of the skin due to exposure to heat or chemicals.
- When the skin is exposed to extreme heat, it causes damage to the skin cells and the surrounding tissue, leading to the formation of a blister.

Clinical features

- The severity of the clinical features depends on the extent of the burn injury.

- Superficial or first-degree burns typically only affect the outermost layer of skin, causing redness and pain.
- Second-degree burns, on the other hand, affect the deeper layers of the skin and can cause blistering.
- Third-degree burns can damage the skin, underlying tissue, and even bone, and may cause extensive blistering or the absence of blisters due to the complete destruction of the skin.

Differential diagnosis

- Herpes simplex virus
- Varicella-zoster virus
- Bullous pemphigoid
- Pemphigus vulgaris
- Epidermolysis bullosa
- Contact dermatitis
- Cryotherapy blister
- Arthropod assault

Diagnostic testing

- The clinical history of a burn at the site of the blister is the key.
- Biopsy is usually not necessary.
- Lesional biopsy for histopathology.

Treatment

- Supportive care is the main therapy for a burn blister and involves keeping the affected area clean and dry, avoiding puncturing the blister, and protecting it with a sterile dressing.

Suction Blister

A suction blister is a blister that is artificially created by applying negative pressure to the skin, which separates the layers of the skin and produces a fluid-filled blister. The process of creating a suction blister involves using a device, such as a suction pump, to generate negative pressure on the skin, usually on the arm or leg. Suction blisters are commonly used in dermatology research for studying the properties of the skin and for grafting purposes.

Pathogenesis

- The pathogenesis of suction blisters involves the disruption of the normal structure and function of the skin due to the application of negative pressure.
- When negative pressure is applied to the skin, it causes the separation of the layers of the skin, including the epidermis and dermis.

Clinical features

- Blisters can be intentionally created by medical procedures such as grafting, particularly for the treatment of stable vitiligo. Alternatively, they can also develop due to unintentional or self-inflicted injuries, particularly in children.

Differential diagnosis

- Bullous pemphigoid
- Pemphigus vulgaris

- Epidermolysis bullosa
- Contact dermatitis
- Impetigo
- Herpes simplex virus
- Varicella-zoster virus
- Bullous erythema multiforme

Diagnostic testing

- Suction blisters are typically diagnosed based on their clinical appearance and history of their formation.

Treatment

- Suction blisters are usually a self-limited condition that will heal on their own within a few days to a week.
- In general, the treatment for suction blisters involves providing supportive care to relieve symptoms and promote healing.

Coma Bullae

Coma blisters may be a result of medications, metabolic disturbances, and stroke, among many other causes. They were originally described in the setting of carbon monoxide intoxication and are most reported in association with barbiturates.[16] They have also been reported following surgical procedures that require general anesthesia.

Pathogenesis

- Pathogenesis is not fully understood; local hypoxia from prolonged pressure has been suggested as the most likely cause.[17]

Clinical features

- Tense blisters that appear on otherwise normal skin.
- Erythematous plaques or patches first appear after about 24 hours of immobilization and progress to dusky plaques with erosions or bullae around 48 hours.

Differential diagnosis

- Trauma bullae
- Neutrophilic eccrine hidradenitis

Diagnostic testing

- Clinical history of coma.
- Lesional biopsy for histopathology.

Treatment

- With appropriate removal of pressure, lesions typically heal within 1 to 2 weeks, with scarring developing in some.

Bullosis Diabeticorum

Bullosis diabeticorum is also known as diabetic bullae or bullous eruption of diabetes mellitus. Lesions in diabetes mellitus are a rare complication of long-standing diabetes mellitus but have been reported as a presenting sign of diabetes. Lesions heal within several weeks without scarring but may recur.

Pathogenesis

- The pathogenesis is unknown.

Clinical features

- Noninflammatory bullae that are tense and vary in diameter from small to very large on the lower extremities of a diabetic patient.

Differential diagnosis

- Pseudoporphyria or porphyria cutanea tarda
- Bullous tinea
- Bullous fixed drug eruption
- Bullous impetigo
- Trauma bullae
- Poison ivy dermatitis

Diagnostic testing

- Clinical history of diabetes.
- Lesional biopsy for histopathology.
- Perilesional biopsy for DIF will be negative.

Treatment

- Glucose control should be optimized. Lesions are usually self-resolving and supportive care should be initiated.

Bullous Fixed Drug Eruption

Fixed drug eruption presents days to 2 weeks after initial drug exposure as sharply demarcated red edematous to dusky plaques on the skin. They are most commonly on the hands, feet, lips, or genitalia. These lesions can blister and become widespread (generalized bullous fixed drug eruption), which can be difficult to differentiate from SJS/TEN. These lesions often heal with post-inflammatory hyperpigmentation, and within 48 hours of drug re-exposure, they present in the same location as before. Other variants include non-pigmented (classically associated with pseudoephedrine) and linear fixed-drug eruption.

Pathogenesis

- It is thought that an antigen from the medication causes the activation of CD8+ cytotoxic T-cells in the epidermis of a fixed area of skin.
- These cytotoxic T-cells are thought to reside in certain locations on the skin or mucous membranes and are stimulated with antigen re-exposure.

Clinical features

- Erythematous macules or patches that develop into a vesicle or bullae minutes to days after drug exposure.
- Recurrence at the same site(s) on re-exposure to the drug.
- The most common sites are the lips, genital area, hands, and feet.

Differential diagnosis

- SJS/TEN
- Erythema multiforme
- Allergic contact dermatitis

- Erosive lichen planus
- Bullous impetigo

Diagnostic testing

- Inducible lesions will appear at previously involved sites with provocation with the possible agent (after allowing for a possible refractory period of weeks to months).
- Lesional biopsy for histopathology.
- DIF is negative.

Treatment

- Mid and high-potency topical corticosteroids can be used for supportive care.
- Drug cessation, if possible, although fixed drug eruption is not a severe cutaneous adverse drug reaction so continuation of medication is not contraindicated if the drug is necessary; although, generalized bullous fixed drug eruption is considered severe and potential culprit drugs should be discontinued.
- Patch testing can be done but must be performed at the site of previous areas of involvement after a refractory period.

Porphyria Cutanea Tarda

Porphyria cutanea tarda (PCT) is the most common porphyria, a group of disorders characterized by dysfunction of the heme biosynthesis pathway. There are 3 types of PCT that can be classified as "familial" or "sporadic" based on the presence or absence of gene mutations of the hepatic enzyme, uroporphyrinogen decarboxylase (UROD). Type 1 (sporadic) accounts for 80% of cases and lacks a UROD mutation.[18] Type 2 (familial) has inherited UROD mutations affecting 1 allele in 20% of cases. Type 3 (familial) does not have an inherited UROD mutation but may have other inherited factors such as hemochromatosis.

Pathogenesis

- Due to decreased activity of UROD.

Clinical features

- Sun-exposed areas of skin with tense vesicles, bullae, erosions, and morpheaform plaques. **Fig. 17.**
- Dorsal hands may have scarring, milia, and hypo/hyperpigmentation in and around active bullae and erosions.
- Delayed photosensitivity with skin fragility.

Differential diagnosis

- Pseudoporphyria
- Epidermolysis bullosa acquisita
- Bullous systemic lupus erythematosus

Diagnostic testing

- First line test is plasma or urinary total porphyrins, PCT will have elevated porphyrins.
- Lesional biopsy for histopathology.

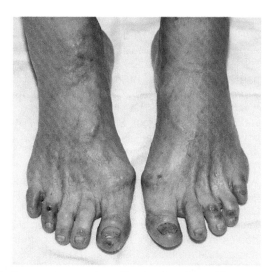

Fig. 17. Vesicles, bullae, erosions, and crusting on dorsal toes. (*Courtesy* of O Sokumbi, MD)

- DIF can show thick and homogenous staining of dermal vessels with IgG, IgA, C3, or fibrinogen. It can show weak granular and linear staining at the basement membrane zone.

Treatment

- First-line therapy is phlebotomy every 2 weeks and/or low-dose antimalarials (ie, hydroxychloroquine 200 mg twice weekly or chloroquine 125 mg twice weekly).
- Encourage the use of sun protection with broad spectrum sunscreens and sun-protective clothing.
- Limit precipitating factors by minimizing or eliminating alcohol consumption and estrogen use.
- Optimize management of comorbidities such as hepatitis or HIV.

CLINICS CARE POINTS

- Bullous dermatoses are primarily categorized by the anatomic level of the split.
- A biopsy for hematoxylin and eosin and direct immunofluorescence may be indicated to render an accurate diagnosis when evaluating bullous dermatoses.
- In older adults, the prevalence of polypharmacy and comorbid conditions complicates diagnosis by adding drug-induced and physical bullous dermatoses to the differential consideration.
- Owing to the relative rarity of these diseases, treatment is based on published evidence, expert opinion, and consensus requiring that physicians fully review all the available data to assist in therapeutic decisions.

REFERENCES

1. Farage MA, Miller KW, Berardesca E, et al. Clinical implications of aging skin: cutaneous disorders in the elderly. Am J Clin Dermatol 2009;10(2):73–86.

2. Deotto ML, Spiller A, Sernicola A, et al. Bullous pemphigoid: an immune disorder related to aging (Review). Exp Ther Med 2022;23(1):50.
3. Wallach D. Intraepidermal IgA pustulosis. J Am Acad Dermatol 1992;27(6 Pt 1): 993–1000.
4. Stanley JR, Amagai M. Pemphigus, bullous impetigo, and the staphylococcal scalded-skin syndrome. N Engl J Med 2006;355(17):1800–10.
5. Kirkham S, Lam S, Nester C, et al. The effect of hydration on the risk of friction blister formation on the heel of the foot. Skin Res Technol 2014;20(2):246–53.
6. Harman KE, Brown D, Exton LS, et al. British Association of Dermatologists' guidelines for the management of pemphigus vulgaris 2017. Br J Dermatol 2017;177(5):1170–201.
7. von Köckritz A, Ständer S, Zeidler C, et al. Successful monotherapy of pemphigus vegetans with minocycline and nicotinamide. J Eur Acad Dermatol Venereol : JEADV 2017;31(1):85–8.
8. Hashimoto K, Hashimoto T, Higashiyama M, et al. Detection of anti-desmocollins I and II autoantibodies in two cases of Hallopeau type pemphigus vegetans by immunoblot analysis. J Dermatol Sci 1994;7(2):100–6.
9. Ellebrecht CT, Payne AS. Setting the target for pemphigus vulgaris therapy. JCI Insight 2017;2(5):e92021.
10. Ouedraogo E, Gottlieb J, de Masson A, et al. Risk factors for death and survival in paraneoplastic pemphigus associated with hematologic malignancies in adults. J Am Acad Dermatol 2019;80(6):1544–9.
11. Paolino G, Didona D, Magliulo G, et al. Paraneoplastic pemphigus: insight into the autoimmune pathogenesis, clinical features and therapy. Int J Mol Sci 2017;18(12). https://doi.org/10.3390/ijms18122532.
12. Mariotti F, Grosso F, Terracina M, et al. Development of a novel ELISA system for detection of anti-BP180 IgG and characterization of autoantibody profile in bullous pemphigoid patients. Br J Dermatol 2004;151(5):1004–10.
13. Prost-Squarcioni C, Caux F, Schmidt E, et al. International Bullous Diseases Group: consensus on diagnostic criteria for epidermolysis bullosa acquisita. Br J Dermatol 2018;179(1):30–41.
14. Samolitis NJ, Hull CM, Leiferman KM, et al. Dermatitis herpetiformis and partial IgA deficiency. J Am Acad Dermatol 2006;54(5 Suppl):S206–9.
15. Fortuna G, Marinkovich MP. Linear immunoglobulin A bullous dermatosis. Clin Dermatol 2012;30(1):38–50.
16. Branco MM, Capitani EM, Cintra ML, et al. Coma blisters after poisoning caused by central nervous system depressants: case report including histopathological findings. An Bras Dermatol 2012;87(4):615–7.
17. Dinis-Oliveira RJ. Drug overdose-induced coma blisters: pathophysiology and clinical and forensic diagnosis. Curr Drug Res Rev 2019;11(1):21–5.
18. Porphyria cutanea tarda (pct). American Porphyria Foundation. https://porphyriafoundation.org/for-patients/types-of-porphyria/pct/. Accessed November 6, 2022.

Diagnosing and Managing Venous Stasis Disease and Leg Ulcers

Sofia Chaudhry, MD[a],*, Kathryn Lee, BA[b]

KEYWORDS

- Venous disease ● Venous insufficiency ● Stasis dermatitis ● Venous ulcers
- Leg ulcers ● Chronic wounds

KEY POINTS

- Chronic venous insufficiency can lead to secondary cutaneous changes that most commonly present as stasis dermatitis but can progress to more serious venous ulcers.
- Venous ulcers are the most common chronic leg wound and account for 80% of lower extremity ulcers.
- The differential diagnosis of leg ulcers is broad and includes venous, arterial, neuropathic, inflammatory, neoplastic, vasculitic, vasculopathic, and infectious ulcers.

INTRODUCTION

Venous insufficiency is a common medical condition that affects many individuals, especially those with advanced age. Chronic venous insufficiency can lead to secondary cutaneous changes that most commonly present as stasis dermatitis (SD) but can progress to more serious venous ulcers.

Venous ulcers are the most common cause of lower extremity ulcers. However, the differential diagnosis of leg ulcers is broad, and clinicians should not establish a diagnosis of venous ulcers without considering other possible causes. The differential diagnoses of leg ulcers include, but are not limited to, arterial, neuropathic, inflammatory, neoplastic, vasculitic, vasculopathic, and primary infectious ulcers. This article will discuss clinical clues to help guide your workup and will review basic clinical evaluation and management of common leg ulcers.

STASIS DERMATITIS

SD, also referred to as venous stasis dermatitis and stasis eczema, is a common inflammatory cutaneous condition due to underlying chronic venous insufficiency. It

[a] Department of Dermatology, Saint Louis University School of Medicine, 1225 South Grand Boulevard, 3rd Floor, Saint Louis, MO 63104, USA; [b] Saint Louis University School of Medicine, 1402 South Grand Boulevard, Saint Louis, MO 63104, USA
* Corresponding author.
E-mail address: sofia.chaudhry@health.slu.edu

Clin Geriatr Med 40 (2024) 75–90
https://doi.org/10.1016/j.cger.2023.09.004
0749-0690/24/© 2023 Elsevier Inc. All rights reserved.

most commonly presents in older adults and affects the lower extremities.[1] The most common nonmodifiable risk factors include advanced age, female sex, and family history of venous disease, whereas common modifiable risk factors include smoking, obesity, prolonged sitting or standing, heart failure, history of venous thrombosis, and pregnancy.[1,2] Chronic venous insufficiency typically leads to pitting edema of the distal lower extremities and development of SD.[1,2]

Venous reflux in the setting of venous hypertension leads to SD.[1,3] The reflux driving venous hypertension is most commonly due to incompetent venous valves, failure of the lower extremity venous muscle pump, and venous outflow obstruction; it can occur in the superficial and/or deep venous systems.[1,2,4] Venous hypertension leads to the extravasation of erythrocytes and accumulation of inflammatory cells, migrating into nearby tissues.[1,2,5] The classic brown and/or blue-gray pigmentation of venous insufficiency is thought to be due to increased hemosiderin deposition and/or melanin deposition.[2]

Clinical Presentation

SD is an eczematous process that classically presents as poorly demarcated itchy, oozing, scaly, erythematous patches and plaques on the lower extremities.[1,2,4] The medial malleolus is the area most frequently and severely involved but it can extend to the knee and foot (**Fig. 1**).[1,4] Symptoms include pruritus, inflammation, and pain/discomfort in the legs. Over time, a brown or blue-gray hyperpigmentation is often observed.[2] Pruritus can lead to chronic scratching, which results in an increased risk of skin infection and lichenification (skin thickening).[1,2]

Caution should be taken before diagnosing a patient with bilateral cellulitis because bilateral cellulitis is exceedingly rare and SD is a much more common cause of bilateral lower extremity erythema and edema.[1,6] It is also important to note that although SD is typically bilateral, it can occasionally occur as a unilateral presentation depending on the underlying pathologic condition, such as a history of deep vein thrombosis (DVT) or venous surgery in one leg.

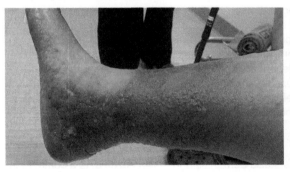
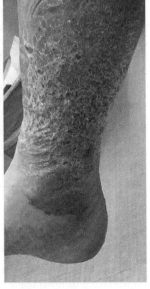

Fig. 1. Stasis dermatitis on the lower extremities.

Diagnosis and Management

SD is often diagnosed by clinical evaluation and medical history. When needed, duplex ultrasonography may be considered to detect venous reflux and/or venous obstruction and assess blood flow directionality.[1,7,8] Although biopsy can demonstrate histologic features of SD, it is often not necessary with classic clinical presentation and is generally avoided due to impaired blood flow in the affected areas, which can lead to poor healing at the biopsy site.[1,7]

Treatment of SD may include multimodal therapies that address the underlying venous insufficiency and manage the lower extremity edema, inflammation, and cutaneous lesions. Mid-to-high-potency topical corticosteroids can be used to manage pruritus, erythema, and scale, although prolonged use may lead to skin atrophy. Compression stockings and compression bandages are the mainstay of treatment because they are used to treat the underlying pathologic condition by reducing ambulatory venous pressures and venous hypertension.[1,5,9] Compression stockings should ideally be at least 30 mm Hg in strength.[10] For more severe disease, multilayer compression bandages, such as Unna boots, can be used.[1,7] Further details on Unna boots are discussed below.

Management with interventional procedures is available to treat the underlying venous reflux. Available minimally invasive procedures include endovenous thermal ablations, ambulatory phlebectomy, and ultrasound-guided foam sclerotherapy.[1]

In addition, SD can be complicated by an allergic contact dermatitis and infection. The patient should be counseled to discontinue any suspected topical allergen, such as neomycin and bacitracin that are common culprits, and cultures can be taken to help guide coinfection treatment.[11]

LIPODERMATOSCLEROSIS

Patients with long-standing venous insufficiency and venous hypertension may develop chronic lipodermatosclerosis (LDS), also known as fibrosing or sclerosing panniculitis. This condition is characterized by fat necrosis and progressive fibrosis.[2] Chronic LDS often manifests as painful, erythematous induration that begins on the lower medial aspect of the lower extremity above the malleolar region.[11,12] The fibrosis may progress to involve the entire lower third of the leg and have the appearance of an "inverted champagne bottle."[11] Chronic LDS may be preceded by an acute phase that presents as painfully firm, warm erythematous plaques, which may be misdiagnosed as cellulitis; however, it is not associated with the systemic features observed with cellulitis.[2,11] Treatment of acute LDS includes the use of non-steroidal anti-inflammatory drugs (NSAIDS), topical and intralesional corticosteroids, fibrinolytic agents, and compression therapy if tolerated.[11]

VENOUS ULCERS

Venous ulcers are a significant complication of long-standing venous disease and are caused by venous reflux through incompetent valves and/or venous thrombosis.[10] Venous ulcers are the most common chronic leg wound and account for 50% to 70% of lower extremity ulcers.[12] Prevalence of this condition increases with age and is more commonly reported in women than in men.[10,11,13] These leg wounds are the result of venous hypertension in the setting of long-standing venous insufficiency. Venous hypertension leads to vessel wall distension, resulting in the leakage of fibrinogen and other macromolecules into the dermis and subcutaneous tissues.[13] Fibrinogen then polymerizes to fibrin that deposit in the vessel walls as "pericapillary perifibrin cuffs" that result in impaired oxygen supply and ulcer formation in the lower extremities.[13]

Clinical Presentation

Patients presenting with venous ulcers often complain of lower extremity edema and aching of the legs that worsens as the day progresses and improves with leg elevation. Venous ulcers most commonly occur near the medial malleolus; however, it can present anywhere over the distal third of the legs and even be circumferential.[1,10,11] The ulceration is often shallow with irregular, poorly defined borders, and a yellow, fibrinous exudate may cover the wound bed.[10,11] Clinical features associated with venous ulcers include varicose veins, hemosiderosis, leg/ankle edema, LDS, SD, and lymphedema.[2,10,11]

Diagnosis and Management

A comprehensive medical history and thorough physical examination should be performed to establish a diagnosis. Patient behaviors, such as smoking, in addition to concerns for anemia, thrombophilia, malnutrition, and hypoproteinemia must be addressed.[14]

Compression therapy is the foundation of venous ulcer treatment. It is a critical component of venous ulcer management because it addresses the underlying pathologic condition of impaired venous return. As in SD, venous ultrasonography can be used to detect venous insufficiency. However, arterial studies should also be performed to assess for commonly associated arterial insufficiency.[14] If significant arterial disease is found, in which the Ankle Brachial Index (ABI) is less than 0.6 or the Toe Brachial Index is less than 0.4, or either index is more than 1.2 (suggesting noncompressible vessels), the patient should be referred to vascular surgery before applying any compression. An ABI of 0.6 to 0.8 may require modified compression therapy; extremities with ABI readings of 0.8 to 1.2 have sufficient arterial perfusion to tolerate treatment with high-strength compression of 40 mm Hg.[14] Compression therapy improves venous flow and oxygenation of the affected tissue while reducing venous reflux and edema.[14,15] Compression therapy can be implemented through 3 possible systems: (1) elastic or inelastic compression bandages, (2) compression stockings, and (3) intermittent pneumatic compression devices.[11]

The Unna boot is a valuable and commonly used multilayer compression bandage that has been shown to promote ulcer healing. It is composed of a zinc-oxide impregnated gauze that is first wrapped over the skin from the base of the toes to the popliteal flexure. The zinc-layer serves as a nonelastic compression bandage. Then a soft cotton gauze is applied circumferentially over the first layer. Finally, an elastic bandage, such as Coban, is wrapped around to provide additional compression. As the bandages are applied, each layer should have a 50% overlap with the earlier layer. Unna boots are usually changed once weekly but more frequently if there is significant exudate.[10]

In addition to compressive therapy, maintaining a moist environment surrounding the wound bed is crucial in managing chronic wounds, such as venous ulcers. Moist occlusive wound dressings have been shown to promote angiogenesis in addition to stimulating collagen synthesis and reepithelialization.[10,11,14] Additionally, occlusive dressings decrease superimposed infections by lowering wound pH and acting as a mechanical barrier that protects against contamination.[9,11] Various dressings exist to promote a moist wound bed. However, if there is drainage from the wound, a more absorbent dressing should be selected to apply over the ulcer. **Table 1** provides an overview of common wound dressings.

Table 1
Overview of basic wound dressings

Dressing Types	Mechanism	When to Use	Therapeutic Benefits	Important Considerations Before Use	Frequency of Dressing Changes
Alginates	• Consist of nonadhesive fibers with strong fiber-integrity • Dissolve and form a hydrophilic gel when in contact with wound exudate, promoting moist healing environment	• Moderate to heavily exudative wounds	• Mildly hemostatic • Highly absorbent	• Can produce fibrous debris	• Can remain on wound until dressing soaked with fluid/exudate
Gauzes	• Loose packing in deep wounds promotes healing from base outward	• Deep wounds • Sinus tracts	• Low cost • Easily accessible	• Poor barrier protection • Drying	• Every 12–24 h
Films	• Promote exchange of water vapor and oxygen between wound bed and environment; semiocclusive, preventing liquid and bacteria from permeating wound	• Superficial wounds • Minimally exudative wounds • Secondary dressing to affix other nonadhesive dressings	• Semiocclusive • Retain moisture • Provide barrier protection, preventing wound contamination • Transparent—can view wound without dressing removal	• May strip skin from freshly reepithelialized skin if applied and removed too frequently • Trap fluid → possible skin maceration • Minimally absorptive	• Can remain on wound for up to 7 d or until fluid leakage from dressing is observed
Foams	• Consist of hydrophobic outer layer that promotes gas exchange; hydrophilic layer in contact with wound bed	• Low to moderately exudative wounds	• Occlusive • Provide thermal insulation • Moderately absorbent	• Can produce malodorous discharge • Opaque—requires dressing removal to monitor	• Every 3 d

(continued on next page)

Table 1
(continued)

Dressing Types	Mechanism	When to Use	Therapeutic Benefits	Important Considerations Before Use	Frequency of Dressing Changes
Hydrocolloids	• Form gel with fluid from wound, maintain most wound environment that promotes healing	• Low to moderately exudative wounds • Shallow wounds	• Occlusive • Provide barrier protection, preventing wound contamination • Absorbent • Can wear for prolonged period	• Can produce malodorous discharge • May strip skin during removal • Trap fluid • Opaque—require dressing removal to monitor • Avoid in heavily exudative wounds→possible periwound maceration	• Can remain on wound for up to 7 d or until fluid leakage from dressing is observed
Hydrogels	• Water-based dressing • Maintain moist wound-healing environment by delivering water molecules into wound bed	• Dry, painful wounds	• Retain moisture • Relieve pain • Nontraumatic removal	• Can overhydrate wound • Avoid in heavily exudative wounds→possible skin maceration	• Every 1–3 d

Reference: Fonder MA, Lazarus GS, Cowan DA, Aronson-Cook B, Kohli AR, Mamelak AJ. Treating the chronic wound: A practical approach to the care of nonhealing wounds and wound care dressings. J Am Acad Dermatol. 2008;58(2):185-206. https://doi.org/10.1016/j.jaad.2007.08.048.

Medical therapies may also aid in the management of chronic venous ulcers. Pentoxifylline, a methylxanthine derivative, has been shown to improve healing by up to 50% and is particularly efficacious in recalcitrant ulcers present for more than 1 year.[14] It has multiple mechanisms of action, such as inhibiting adhesion and activation of neutrophils in addition to promoting fibrinolysis and increasing erythrocyte deformability.[11,14] Typical dosage and frequency is 400 mg taken thrice daily; however, lower dosages are recommended for patients with renal failure. It is contraindicated in patients who are intolerant of methylxanthine derivatives and those with significant cardiac disease.[14] Doxycycline has also been shown to display anti-inflammatory, antiapoptotic, and anti-antigenic properties.[14] Doxycycline 100 mg taken twice daily in conjunction with compression therapy may improve healing in venous ulcers.[16]

It is common for chronic wounds to be colonized with bacteria. However, once bacterial loads exceed 10^5 organisms per gram of tissue, bacterial toxins can damage tissue and impair wound healing. Topical antiseptics, such as Dakin solution 0.025%, and topical antimicrobial dressings, such as silver sulfadiazine 1%, can be used to the ulcer to decrease bacterial load. However, if the wound becomes clinically infected, this requires systemic antibiotic treatment. Signs of an active infection include increased pain, erythema, and edema. In addition, the presence of yellow, green, and/or malodorous exudate is suggestive of overlying infection.[14] Wound cultures should be obtained in cases where clinical suspicion for infection is high to guide antibiotic selection. Culture samples should ideally be obtained from deeper tissues within the wound bed and colony count per gram of tissue should be quantified to prevent misinterpretation of positive cultures that may be due to colonization of the superficial wound bed.[14]

Although regular debridement of venous ulcers is not supported by current studies, existing literature suggests that the removal of debris from the wound bed may be beneficial.[17,18] Sharp debridement is the most precise method to remove necrotic tissue and debris—the wound is debrided until reaching well-vascularized, normal tissue.[14] Debridement is efficacious in transforming chronic wounds to acute wounds with improved blood supply and healing response, promoting macrophage and neutrophil recruitment.[11,14]

Procedural interventions for the management of venous ulcers may be beneficial for some patients. Referral to vascular surgery can aid in patient evaluation and management. Similar to the treatment of SD, minimally invasive, percutaneous techniques such as radiofrequency therapy, endovenous laser ablation, and ultrasound-guided foam sclerotherapy can be considered.[11]

Differential Diagnoses

Although venous disease is the most common cause of lower extremity ulcerations, the differential diagnosis of leg ulcers is broad (**Table 2**). Therefore, a thorough differential should be considered when evaluating a patient with a leg ulcer. For example, given that a significant proportion of patients may present with a mixed clinical picture involving both venous and arterial insufficiency, arterial insufficiency should be excluded before initiating treatment. Patients who report a history of recurrent deep vein thrombosis or those with examination findings consistent with livedoid vasculopathy (see later discussion) should be further evaluated for hypercoagulability.[9] Additionally, biopsy of long-standing, nonhealing ulcerations is recommended to rule out other entities such as inflammatory, neoplastic, vasculitic, and infectious causes. An additional biopsy for pan tissue culture can be helpful when evaluating for infection. In the following sections, we will review the clinical presentations of select key differential diagnoses of leg ulcers beyond venous ulcers.

Table 2
Common causes of leg ulcers

Ulcer Type	Associated Conditions
Primary infectious	*Bacterial infections*: Ecthyma gangrenosum, bullous erysipelas, bartonellosis, meningococcemia, necrotizing fasciitis, *Treponema*, *Staphylococcus*, and *Bacillus anthracis* *Atypical mycobacterium*: *Mycobacterium ulcerans* (Buruli ulcer) *Viral infections*: Herpes simplex virus, varicella zoster virus, and cytomegalovirus *Fungal infections*: Blastomycosis, eumycotic mycetoma, histoplasmosis, sporotrichosis, coccidiomycosis, and paracoccidioidomycosis *Protozoal infections*: Leishmaniasis and amebiasis
Neoplastic	SCC, BCC, melanoma, cutaneous lymphoma, cutaneous metastases of other malignancies, Kaposi sarcoma, and Merkel cell carcinoma
Inflammatory skin diseases	PG, sarcoidosis, necrobiosis lipoidica, autoimmune bullous diseases (ie, bullous pemphigoid), and panniculitis
Substance abuse-related	Injection site reactions and cocaine-induced vasoconstriction
Systemic diseases	Diabetes mellitus Inflammatory bowel disease: Metastatic Crohn disease *Autoimmune connective-tissue disease-associated vasculitis*: Lupus erythematosus, Sjögren syndrome, dermatomyositis, and rheumatoid arthritis *Hematologic disease*: Sickle cell disease, polycythemia vera, and thrombocytopenias *Hypertensive disease*: Arterial hypertension (Martorell's ulcer) *Neuropathic*: Tabes dorsalis, multiple sclerosis, and paraplegia *Nutritional deficiencies*: Vitamin C, zinc, Vitamin B1, Vitamin B6, Vitamin B12, thiamine, and niacin
Trauma-induced	Pressure-induced, postprocedural, burns, and arthropod bites (ie, brown recluse spider bite)
Vascular	*Arterial disease*: Arterial insufficiency *Venous disease*: Chronic venous insufficiency, mixed venous-arterial or venous-lymphatic insufficiency, and arteriovenous malformation
Vasculitic	*Small vessel vasculitides*: Cutaneous small vessel vasculitis, microscopic polyangiitis, granulomatosis with polyangiitis, eosinophilic granulomatosis with polyangiitis, mixed cryoglobulinemia, and immunoglobulin A vasculitis (Henoch-Schonlein purpura) *Medium vessel vasculitides*: Polyarteritis nodosa, Buerger disease (thromboangiitis obliterans)
Vasculopathic	Calciphylaxis, DIC, livedoid vasculopathy, purpura fulminans, cholesterol emboli, hypercoagulable disorders (ie, antithrombin deficiency, factor V leiden, and protein C or S deficiency), and platelet-related thromboses (ie, HUS, TTP)
Drug-induced	Chemotherapy, warfarin, methotrexate, and hydroxyurea

Reference: Abbade LPF, Frade MAC, Pegas JRP, et al. Consensus on the diagnosis and management of chronic leg ulcers - Brazilian Society of Dermatology. An Bras Dermatol. 2020;95 Suppl 1(Suppl 1):1-18. https://doi.org/10.1016/j.abd.2020.06.002.

ARTERIAL ULCERS

Arterial ulcers comprise approximately 25% of leg ulcers.[12] They are due to inadequate blood supply to affected tissues, leading to tissue necrosis and wound healing impairment.[10,14] Atherosclerotic disease, such as peripheral arterial disease, is the most common cause of ischemic ulcers; however, thromboembolic disease may also induce ulcer formation. The risk factors for arterial ulcer formation include smoking, diabetes, advanced age, and observed arterial disease affecting other parts of the body. Patients with arterial insufficiency commonly report symptoms of intermittent claudication worse with rest and relief when in a dependent position.[10,14]

Arterial ulcers often present as round lesions with sharply demarcated borders and occur over distal bony prominences, anteriorly on the leg, or sites of pressure (distal toes, heel, malleoli, and shin).[11] The skin surrounding the ulceration may be shiny, atrophic, and hairless.[10,11] Significant pain that worsens with limb elevation is often associated with arterial ulcers. Physical examination findings associated with arterial insufficiency include weak pedal pulses, cool feet, and delayed capillary toe refill. Doppler ultrasonography may be used to evaluate distal pulses, and ABIs may be performed to assess for insufficient arterial supply in the extremities. An ABI less than 0.9 indicates arterial stenosis and peripheral arterial disease.

Restoration of peripheral arterial perfusion by means of endovascular procedures (ie, stent placement and percutaneous angioplasty) or by surgical techniques, such as a femoral popliteal bypass may be performed.[10,11] Moist occlusive wound dressings can be used for localized treatment of arterial ulcers. Additionally, interventions such as smoking cessation and antiplatelet medications such as cilostazol, and management of medical comorbidities (ie, hypertension, diabetes, and hyperlipidemia) are recommended where applicable.[11] Sharp debridement should be performed with considerable caution or avoided to prevent further necrosis of the affected skin and worsening of the ulceration.

NEUROPATHIC ULCERS

Neuropathic ulcers (NUs) are the result of peripheral neuropathy, with diabetes being the most common cause. Other possible causes include human immunodeficiency virus (HIV), leprosy, vitamin deficiencies, sarcoidosis, and alcoholic neuropathies.[19,20] It is important to note that clinical symptoms associated with NUs may develop before ulcer formation. Reductions in pain and proprioception, along with possible gait alteration and paralysis, can lead to callus formation at support points that withstand continuous mechanical stress and pressure; repetitive mechanical stress may lead to traumatic injury and ulcer development at the callus sites.[19]

NUs commonly occur in support points that sustain frequent mechanical stress, such as the calcaneus, metatarsals, and plantar surfaces of the toes.[19] The NU is often surrounded by a hyperkeratotic rim; local tissue necrosis and hemorrhagic areas indicative of trauma may also be present.[19] Clinicians should assess for structural deformities, such as claw toes and Charcot arthropathy, during physical examination. A comprehensive history related to onset of NU signs and symptoms is also necessary to establish a diagnosis.

The type of nerve fiber involvement and neuropathy can be telling of the diagnosis. Monofilament testing to assess for tactile sensation, vibration testing using a 128-Hz tuning fork, and pinprick testing to assess sensitivity to pain may be performed.[19] Evaluation for hyporeflexia and decreased muscle tone may also be indicated. More invasive testing, such as electromyography and nerve conduction studies, may also be considered for certain patients.[20] Finally, the evaluation of limb perfusion, particularly in patients with diabetes, should be performed given the association of NUs and ischemic ulcers. Patients with diabetes have a 15% to 25% risk of developing a foot ulcer because of diabetic peripheral neuropathy or associated vascular disease.[10,11,21]

The primary complications associated with NUs include localized cutaneous infections and osteomyelitis.[10,19] Signs of local infection include presence of a malodorous green/yellow exudate, erythema, warmth, and pain. Conversely, the onset of osteomyelitis may be clinically silent and present as an exudative, nonhealing wound.[19] Microbial culture of the wound bed, complete blood count (CBC), erythrocyte sedimentation rate (ESR), and c-reactive protein (CRP) level should be ordered in cases with high clinical suspicion for infection. Imaging modalities, such as radiography, bone scintigraphy, CT, and MRI, can be performed to evaluate for infection of the deep soft tissue or bone. Bone biopsy remains the gold standard for diagnosis of osteomyelitis.[11]

Management of Neuropathic Ulcers

Conservative management of NUs includes off-loading interventions to lessen acute trauma caused by repetitive mechanical stress on the ulcers. Use of therapeutic shoes, walkers, crutches, and wheelchairs can assist in reducing the stress placed on NUs.[11] Cleansing of the wound bed and proper debridement of the callus and surrounding necrotic tissue is also an important component of management. Moist occlusive dressings may be used to treat diabetic ulcers; however, this therapy should be used cautiously to prevent maceration of the surrounding skin.[11] Preventative measures—such as daily foot washing, regular inspection of the feet for cutaneous changes along with neurologic and vascular status, use of appropriate footwear, skin moisturization, and treatment of nail and foot fungal infections—is crucial. For patients with diabetes, strict glycemic control, smoking cessation, and management of cholesterol/lipid levels are critical.[11,19]

PYODERMA GANGRENOSUM

Pyoderma gangrenosum (PG) is a chronic inflammatory, ulcerative cutaneous disease with distinct morphology. Although uncommon, PG is a neutrophilic dermatosis that more commonly affects women aged between 20 and 50 years.[11] Although diagnosis depends on the characteristic clinical appearance, history, and supportive histologic findings, PG is a diagnosis of exclusion, and therefore, a biopsy of the ulcer's intact edge should be done to rule out other possible diagnoses. PG is often associated with systemic diseases, most commonly inflammatory bowel disease, rheumatoid arthritis, hematologic disorders (ie, myelodysplasia, acute myelogenous leukemia, and IgA monoclonal gammopathy), and malignancies.[10,11] Classic PGs are typically painful, and most are located on the lower extremities, specifically the pretibial region. However, they can occur at other sites (ie, peristomal areas and mucous membranes).[11]

PGs often first present as an erythematous tender papulopustular lesion or nodule. The lesions necrose and develop into a central shallow or deep ulcer, potentially even exposing underlying connective tissue.[11] In later disease stages, the ulcers will present with a purulent wound bed, surrounded by irregularly shaped, undermined borders that seem "gunmetal gray" in color (**Fig. 2**).[10,11] The pathogenesis of PG is not well understood, and diagnosis is made based on examination findings and clinical history. Ulcer severity may be associated with severity of the associated systemic

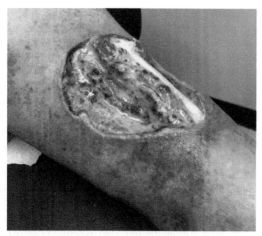

Fig. 2. Pyoderma gangrenosum on the lower extremity.

disease, and treatment of the underlying condition can lead to ulcer improvement.[10] Specific treatments depend on the associated condition but include intralesional steroids, dapsone, cyclosporine, and tumor necrosis factor (TNF)-alpha inhibitors.

NEOPLASTIC ULCERS

When assessing ulcers, clinicians must also consider neoplastic causes. Ulcers associated with basal cell carcinoma (BCC) and squamous cell carcinoma (SCC) occur more commonly than ulcers associated with other primary cutaneous cancers, cutaneous T-cell and B-cell lymphomas, and cutaneous metastases of other malignancies.[11]

BCC-associated ulcers typically occur in sites of chronic sun exposure and are most commonly associated with the nodular subtype.[11,22] Nodular BCC is the most common variant and accounts for 50% to 80% of BCCs.[23] Advanced nodular BCCs can enlarge and ulcerate (referred to as rodent or phagedenic ulcers).[11,23] Clinical cues that point toward a diagnosis of BCC is the presence of rolled borders surrounding the lesion.

Invasive cutaneous SCC most commonly occurs in areas of chronic sun damage and can ulcerate.[22,23] Marjolin ulcer refers to the development of an ulcerating SCC in areas of chronic inflammation, long-standing ulcers, oncogenic human papillomavirus (HPV) infection sites, and old scars.[10] Invasive SCC clinically presents as an erythematous papulonodule or plaque with overlying scale and may demonstrate crusting along with ulceration.[22]

Biopsy is essential in establishing diagnosis of neoplastic ulcers. Complete treatment depends on tumor stage and presence of any high-risk features but typically involves surgical management.[24]

VASCULITIC ULCERS

Deposition of immune complexes within vessel walls leads to activation of the inflammatory cascade, inducing vessel inflammation and necrosis.[10,25] The cutaneous manifestations of vasculitis depend on the size of the vessel affected. Cutaneous small vessel vasculitis (CSVV), histologically referred to as leukocytoclastic vasculitis, classically presents as palpable purpura. Secondary bullae, necrosis, and ulceration are less common but can sometimes be seen.[26] Examples of CSVV include immunoglobulin A vasculitis (such as Henoch-Schönlein purpura); urticarial vasculitis; type II and III cryoglobulinemic vasculitis; and secondary causes such as drugs, infections, autoimmune diseases, and malignancy. Medium-sized vessel vasculitis, such as polyarteritis nodosa and thromboangiitis obliterans (Buerger disease), affects vessels in the deep reticular dermis or subcutis. Clinically, this leads to livedo racemosa, retiform purpura, subcutaneous nodules, and ulcerations. Certain vasculitides (ie, microscopic polyangiitis, granulomatosis with polyangitis, and eosinophilic granulomatosis with polyangiitis) can have a mixed clinical picture, and that affects both small-sized and medium-sized vessels.[11] Takayasu arteritis, a large-vessel vasculitis, can affect the lower extremities and presents with erythematous subcutaneous nodules and ulcerations, including PG-like ulcers.[11]

Cutaneous ulceration in the setting of livedo racemosa and subcutaneous nodules is a clinical clue strongly suggesting a medium-vessel vasculitis. If suspecting a cutaneous vasculitis, a comprehensive history and thorough review of systems to screen for systemic involvement is essential, along with a full physical examination. Skin biopsy is necessary to exclude conditions that can appear similar to cutaneous vasculitis and to identify the vessel size involved.[11] Excisional or deep incisional biopsy that captures subcutaneous tissue should be performed if there is clinical suspicion for medium-sized vessel involvement; biopsies taken from subcutaneous nodules, when present, often provide the highest diagnostic yield.[11] Ulcer beds should not be biopsied because ulcers can display a nondiagnostic incidental vasculitis but rather the ulcer edge and peripheral inflammation should be biopsied.[11] In addition, a biopsy for direct immunofluorescence should be performed to evaluate for vascular deposition of immunoglobulins and complement to aid in diagnosis. Laboratory evaluation of vasculitis should always include a complete urinalysis, CBC and complete metabolic panel (CMP). However, if there is recurrent or chronic disease, suspicion for medium vessel involvement, or concern for systemic causes, a more thorough laboratory investigation is warranted to include antineutrophilic cytoplasmic antibodies (ANCAs), cryoglobulins, antistreptolysin O (ASO), hepatitis panel, rheumatoid factor, antinuclear antibody (ANA), anti-extractable nuclear antigen (ENA) antibodies, and HIV. In older patients, or in the correct clinical setting, a serum and urine protein electrophoresis and immunofixation should be checked.[11] Treatment depends on the severity of cutaneous and systemic vasculitic involvement.

VASCULOPATHIC ULCERS

Vasculopathic ulcers are the result of vaso-occlusive processes that lead to ulcer formation secondary to reduced vascular supply and tissue ischemia. A variety of disease processes can lead to the occlusion of cutaneous vessels. Examples include uremic and nonuremic calciphylaxis (**Fig. 3**), hypercoagulable states (ie, disseminated intravascular coagulation [DIC], antiphospholipid antibody syndrome, protein C/S deficiency, factor V leiden, and prothrombin III mutation), embolic processes (ie, cholesterol, septic, fat, and air emboli), platelet-related thromboses (hemolytic uremic syndrome [HUS], thrombotic thrombocytopenic purpura [TTP], heparin-induced thrombocytopenia and thrombosis), angioinvasive infections, and temperature-related vasculopathy (ie, type I cryoglobulinemia).[19,27,28] Livedoid vasculopathy is an example of a vasculopathy that favors the ankles and distal lower extremities that occurs in the setting of thrombophilia. It presents with painful punched-out ulcerations due to tissue infarctions and can have surrounding retiform purpura and brown hyperpigmentation. This condition is characterized by atrophie blanche, which is white, stellate atrophic scars with surrounding telangiectasias.[2,10]

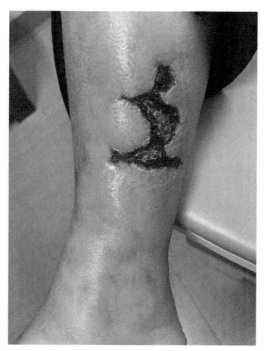

Fig. 3. Calciphylaxis ulcer of the lower extremity.

Clinical clues that may indicate an ulcer secondary to vasculopathy is the presence of retiform purpura bordering the ulcer. Retiform purpura seems as nonblanching, red-to-purple patches with a characteristic peripheral branching and central purpura, necrosis, or ulceration.[25] The angulated appearance of retiform purpura is in contrast to livedo reticularis, which demonstrates a classic "net-like pattern of rings" and does not have central necrosis.[27] Retiform purpura is typically persistent and may be painful due to obstruction of blood flow, which produces the ischemic cutaneous changes.

In an emergent setting, where the patient presents with retiform purpura and seems to be severely ill with organ failure and/or signs and symptoms of septic shock, a workup should be discussed with a multidisciplinary team of providers. Urgent skin biopsy should be performed for H&E histology, tissue culture, and direct immunofluorescence; antibiotic and antifungal therapies should be started immediately in immunocompromised or septic patients while waiting for tissue culture results and antimicrobial sensitivities.[27] Laboratory results such as CBC and coagulation studies should also be performed. Additionally, a review of patient medications should be promptly conducted to determine whether the patient is taking any high-risk medications, such as heparin or coumadin.

Clinicians should also take great care in obtaining a detailed medical history from the patient. Questions should be focused on the location and acuity of the ulceration and skin changes, assessing for recent or active infections, exposure to new medications/illicit drugs, and recent procedures.[27] Full-body skin examination is crucial as morphology, extent of erythema, and location can be telling of the diagnosis. A complete physical examination should also be performed for associated clinical findings.

INFECTIOUS ULCERS

Ulcers may also be the result of a primary infection due to bacterial, mycobacterial, viral, and deep fungal organisms (further detailed in **Table 2**). Clinical suspicion for infectious ulcers increases in the setting of an immunocompromised patient. Ulcers associated with a primary infection are often present on exposed bodily sites; infectious ulcers specifically associated with leprosy and tertiary syphilis tend to occur at pressure sites.[11] Clinicians should obtain tissue culture as well as skin biopsy for H&E histology to aid in diagnosis and management. Tissue culture from the skin may identify the infectious microbe and provide sensitivities that can guide treatment with antimicrobial therapies.

DISCUSSION

Venous disease and chronic leg ulcers are common medical conditions that affect a significant proportion of the population, leading to increased morbidity and mortality and imposing high economic burden. Thus, prompt diagnosis and effective management is necessary to minimize disease burden and preserve patient quality of life. This article detailed the clinical clues to aid diagnostic workup, clinical evaluation, and management of lower extremity venous disease and ulcers.

CLINICS CARE POINTS

- Venous insufficiency is a common medical condition in the older adult population that leads to cutaneous complications of SD, LDS, and venous leg ulcers.
- SD and LDS can be misdiagnosed as bilateral cellulitis.
- Vascular studies, including screening for concurrent arterial insufficiency, are important.
- Compression treatment is essential in the treatment of skin diseases from venous insufficiency, with Unna Boots being particularly helpful.
- Medical therapies, wound care, and interventional procedures are beneficial in treating venous disease and leg ulcers.
- The differential diagnosis of leg ulcers is broad and includes venous, arterial, neuropathic, inflammatory, neoplastic, vasculitic, vasculopathic, and infectious causes.
- Clinical presentation can help differentiate the various pathologic conditions of a leg ulcer but skin biopsies are often necessary to establish a diagnosis.
- Leg ulcers and associated cutaneous findings can be a sign of more serious systemic disease necessitating prompt evaluation and management.

DISCLOSURE

The authors have no financial disclosures.

REFERENCES

1. Yosipovitch G, Nedorost ST, Silverberg JI, et al. Stasis dermatitis: an overview of its clinical presentation, pathogenesis, and management. Am J Clin Dermatol 2023;24(2):275–86.
2. Kumar P, Khan IA, Das A, et al. Chronic venous disease. Part 1: pathophysiology and clinical features. Clin Exp Dermatol 2022;47(7):1228–39.

3. Sundaresan S, Migden MR, Silapunt S. Stasis dermatitis: pathophysiology, evaluation, and management. Am J Clin Dermatol 2017;18(3):383–90.
4. Bergan JJ, Schmid-Schönbein GW, Smith PD, et al. Chronic venous disease. N Engl J Med 2006;355(5):488–98.
5. Takase S, Pascarella L, Lerond L, et al. Venous hypertension, inflammation and valve remodeling. Eur J Vasc Endovasc Surg 2004;28(5):484–93.
6. Nedorost S, White S, Rowland DY, et al. Development and implementation of an order set to improve value of care for patients with severe stasis dermatitis. J Am Acad Dermatol 2019;80(3):815–7.
7. Rzepecki AK, Blasiak R. Stasis dermatitis: differentiation from other common causes of lower leg inflammation and management strategies. Curr Geriat Rep 2018;7(4):222–7.
8. Zygmunt JA. Duplex ultrasound for chronic venous insufficiency. J Invasive Cardiol 2014;26(11):E149–55.
9. Mosti G, Picerni P, Partsch H. Compression stockings with moderate pressure are able to reduce chronic leg oedema. Phlebology 2012;27(6):289–96.
10. Fonder MA, Lazarus GS, Cowan DA, et al. Treating the chronic wound: a practical approach to the care of nonhealing wounds and wound care dressings. J Am Acad Dermatol 2008;58(2):185–206.
11. Hafner A, Sprecher E. Chapter 105: Ulcers. In: Bolognia JL, Schaffer JV, Cerroni L, et al, editors. *Dermatology*. 4th edition. Elsevier; 2018. p. 1828–46.
12. Morton LM, Phillips TJ. Wound healing and treating wounds: differential diagnosis and evaluation of chronic wounds. J Am Acad Dermatol 2016;74(4):589–606.
13. Kirsner RS, Vivas AC. Lower-extremity ulcers: diagnosis and management. Br J Dermatol 2015;173(2):379–90.
14. Alavi A, Sibbald RG, Phillips TJ, et al. What's new: management of venous leg ulcers: approach to venous leg ulcers. J Am Acad Dermatol 2016;74(4):627–42.
15. de Araujo Tami, Valencia Isabel, Federman Daniel G, et al. Managing the patient with venous ulcers. Ann Intern Med 2003;138:326–34 [Epub 18 February 2003].
16. Sadler GM, Wallace HJ, Stacey MC. Oral doxycycline for the treatment of chronic leg ulceration. Arch Dermatol Res 2012;304(6):487–93 [published correction appears in Arch Dermatol Res. 2012 Aug;304(6):495. Dosage error in published abstract; MEDLINE/PubMed abstract corrected].
17. Lebrun E, Kirsner RS. Frequent debridement for healing of chronic wounds. JAMA Dermatol 2013;149(9):1059.
18. Wilcox JR, Carter MJ, Covington S. Frequency of debridements and time to heal: a retrospective cohort study of 312 744 wounds. JAMA Dermatol 2013;149(9):1050–8 [published correction appears in JAMA Dermatol. 2013 Dec;149(12):1441].
19. Abbade LPF, Frade MAC, Pegas JRP, et al. Consensus on the diagnosis and management of chronic leg ulcers - Brazilian Society of Dermatology. An Bras Dermatol 2020;95(Suppl 1):1–18.
20. Eastman DM, Dreyer MA. Neuropathic Ulcer. (Updated 2022 Sep 28). In: StatPearls (Internet). Treasure Island (FL): StatPearls Publishing; 2023 Jan-. Available at: https://www.ncbi.nlm.nih.gov/books/NBK559214/.
21. Singh N, Armstrong DG, Lipsky BA. Preventing foot ulcers in patients with diabetes. JAMA 2005;293(2):217–28.
22. Bolognia JL, Schaffer JV, Cerroni L, et al. Actinic keratosis, basal cell carcinoma, and squamous cell carcinoma. In: Dermatology. Elsevier; 2018. p. 1872–93.
23. Cameron MC, Lee E, Hibler BP, et al. Basal cell carcinoma: epidemiology; pathophysiology; clinical and histological subtypes; and disease associations. J Am

Acad Dermatol 2019;80(2):303–17 [published correction appears in J Am Acad Dermatol. 2021 Aug;85(2):535].

24. Que SKT, Zwald FO, Schmults CD. Cutaneous squamous cell carcinoma: incidence, risk factors, diagnosis, and staging. J Am Acad Dermatol 2018;78(2): 237–47.

25. Wetter DA, Dutz JP, Shinkai K, et al. Chapter 24: Cutaneous Vasculitis. In: Bolognia JL, Schaffer JV, Cerroni L, et al, editors. *Dermatology*. 4th edition. Elsevier; 2018. p. 409–39.

26. Russell JP, Gibson LE. Primary cutaneous small vessel vasculitis: approach to diagnosis and treatment. Int J Dermatol 2006;45(1):3–13.

27. Georgesen C, Fox LP, Harp J. Retiform purpura: a diagnostic approach. J Am Acad Dermatol 2020;82(4):783–96.

28. Piette WW. Chapter: 23: Cutaneous Manifestations of Microvascular Occlusion. In: Bolognia JL, Schaffer JV, Cerroni L, et al. *Dermatology*. 4th edition. Elsevier; 2018: 390-408.

Evaluation and Management of Pruritus and Scabies in the Elderly Population

Shakira Meltan, BS[a], Bharat Panuganti, MD[b],
Michelle Tarbox, MD[c],*

KEYWORDS

- Pruritus • Systemic etiology underlying pruritus • Neurogenic pruritus
- Phototherapy • Pharmacologic treatments of pruritus • Elderly

KEY POINTS

- Pruritus is a common skin complaint in elderly patients, a unique subsection of the patient base that requires a similarly unique clinical approach.
- Pruritus may have considerable effects on the quality of life.
- Pruritus in nursing home patients or recently hospitalized patients may be due to scabies.

INTRODUCTION: NATURE OF THE PROBLEM

Pruritus is the most common dermatologic complaint in the geriatric population.[1] Its growing prevalence coincides with the rapid growth of the elderly population (>65 years of age) in the United States. According to the US Census Bureau, 16.9% of the population, or more than 56 million adults 65 years and older, lived in the United States in 2022.[2] Pruritus is a condition that accompanies a diverse array of underlying etiologic factors. The mechanism of normal itch impulse transmission has been recently elucidated. The itch sensation originates from epidermal/dermal receptors connected to unmyelinated, afferent C-fibers that transmit the impulse from the periphery. After reaching the neuronal cell bodies in the dorsal horn of the spinal cord, the itch impulse continues through the central nervous system in the lateral spinothalamic tracts before it synapses in the ventral posterolateral nucleus of the thalamus and in the primary somatosensory cortex in the forebrain. The primary somatosensory neurons that detect and transmit the itch sensation are tonically inhibited by the more

[a] School of Medicine, Texas Tech University Health Sciences Center, TX, USA; [b] University of Alabama at Birmingham Hospital, MA, USA; [c] Department of Dermatology, Texas Tech Health Science Center, 3601 4th Street, Stop 9400, Lubbock, TX 79430, USA
* Corresponding author. Department of Dermatology, Texas Tech Health Science Center, 3601 4th Street, Stop 9400, Lubbock, TX 79430.
E-mail address: Michelle.Tarbox@TTUHSC.edu

Clin Geriatr Med 40 (2024) 91–116
https://doi.org/10.1016/j.cger.2023.09.010
0749-0690/24/© 2023 Elsevier Inc. All rights reserved.

common myelinated and nociceptive spinal cord neurons. This tonic inhibition is impeded by opioids acting on the central nervous system. The intimate relationship between the propagation of itch and pain sensations has considerable value clinically.[3] Histamine is the primary mediator of the itch sensation, although several other neurotransmitters and neuropeptides are also implicated.[4] The process of identifying the ideal course of treatment is inextricable from the elucidation of the etiology of the pruritus and, hence, the specific mediator involved. Based on a study on 389 healthy blood donors at the Mayo Clinic, normal aging is associated with increased Th2 cells. This is due to a shift in the balance of T helper cell subsets, with a decrease in Th1 and an increase in Th2 cells. This shift is driven by changes in the cytokine environment, with an increase in IL-4 and IL-10, which promote Th2 differentiation and inhibit Th1 differentiation.[5] Chronic pruritus is a potentially debilitating condition that can have a significant impact on an elderly patient's quality of life. Sufferers of pruritus are often plagued by a lack of sleep and a sense of helpless desperation that may culminate in a state of clinical depression. The elderly constitute a particularly vulnerable demographic, as the regression in the integrity of the human integumentary system over time is well-documented. These changes include a loss in skin hydration, a pro-inflammatory immune system, a loss of collagen, and a higher incidence of dry skin secondary to a reduction in the concentration of epidermal lipids and sweat/sebum production.[6]

PATIENT HISTORY

A detailed patient history is imperative for an accurate explanation of geriatric pruritus, considering the multiplicity of possible underlying causes and the higher incidence of comorbid conditions in the elderly population. The following points offer a road map for a clinician to abide by when an elderly patient presents with pruritus.

One should obtain information pertaining to the onset of pruritus (abrupt vs progressive), the location of the itch (generalized or localized), and the duration of the pruritus (<6 weeks or acute vs >6 weeks or chronic). Other helpful historical elements include the character of the itch (severity, intensity, and quality, including such descriptors as burning, tingling, numbness, or pain) and the determination of factors that aggravate or alleviate the rash (ie, warm or cold temperatures, sweating, low or high humidity, types of clothing, activities, emotions, topical skin care products, detergents, time of day). The presence or absence of a rash is an important historical point. If a rash is present, it is critical to elucidate whether the rash appears before it is scratched or if the itch precedes the development of the rash. Finally, evaluating the patient's treatment history for their pruritus is vitally important. All treatments, including over-the-counter (OTC) products, prescription treatments, physical remedies, and nontraditional treatments, should be discussed as to their effect on the condition and degree of benefit or worsening obtained from each. It is not unusual for a patient's attempts at treating pruritus to worsen the underlying skin disorder, and neglecting this part of the history could result in missing a potentially helpful therapeutic intervention. An expanded history is undoubtedly advisable in cases of elderly patients with pruritus and could include that patient's social history (sexual activity and drug abuse), prescription and OTC drug use, surgical history, travel history, other medical comorbidities, and any unusual dietary restrictions.

Systemic or endogenous causes of pruritus typically manifest gradually, worsening over time. This clinical course stands in stark contrast to acute-onset pruritus that may be associated with drug interactions or infestations among other clinical entities. Opiates, prescribed to elderly patients to manage pain, incite mast cells to release histamine, which induces a rapid onset of pruritus. When inquiring about the duration of itch, it is strategic to identify any lifestyle or environmental changes that were coincidental with the onset of pruritus.

Hygiene and Grooming

The elderly population may neglect everyday grooming practices because of a lack of resources, cognitive impairment, depression, or physical disability. As such, it is important for a clinician to inquire about the patient's daily hygiene routines to reveal any practices that might predispose the patient to itch. Hot showers, for example, tend to dry out the skin as the water evaporates after bathing and affect the surface concentration of sebum. Xerosis is recognized as the most common cause of pruritus in elderly patients, so the elimination of such easily avoidable habits such as the use of hot showers has significant clinical value.[7] It is similarly prudent to ask the patient if they use hot tubs to investigate the possibility of hot water or *Pseudomonas* dermatitis/folliculitis as the grounds for pruritus.[8] Clinicians should also become familiar with the types of soaps, detergents, moisturizers, and topical medications used by the patient. Alkaline cleansers and formulas containing alcohol tend to dry the skin, whereas mild moisturizers and soaps containing lanolin and glycerin are less likely to incite skin irritation.[9] Moisturizers containing ceramide have been found to be of particular benefit to xerotic skin, significantly improving skin hydration and barrier function.[10] Neglect of routine hygiene may facilitate bacterial or yeast overgrowth, which can result in skin infections and secondary dermatoses.

Distribution of Pruritus

The location and extent of pruritus, evaluated together with other qualifying information, can be very revealing about the underlying etiology of itch. Initially, a clinician should assess whether the patient's itch is generalized or localized to a particular region of the body.

Generalized pruritus: Etiology
As previously indicated, xerosis is the most common cause of pruritus (particularly generalized pruritus) in the elderly population. Cases of dry skin may be exacerbated by hypolipidemic agents.[11] Generalized pruritus accompanied by characteristic collections of superficial burrows in the epidermis (created by the mite *Sarcoptes scabiei*) and the tendency to worsen at night may indicate scabies infestation, a condition discussed later in more detail. Elderly patients residing in communal institutions (nursing homes, assisted living facilities, or hospitals) are more likely to contract scabies, owing to the close proximity of residents and the easily transmissible nature of the infestation.[10] Paraneoplastic syndromes have also been implicated in cases of chronic, generalized pruritus. Pruritus following Hodgkin lymphoma is generally considered to be the prototype of paraneoplastic itch and can be one of the first presenting signs of this malignancy.[12] In fact, approximately 50% of patients who have Hodgkin lymphoma may present with pruritus, a symptom regarded as a bad prognostic sign.[13] Concomitant itch and rapid weight loss warrant the inclusion of occult malignancy in the differential diagnosis. Generalized itch is indeed an essential clinical sign in a series of paraneoplastic dermatologic syndromes, including malignant acanthosis nigricans and dermatomyositis.[14] Clinicians should ensure that any patient presenting with generalized pruritus has undergone the recommended, age-appropriate cancer screenings.

Generalized pruritus is also associated with a series of system-specific maladies. Metabolic causes should be considered highly in patients with minimal surface lesions, excluding excoriations.[15] In fact, 90% of patients suffering from renal failure or uremia treated by dialysis report symptoms of pruritus.[16] In the United States, hepatitis C infections have been reported with peak prevalence in individuals between the ages of 45 and 54 years.[17] Although the total incidence of hepatitis C in the country has steadily decreased, the medical complications that accompany long-term liver damage in an aging population will present a public health issue that will have to be addressed. A significant portion of patients infected with hepatitis C report pruritus as a manifesting symptom of the disease.[18] Although the pathogenesis of itch related to hepatitis C infection has not been definitively proven, the accumulation of bile acid in the skin and nerves has been offered as an explanation. The pruritic potential of hepatitis C and human immunodeficiency virus (HIV) infections necessitates inquiry about the patient's possible drug abuse and sexual history.

Patients suffering from nonalcoholic steatohepatitis, another etiologic factor underlying chronic liver damage, may suffer from pruritus for similar reasons. Cholestatic pruritus is typically more pronounced at night and affects the palms and the soles with greater severity. Current speculation about the mechanism of itch caused by cholestasis involves the enzyme autotaxin, which releases the lipid-signaling molecule lysophosphatidic acid (LPA). Serum levels of autotaxin or LPA can be measured to assess cholestasis.[19,20] It is important to remember that a potential side effect of certain prescription drugs (statins, tamoxifen, erythromycin, and other macrolides, and ibuprofen) is cholestasis 60.

Endocrine comorbidity. Conditions affecting the endocrine system have also been implicated in generalized itch. Diabetes mellitus results in progressive nerve damage that may become apparent as neuropathic itch. Cases of hyperthyroidism and hypothyroidism have been linked to generalized itch. The extensive systemic influence of the thyroid on the human body enables broad speculation about the pathophysiologic basis of thyroid-related itch. Most cases can be explained by a higher relative concentration of antithyroid antibodies.[7] In patients suffering from hypothyroidism, pruritus is generally secondary to xerosis or to widespread urticaria, as in the case of Hashimoto disease.[21–23]

Neurologic comorbidity. Neurologic dysfunction is a prominent feature of the aging process that must certainly be considered during an evaluation of generalized pruritus in an elderly patient. After a stroke, damage to the thalamus (likely the ventral posterolateral nucleus in cases of systemic pruritus) or the parietal lobe can result in neurogenic pruritus in the absence of peripheral stimuli.[24] Other nerve-related conditions, including multiple sclerosis and neuromuscular junction disorders (ie, Lambert-Eaton syndrome and myasthenia gravis), may similarly cause neuropathic itch. Generalized pruritus has more rarely been reported in progressive neurodegenerative disorders such as Creutzfeldt–Jakob disease.[25]

Psychiatric comorbidity. Psychogenic itch is another crucial consideration to make, as psychiatric conditions are common in patients suffering from chronic itch.[26] Depression, obsessive-compulsive disorder, anxiety, somatoform disorders, mania, psychoses, and substance abuse have all been correlated with itch.[27] Several studies have suggested that depression is the most important mood disorder underlying psychogenic pruritus.[28] Patients who have schizophrenia seldom report physical ailments, creating a problematic situation for clinicians in cases of psychogenic pruritus.[29] Mental decline in elderly patients can be a clinical roadblock under any circumstances and can make it challenging to obtain an accurate patient history. The patient's pharmacy, family members, and caretakers may be helpful sources of missing information.

Physicians should be careful to properly obtain the patient's consent to contact others about their care.

Hematologic comorbidity. Patients with hemochromatosis have presented with diffuse pruritus, presumably due to widespread nerve injury by iron deposition.[21] Iron-deficiency anemia is perhaps a more common iron-related cause of generalized pruritus, constituting the single most prevalent cause of itch in one retrospective study of elderly dermatologic patients.[22]

Generalized pruritus secondary to dermatologic disease. Pruritus is often associated with primary dermatologic diseases. For example, the appearance of urticaria and angioedema can be the presenting symptoms of a severe drug reaction and should be treated as such.[30] Transient urticarial outbreaks are generally the manifestations of allergic reactions. Bullous pemphigoid is a relatively common autoimmune subepidermal bullous disease that occurs with the greatest frequency in elderly patients. The disease predominates over anatomic flexures as tense blisters overlying regions of urticaria and pruritus.[31] Contact dermatitis is induced more easily in an elderly population plagued by skin-barrier insufficiency and a pro-inflammatory immune system. Atopic dermatitis (eczema) is typically more pronounced in younger demographics but does persist through adulthood in some cases. Some patients will experience new-onset atopic dermatitis as the immune system shifts toward a Th2 response with age.

Localized pruritus: Etiology
Localization of pruritus in an elderly patient suggests a different array of underlying causative factors. For example, seborrheic dermatitis is localized to surfaces rich in sebaceous glands, including the nasolabial folds and the scalp. The disease is characterized by alternating periods of significant erythema/skin flaking and relief, affecting a broad spectrum of ages. *Malassezia*, a genus of fungus that metabolizes fat, is primarily implicated in cases of seborrheic dermatitis. Dermatomyositis may present initially with signs and symptoms resembling seborrheic dermatitis before the onset of active muscular involvement. In fact, one recent study found that dermatomyositis in 14 of 17 patients initially manifested as seborrheic dermatitis-like scalp lesions.[32] In cases of temporal arteritis, a vasculitis that preferentially affects branches of the external carotid artery, patients may suffer from pruritus localized to the scalp. Forms of neuropathic itch affect the head and neck areas with greater frequency.[33] The prime example of this is the predominance of postherpetic itch of the head and neck following shingles. Trigeminal neuralgia, which can be a component of postherpetic neuralgia or the result of trauma, has also been associated with localized pruritus. It is important to note that postherpetic itch manifests within dermatomes previously involved by herpes zoster infection. Various dermatoses are essential to consider in the elderly patient population due to the poor skin barrier function and pro-inflammatory immune function inherent in this patient base. Irritant contact dermatitis is a nonspecific inflammatory reaction to a chemical insult that is often localized on the hands. Elderly patients are particularly susceptible to cleaning agents used for bedding and clothing in institutionalized settings. Allergic contact dermatitis (ACD) is an immunologic response to one or more harmless allergens that come into contact with the skin. The best treatment for this condition is avoidance of these allergens. Nickel, cobalt, and fragranced skin products are the most prevalent causative agents for older adults.[34]

Itch localized to the region of the thigh may be the result of meralgia paresthetica, a condition brought on by irritation of the lateral femoral cutaneous nerve (branch of the lumbar plexus). Meralgia paresthetica can be a function of diabetic neuropathy or compression by clothing/belting enabled by the deterioration of protective layers of adipose tissue in the elderly.[35,36] Notalgia paresthetica commonly manifests as pruritus and hyperpigmented patches at the interscapular region, with occasional associated pain, paresthesia, or burning. The presumed pathophysiology includes spinal nerve impingement.[37] It is known, however, that notalgia paresthetica is a common neuropathic condition in elderly patients that can be treated with capsaicin or with one of several empirically efficacious neuroleptic agents (gabapentin and pregabalin).[38] Kyphosis may also be revealed in patients with notalgia paresthetica on physical or radiologic examination.

Physical Examination

Arriving at a definitive diagnosis in a pruritic elderly patient, particularly one that is cognitively impaired, may be difficult for any clinician. A thorough physical examination, following a meticulous history of present illness, is strategic in determining the underlying causes of itch. Clinicians should also collect information about the patient's general appearance to gauge the patient's grooming behavior and cleanliness. Signs of depression or psychiatric illness may suggest psychogenic pruritus. The focus of the physical examination should be the skin. However, clinicians should palpate the abdomen, thyroid, and major lymph node basins for signs of organomegaly or lymphadenopathy. Vital signs and other basic physical information should be obtained to assess the possibility of pruritus caused by an infectious process (high fever) or malignancy (significant weight loss).

The cutaneous examination is multifaceted. Clinicians should observe any significant skin discoloration, as would be present in the case of a jaundiced patient experiencing generalized pruritus caused by excessive bile acid deposition around nerves responsible for the transmission of the itch sensation. The presence of erythema in localized areas of pruritus may suggest an infectious origin.[20] It is imperative that clinicians carefully look for primary and secondary lesions. Clinicians should observe the patient's skin for primary cutaneous lesions, including urticarial wheals and dermatitic plaques (suggestive of one of the aforementioned dermatoses). Of note, secondary lesions due to excoriations or lichenification, significant thickening of the skin induced by a protracted period of itching, often camouflage primary lesions.[39] Blisters (vesicles and bullae) may be the result of contact dermatitis, drug reactions, or autoimmune disease (bullous pemphigoid).[20] Excoriations seldom accompany primary dermal processes, such as urticaria, and suggest a great deal about the intensity of the pruritus.[39] Excoriations can further compromise the integrity of the skin's barrier function, increasing the patient's susceptibility to infection. The observed distribution of the lesions, generalized or localized, also lends significantly to the clinical diagnosis. Physicians should be thorough, inspecting the genitalia, axillae, areolae, and web spaces for signs of scabies infestation. Xerosis, the most frequent culprit in cases of elderly pruritus, can easily be observed as scaly or cracked skin.

Laboratory and Additional Testing

Laboratory tests complement the information obtained by the patient's history and physical examination and are of particular value when a systemic disease process is suspected in a pruritic patient. Clinicians can obtain a complete blood count to assess the white blood cell count (evaluating for chronic lymphocytic leukemia, leukocytosis in the setting of bacterial infection, or other leukocyte abnormalities) and to reveal abnormalities of red blood cell numbers (including anemia, polycythemia, macrocytosis, and microcytosis). Laboratory signs of iron-deficiency anemia should prompt an investigation of potential blood loss. Eosinophilia may indicate an underlying malignancy or parasitic infection.[15] A complete metabolic panel (including blood urea nitrogen, creatinine, alkaline phosphatase, direct and indirect bilirubin, alanine aminotransferase, asparagine aminotransferase, and albumin) can provide information about renal function, hepatic function, and nutritional status and can also help evaluate for possible cholestasis. Abnormalities in liver enzymes could suggest possible infectious, drug-related, alcoholic, or inflammatory hepatitis or could be the first indicator for nonalcoholic steatohepatitis, which is vital to consider, particularly in the obese, elderly patient. Thyroid studies (thyroid-stimulating hormone, T4) and a fasting glucose test can detect abnormalities of endocrine origin. Patients should be up to date on age-appropriate cancer screenings, but occult malignancy tests are indicated in patients suspected to have pruritus of cancerous or paraneoplastic origin. These tests include serum protein and urine protein electrophoreses for the detection of multiple myeloma or chronic inflammatory disease (abnormal gamma-globulin concentrations). Fecal occult blood tests can be obtained to screen for gastrointestinal malignancies. Antibody levels may be measured to detect an autoimmune condition or to document exposure to a foreign antigen or foreign agent. An infection/infestation workup for hepatitis C and HIV and *S scabiei* using a mineral oil prep at the bedside can be conducted in appropriately selected patients. Stool studies for ova and parasites could be beneficial in patients with hypereosinophilia, concomitant gastrointestinal complaints, or those with social or travel histories that suggest risk for acquisition of helminthic infection. If primary lesions are present on physical examination, a skin biopsy can aid in the diagnosis of such conditions as *S scabiei* infestation, urticaria, the urticarial stage of bullous pemphigoid, ACD, or drug eruption. In patients with a history of present illness and physical examination suggestive of ACD, patch testing can be used to great effect, helping to determine which potential allergens could be contributing to the patient's eruption.[20,39]

Section Summary

Pruritus is a common skin complaint in a rapidly growing elderly population. Hence, primary care physicians and dermatologists should have a working knowledge of recommended diagnostic and treatment protocols. Chronic itch is a potentially debilitating condition affecting a significant proportion of an elderly demographic that also suffers from a higher relative rate of comorbidities. This situation makes the diagnosis of pruritus increasingly difficult, particularly in patients with cognitive deficits. Chronic itch can have a significant impact on a patient's quality of life, sleep schedule, mental state, and mood and therefore warrants a thorough investigation and a carefully thought-out individualized treatment plan focused on improving symptoms while minimizing iatrogenic side effects.

MANAGEMENT OF PRURITUS IN THE ELDERLY

Clinicians should abide by a cohesive set of management goals when addressing the complaint of pruritus in an elderly patient to minimize the risk of complications and to ensure improvement in the patient's quality of life. It is integral, however, that clinicians tailor their treatment plans according to each individual patient's unique cognitive and physical characteristics (ie, the severity of pruritus, susceptibility to falls, dementia, mobility, and concurrent medications). Elderly patients are often discouraged because of the inability to sleep through intense itching. Clinicians must address the cause of pruritus to avoid future sleep disturbances. It is important to counsel elderly patients about appropriate skin and scalp hygiene to help ensure the longevity of itch relief.

This step includes recommendations about skin moisturizers that have a low pH and contain ceramides, lanolins, and glycerin. If pruritus in elderly patients is due to atopic dermatitis, a trial of Gladskin cream might be an effective OTC treatment. Atopic dermatitis is associated with an imbalance of the microbiome and over-colonization with *Staphylococcus aureus*. Gladskin cream, which contains *S aureus*-targeting endolysin, treats skin microbiome dysbiosis, and can reduce symptoms by 48% as early as 7 days following treatment; however, this medication is expensive.[40] Dermeleve, a novel OTC lotion containing strontium salt, has been demonstrated to alleviate pruritus in a variety of skin conditions by interfering directly with the synaptic transmission of C-nerve fibers. This strontium salt contains ions such as Sr^{+2}, which enter synaptic clefts via calcium channels and prevent C-type nerve neurons from depolarizing due to calcium. In a clinical trial, compounds containing strontium salt reduced both the severity and duration of pruritus.[41]

A simple non-pharmacologic step to diminish xerosis and possibly pruritus is counseling patients to avoid lengthy and hot showers. Moisturizers should be administered immediately after showers to maintain skin hydration. Moisturizers such as Cerave, Cetaphil, or Vaseline petroleum jelly are excellent choices because not only are they widely available but they are also reasonably priced.

Polypharmacy is common in the elderly demographic. Physicians must limit the iatrogenic risk of therapy. For example, the use of systemic antihistamines may have significant anticholinergic and sedative effects. Indeed, it has been suggested that the effectiveness of systemic antihistamines in certain common pruritic conditions (eczema and psoriasis) stems from the drugs' sedative properties.[42] In patients who present with excoriations, clinicians should acknowledge the possibility of infections acquired through a compromised skin barrier and advise against excessive scratching. In fact, cutaneous inflammation brought on by excessive scratching may worsen the intensity of itch.[43] Many dermatologic conditions are exacerbated by sweat and skin irritation brought on by tight clothing. Specialized fabrics designed to minimize skin irritation have been developed to help address this aspect of skin care. Several research studies have revealed that silver and chitosan have antibacterial properties. Antibacterial therapeutic clothing is meant to prevent skin colonization by *S aureus* to treat atopic dermatitis. Despite this, the efficacy of antibacterial therapeutic clothing for people with atopic dermatitis is still being researched, with little evidence to back it up.[44] A 2019 study investigated the effect of Merino wool clothing on atopic dermatitis. Merino wool clothing reduces the severity of atopic dermatitis and improves patients' quality of life.[45] MICROAIR Dermasilk (Alpretec, San Dona di Piave, Italy) is a prototypical fabric meant to alleviate undue irritation secondary to irritating or coarse clothing fibers. Dermasilk has been recommended with confidence in cases of atopic dermatitis, but silk fabrics have utility in many cases of pruritus. Silk fabrics allow the skin to "breathe," regulating body temperature and minimizing the moisture loss that worsens xerotic skin.[45]

TREATMENT
Topical Steroids

A series of pharmacologic strategies may be indicated in cases of pruritus that cannot be managed by non-pharmacologic measures. Topical corticosteroids are effective in treating pruritic conditions with inflammatory and immunologic origins, including a variety of dermatoses (eczema, atopic, and seborrheic dermatitis), psoriasis, and bullous pemphigoid. Although topical steroids can help treat secondary pruritus produced by disorders like atopic dermatitis, they are less effective in treating generalized pruritus with no skin manifestation. Clinicians should exercise caution in prescribing topical corticosteroids to elderly patients because of their increased vulnerability to local and systemic toxicity. This increased risk is correlated with a higher surface area to body weight ratio and diminished skin barrier function. Whereas high-potency topical corticosteroids may be appropriate for use on regions with small surface areas and thick stratum cornea (palms of hands and soles of feet), lower potency steroids should be considered in elderly patients with generalized pruritic conditions. Penetration and absorption of topical steroids is 300 times less effective on the soles of the feet than on areas with thin stratum cornea (eyelids).

Hydrocortisone is classified as a low-potency topical steroid, whereas triamcinolone serves as an example of a medium-potency corticosteroid and clobetasol is regarded as a high-potency corticosteroid.[46] Their efficacy also varies depending on the vehicle in which they are prepared. Different vehicles are also used for different sections of the body. Because it can induce maceration and folliculitis, the ointment should not be used in hairy areas. For dry and hyperkeratotic skin, ointments are suggested.[46] If the patient's skin is not dry, cream vehicles that are less oily and can be used in intertriginous areas such as the groin and axilla are recommended.[46] Low-potency steroids, on the other hand, are indicated for these locations. Shampoos and foams are effective treatments for itchy scalp. The foams, on the other hand, are more expensive.[46]

The potential systemic and local adverse effects of topical corticosteroids include hypertension, hypothalamic–pituitary–adrenal axis suppression, telangiectasia, acne, and, possibly, tachyphylaxis.[47] Tachyphylaxis describes an acute tolerance to the vasoconstrictive effects of topically applied corticosteroids, but its importance as a side effect has been disputed.[48] Last, studies have been conducted to demonstrate the efficacy of topical corticosteroids used in conjunction with wet wrap dressings, particularly in cases of exacerbated atopic dermatitis.[49]

Topical Anti-itch Agents

Capsaicin, the main capsaicinoid in chili peppers, has been used to treat cases of neuropathic and dermatologic pruritus. Capsaicin has demonstrated considerable efficacy in the treatment of postherpetic neuralgia, prurigo nodularis, and brachioradial pruritus (BRP).[50–52] BRP is a type of localized neuropathy that mostly affects the dorsolateral upper extremities of middle-aged white women, especially in the summer when it is warmer.[53]

Prurigo nodularis consists of severe itching nodules characterized by collagenous fibrosis and inflammatory infiltrates.[54] Topical capsaicin (0.025%) was shown to exert a suppressive effect on histamine, substance P (SP), and protease activated receptor-2 (PAR-2) agonist-derived itch responses.[55] The most prominent untoward effects of capsaicin treatment, burning and stinging at the site of application, can be avoided with topical anesthetic cream (EMLA: lidocaine 2.5%/prilocaine 2.5%) application 60 minutes before the administration of topical capsaicin.[56] Even with the administration of a topical anesthetic, capsaicin can be difficult to tolerate on broken skin. Clinicians should discuss the nature of capsaicin with patients beforehand to ensure adherence and warn of possible discomfort. Pramoxine is a topical medication that works by stabilizing the membrane of sensory neurons and preventing itch perception.[57] Camphor extracted from camphor tree is a natural topical treatment for pruritus that produces a cooling sensation and has calming properties.[58]

Antihistamines

Orally administered antihistamines have notable value in the treatment of pruritus arising from the stimulation of histamine receptors, as in urticaria. Although histamine is generally considered to be the primary mediator of itching, not all forms of pruritus respond to antihistamine therapy, suggesting the involvement of other mediators, such as serotonin (5-hydroxytryptamine) and acetylcholine.[20] Topical antihistamines are of little benefit and may induce ACD.[59] The use of topical antihistamine may also result in systemic absorption and possible toxicity caused by an impaired epidermal barrier in the debilitated integument of the elderly.[60] Antihistamines work by blocking histamine receptors. First-generation antihistamines such as diphenhydramine have many anticholinergic and sedative effects and are not recommended for older adults. Second-generation antihistamines are nonsedative and have no significant side effects. Fexofenadine, a nonsedative antihistamine, is often used to treat pruritus due to atopic dermatitis. The suggested daily dose is 180 mg in the morning. Cetirizine is a nonsedative antihistamine that is extensively used in the treatment of atopic dermatitis. The recommended daily intake is 10 mg.[61]

Naltrexone and Cholestatic Pruritus

Naltrexone has been demonstrated to be a viable treatment option for cholestatic pruritus, particularly in patients who are unresponsive to other traditional treatments (rifampin and cholestyramine).[62] Under these circumstances, clinicians should ensure the compatibility of the patient's prescribed drugs. For example, naltrexone is contraindicated in patients with chronic narcotic analgesic use to prevent precipitating acute withdrawal symptoms. The clear benefit of opioid antagonists in the treatment of pruritus stems from the role played by nociceptive neurons in the tonic inhibition of itch fibers.[39]

Cyclosporine

Cyclosporine, administered orally, is an immunosuppressive drug that effectively palliates itch related to atopic dermatitis, chronic idiopathic urticaria, and prurigo nodularis.[54,63,64] Cyclosporine diminishes T-cell activity by inhibiting calcineurin phosphorylase 64. One study aimed at elucidating the value of cyclosporine in the treatment of "essential senile pruritus" demonstrated the drug's efficacy in all 10 of the patients assessed. The age range of the 10 patients was 59 to 72 years, and all were suffering from generalized pruritus for between 6 and 11 months. The cohort was universally resistant to antihistamine therapy, topical or oral corticosteroids, and topical emollients. Eight patients reported the complete disappearance of pruritus by the 14th week of treatment without experiencing significant side effects. The adverse effects of cyclosporine, including nephrotoxicity, hepatotoxicity, gingival hypertrophy, tremor, and elevated blood pressure, limit its application.[65]

Tricyclic Antidepressants

Tricyclic antidepressants (TCAs) offer the unique therapeutic advantage of being H1-receptor antagonists, a pharmacologic property that is presumably independent of the drugs' antidepressant potential. It has been suggested, however, that the magnitude of a patient's depression is directly correlated with the severity of itch. Therefore, the administration of TCAs is doubly efficacious in the management of depression affecting patients with concomitant psoriasis, atopic dermatitis, and chronic idiopathic urticaria.[66] TCAs also have empirical value in the treatment of pruritus in patients without depressive symptoms.[67] For example, amitriptyline has been reported to aid the resolution of poststroke pruritus 24. Doxepin may improve pruritus in endstage renal patients who do not respond to traditional antihistamines and can be administered to attenuate chronic idiopathic urticaria.[67,68] Topical 5% doxepin has also been used in the treatment of atopic dermatitis.[69] The TCA trimipramine has considerable antihistaminic properties and has been prescribed to mitigate pruritus of atopic dermatitis.[70]

Thalidomide

Thalidomide helped one patient with severe Hodgkin-associated paraneoplastic pruritus[71] and has demonstrated value in the treatment of prurigo nodularis. In a study involving 22 patients with prurigo nodularis, 20 reported a significant immediate relief from itch and showed a marked reduction in the size of lesions after 1 to 2 months of taking thalidomide.[72] Thalidomide has also been used in the treatment of refractory uremic pruritus, although the mechanism of the drug's efficacy in this setting has not been elucidated. Fifty-five percent of the patients in the thalidomide study reported reductions in pruritic symptoms by 78% to 81%. Thalidomide's use extends to cases of pruritus associated with lupus erythematosus and lichen planus.[73] Birth defects, sensorimotor peripheral neuropathy, somnolence, rash, tiredness, and constipation are the most serious side effects of thalidomide.[74] The US Food and Drug Administration has established the Thalidomide Risk Evaluation and Mitigation Strategy to prevent pregnant women from using thalidomide. The program ensures that pregnant women do not use thalidomide and that women who are taking thalidomide do not become pregnant.[74]

Dupilumab

Despite being a common condition, pruritus can be challenging because many drugs fail to give long-term relief. In several clinical trials, dupilumab has shown excellent results in suppressing pruritus, making it a practical treatment choice for people suffering from these distressing symptoms. Dupilumab is a human monoclonal antibody that blocks the signaling of two interleukins, interleukin (IL)-4 and IL-13, which are essential in developing pruritus. It binds to the IL-4 receptor alpha subunit, inhibiting both IL-4 and IL-13 signaling.[75] A 2016 study found that dupilumab, compared with a placebo group, successfully lowered pruritus severity in patients with atopic dermatitis within 2 weeks of treatment. The patients achieved symptom alleviation during the 16-week therapeutic experiment, with no substantial severe side effects recorded.[75]

Another clinical trial completed in 2019 verified the efficacy of dupilumab for the treatment of pruritus in patients with chronic renal disease. Those who received dupilumab experienced a significant reduction in pruritus severity when compared with the placebo group. The patient's quality of life significantly improved, and they experienced decreased sleep disruption.[76] Dupilumab, despite its efficacy, can induce side effects such as conjunctivitis (eye inflammation), injection site reaction, and upper respiratory tract infections. Although dupilumab might have adverse effects, they are usually minimal and outweighed by the benefits.[77]

Janus Kinase Inhibitors

Janus kinase is an intercellular signal transducer that serves as a transcription pathway activator and regulates gene expression via the stand for the janus kinase-signal transducer and activator of transcription (JAK-STAT) pathway. Numerous clinical trials and case reports have demonstrated that Janus kinase inhibitors, which have been evaluated and used to treat a variety of autoimmune disorders, are also useful in the treatment of pruritus. Janus kinase inhibitors have the potential to be a good therapy choice for a wide range of illnesses. Janus kinase inhibitors have been used to treat pruritus in atopic dermatitis, psoriasis, and other disorders such as prurigo nodularis and lichen planus, delivering faster itch alleviation than traditional treatments. The most common side effects recorded include nasopharyngitis, acne, and increased blood creatine phosphokinase levels. Janus kinase inhibitors are currently labeled with a risk of cancer and cardiovascular problems in geriatric patients.[78]

Phototherapy

Generalized pruritus may be successfully treated with ultraviolet B (UVB) phototherapy, which has widespread anti-inflammatory cutaneous activity. Broadband UVB phototherapy is the treatment of choice in patients with moderate to severe uremic pruritus.[60] Phototherapy, when administered judiciously, is an effective clinical measure against pruritus that avoids the side effects associated with systemic drugs. This consideration is a particularly important one to make in cases of polypharmacy. The efficacy of phototherapy in the treatment of itch has been established in a series of randomized controlled trials.[79,80] Phototherapy may even have diagnostic value. Treating a severe case of generalized pruritus may ameliorate the generalized itch to reveal a previously hidden localized itch.[39] Ward and Bernhard hypothesize that in conditions such as BRP and stasis dermatitis, the presence of intense localized itch reduces the threshold for itch throughout the rest of the body by neurologic and/or psychogenic mechanisms, resulting in a process known as secondary autoeczematization.[39] In addition, phototherapy for the treatment of pruritus is typically well covered by Medicare, making it both an effective and attainable therapeutic option for elderly patients. Obstacles to phototherapy may include difficulties with transportation and adherence to a schedule in the elderly population.

Cognitive Behavioral Therapy

Cognitive behavioral therapy may be of utility in mildly demented and depressed patients suffering from pruritus. It should also be administered to break the "itch-scratch cycle,"[80] described earlier as a progressive succession of itching and scratching that culminates in excoriations and increasingly intense itch sensations. It has been suggested that certain psychogenic forms of itch may resolve in response to verbal cues or physical diversions. For example, a patient with chronic "neurotic excoriations" who is habituated to scratching when distressed or bored may be able to address this impulse by verbally saying "stop." Similarly, patients may be able to divert nervous energy into a physical activity such as knitting or playing cards or even lightly snapping a rubber band worn around their wrist in lieu of scratching or picking at their skin. Cognitive therapy might ultimately develop into a therapy that is able to adjust a patient's expectations of itch to treat their pruritus.[81]

MANAGEMENT OF MEDICATIONS

Pruritus may also originate as a side effect of prescription or recreational drug use.

Clinicians should consider polypharmacy in the elderly demographic when prescribing additional medications but also when they are searching for a possible cause of pruritus. Management of pruritus in the elderly may simply require curtailing or modifying a patient's daily drug regimen. For example, an infrequent side effect of systemic statin use is itch, presumably due to a decrease in skin cholesterol concentrations. Studies have established that measured changes in skin cholesterol may simply be the result of natural fluctuations.[82] Other studies have also refuted the association between statin use and transepidermal water loss.[83,84] Nevertheless, clinicians can attempt to ameliorate pruritic symptoms with omega-3 fatty acid supplementation. Daily flaxseed oil supplements, a nutritional asset for its high concentration of alpha-linolenic acid, have been shown to minimize skin sensitivity, roughness, and scaling while increasing integumentary smoothness and hydration.[85] The specific value of concomitant statin and omega-3 fatty acid use, however, has yet to be studied extensively. Opioids form a class of drugs that cause pruritus by a centrally mediated mechanism, or by the release of histamine, in 2% to 10% of patients who take those 20. Diuretics, the most commonly prescribed class of drugs in the elderly, are often implicated in cases of dermatologic problems.[86] Cases of diffuse urticarial pruritus have been reported as a manifestation of hypersensitivity reactions to furosemide.[87] Diuretics may also induce inadequate skin hydration and cause xerosis.[88] Hyperuricemia has been established as a possible adverse event following the administration of thiazides and has been implicated as a causative factor underlying profuse, generalized itch.[87]

One 2006 study measured the adverse cutaneous drug reactions caused by antihypertensive drugs in a cohort of 1176 subjects, finding that beta-blockers were the most frequent culprit, with calcium-channel blockers implicated as the next most frequent. The most common skin manifestations included urticaria and lichenoid drug eruptions.[89] Another investigation estimated that 10% to 60% of all adverse events with antihypertensive drugs were dermatologic.[90]

SUMMARY

Treating chronic pruritus in elderly patients represents a therapeutic challenge due to often complex medical background of these patients and potentially difficult social and economic constraints. The edict of "First do no harm" must be exercised when choosing therapeutic interventions for elderly patients, and topical treatments or environmental modification should be attempted first to help avoid possible side effects of medication and drug–drug interactions. The potential medical frailty of elderly patients should remain a consideration when discussing therapeutic options with patients, their families, and possibly other members of their care teams. However, it is also important to consider the significant morbidity that can be associated with chronic pruritus in elderly patients and the deleterious effects that chronic itch can have on their quality of life. Appropriate steps up to a carefully thought-out therapeutic ladder can help to ensure symptom relief while minimizing potential adverse events. Specific patient characteristics such as chronic kidney disease, cholestasis, or other medical comorbidities should also be considered, because certain therapies may be more beneficial for one group of patients than for another.

SCABIES EVALUATION AND TREATMENT
Overview

Scabies, known colloquially as the "7-year itch," is a contagious dermatologic condition caused by the parasitic arthropod *Sarcoptes scabiei* var hominis. Scabies infestation typically presents as a characteristic set of symptoms mediated through inflammatory and allergy-like reactions that result in severe pruritus affecting the wrists, elbows, back, buttocks, external genitalia, and the webbing between the fingers. Scabies is particularly prominent in nursing homes and assisted living communities, affecting an immunologically impaired population living in close quarters.[91] The possibility of secondary infections by group A streptococci and *S aureus* through excoriations and the potentially debilitating effects of severe generalized pruritus necessitate a comprehensive explanation of the diagnostic and management protocols for scabies in the elderly population.[92]

Introduction

Scabies is a condition caused by the itch mite, *S scabiei*, an obligate ectoparasite that burrows into the host stratum corneum to incite a strong pruritic allergic response.[92,93]

In fact, the irritating qualities of the scabies mite were documented as far back as the fourth century BCE by Aristotle, who described them as "lice in the flesh."[92] The mite is approximately a third of a millimeter long and has a flattened oval body with eight legs. The S scabiei mite leaves behind eggs and fecal pellets, allergens that broaden the potential for a widespread immunologic response by the human body. The larvae typically hatch after 2 to 3 days to survive for upward of 2 months, mating and producing offspring every 10 to 17 days.[93] Adult mites emerge on the surface of the skin after 2 weeks to either reinfect the host or spread to a new host.[94]

The primary mode of transmission is skin-to-skin contact with affected individuals, the likelihood of which may increase significantly in close quarters.[92,94] Contacted bed sheets and undergarments can also be vehicles of transmission for a limited period of time following exposure. In fact, the importance of fomites as a transmission mechanism has been demonstrated internationally in hospital and nursing home settings.[95]

The gravity of transitory skin-to-skin contact and fomites increases in cases of crusted (Norwegian) scabies, a more severe variant of the traditional scabies infection characterized by the widespread crusty lesions and a much more significant mite burden. The risk of developing scabies and especially crusted scabies is particularly prominent in individuals affected by T-cell deficiencies, systemic autoimmune disorders (systemic lupus erythematosus or rheumatoid arthritis), leprosy, or leukemia. The elderly population typically has a pro-inflammatory immune system 6 that is debilitated by varying degrees, making the aged patient base uniquely vulnerable to exaggerated cases of scabies (or crusted scabies).

The debilitating effects that scabies-induced pruritus may have on a patient's quality of life are considerable. Scabies has an excellent prognosis when managed promptly and appropriately. As such, it is essential for clinicians to immediately recognize the possibility of scabies in elderly patients suffering from diffuse persistent pruritus. Risk factors and treatment recommendations are expounded on here.

Patient History

Scabies should be considered part of the differential diagnosis if a patient presents with generalized pruritus that worsens at night. Scabies is frequently transmitted among family members, owing to their regular proximity. Therefore, the clinician should inquire about the patient's family or residential history of scabies. The high incidence of transmission in institutionalized settings should prompt the clinician to ask about the patient's living conditions.[91] Nursing homes and assisted living communities offer the ideal environment for the extensive spread of S scabiei. Populated densely by a demographic largely plagued by aged, naturally debilitated immune systems, residential institutions are rife with fomites (ie, bed sheets) that act as modes of transmission. In fact, mites removed from their human host can survive potentially for 24 to 36 hours at room temperature and normal to low humidity.[92] Lower temperatures and high humidity enable greater mite longevity. Clinicians should also inquire about the patient's past and current medication use. Topical or oral steroids prescribed for dermatologic comorbidities may compromise the efficacy of the immune system, increasing the patient's susceptibility to a scabies infestation. It is also important for clinicians to investigate medical histories to identify any immunosuppressive disorders, although elderly patients with relatively intact immune systems are still susceptible.

Clinical diagnosis of scabies is difficult without a comprehensive physical examination and the use of appropriate laboratory tests. The similarity between scabies and other pruritic conditions of noninfectious origin broadens the margin of error in clinical diagnoses.[96]

Physical Examination

Clinicians should administer a thorough physical examination in cases of suspected scabies infestation. Pruritic papules are typically localized to the webs of the fingers, the flexor and extensor aspects of the elbow, wrists, buttocks, axillae, external genitalia, and the periareolar region (in women).[92] The unique immunologic/inflammatory response demonstrated by each individual patient enables some diversity in the physical presentation of the disease. However, the most prominent visible characteristic feature of *S scabiei* infestation is the aforementioned epidermal burrows (**Fig. 1**).

The burrow tracks are generally linear, presenting in groups of four or more closely aligned frequently crusted lesions that are approximately 5 mm in length. These burrows may not be immediately evident and may be camouflaged by excoriations.[97] After all, the elderly population is susceptible to a range of dermatologic conditions due to the decreasing integrity of the integument that coincides with age. Crusted scabies, or Norwegian scabies, has a much more extreme presentation characterized by thick-crusted, scaly, hyperkeratotic lesions that blanket almost the entire integument (head, chest, back, arms, legs, groin, hands, and feet). Scales may reveal extraordinary numbers of mites and eggs (millions in severe cases).

Laboratory Tests and Other Diagnostic Mechanisms

A definitive diagnosis of scabies depends on detection by light microscopy of mites, their remnants, fecal matter (scybala), eggs, or eggshells in a skin scraping. Several drops of mineral oil are typically applied to the scabietic lesion before being scraped. Most scabies patients are infested with approximately 11 mites.[91] As such, a simple skin scraping may not necessarily expose sufficient evidence to declare a diagnosis of scabies. Samplers may have to retrieve several scrapings and must be adequately experienced in identifying mites. Given the challenging nature of microscopic identification of mites and their remnants, a negative result from a skin scraping does not indicate invariably that the patient does not have scabies. However, a positive result from a skin scraping can be corroborated by histologic analysis of cutaneous tissue. The stratum corneum should appear significantly thicker, and there is a perivascular lymphocytic infiltrate with eosinophils in the dermis (**Fig. 2**).

Immunoglobulin E serum antibody concentrations are directly correlated with the intensity of the skin reaction.[98] If scabies is suspected, treatment may be started for diagnostic purposes in situations where an alternative is not available. However,

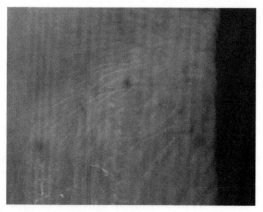

Fig. 1. Acral skin demonstrating a scabies burrow.

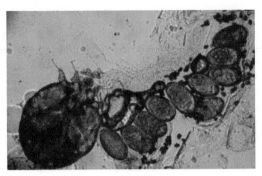

Fig. 2. Positive mineral oil prep demonstrating scabies mite, eggs, and scybala.

this method of evaluation is complicated by the diversity in treatment responses and mutable time frames for symptom resolution in different patients. More importantly, persistence of symptoms following treatment does not necessarily signify an incorrect diagnosis. Resistant mites and insufficiently potent treatment are equally valid explanations. After staining potentially infested skin with India ink, dermatoscopy can also be used to identify superficially situated mites in their burrows.[99] The "delta-wing sign" is the hallmark sign of the scabies mite in a dermoscopic image (**Figs. 3** and **4**).

However, the delta-wing sign is difficult to observe in pigmented skin, and mites may be confused with natural artifacts (eg, crusts or even small pieces of dirt).[97] Studies have been conducted to evaluate the efficacy of dermatoscopy as a diagnostic tool when compared with the adhesive tape test. The adhesive tape test is carried out by cutting pieces of transparent tape to the size of a microscope slide, applied to a scabietic lesion, and rapidly removed. The sample adhering to the tape is transferred to a microscope slide and stored in exceptionally cool conditions until it is read. The sensitivity of dermatoscopy was found to be significantly higher than that of the adhesive tape test and was revealed to increase according to the severity of the disease.[100]

Several trials have also shown that the sensitivity of dermatoscopy (0.86) is significantly higher than that of skin scraping (0.46). In fact, in one study, only 18% of 151 positive skin-scraping tests were representative of true scabies infestations.[101] Thus, empirical evidence constitutes a reason to consider dermatoscopy as a viable diagnostic method, despite its previously described limitations.

Treatment

The treatment protocol for scabies has advanced over time and will continue to develop as the *S scabiei* mite demonstrates progressive resistance to currently prescribed insecticides. Topical lindane (gamma benzene hexachloride) was previously accepted as the standard of care for most cases of scabies before evidence of central neurotoxicity was revealed. Permethrin 5% is the recommended antiscabietic treatment option in the United States and most other developed countries. Permethrin selectively affects the eggs, lice, and mites through its action on sodium transport across neural membranes in arthropods, resulting in depolarization. Consequently, the arthropod experiences respiratory paralysis. Permethrin undergoes rapid metabolism by ester hydrolysis, resulting in the formation of metabolites that lack biological activity. These metabolites are predominantly eliminated from the body through urinary excretion.

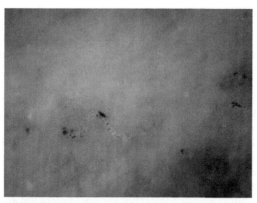

Fig. 3. Dermoscopic image with multiple positive "delta-wing" structures corresponding to scabies mites and demonstrating a mite within a burrow containing scybala. (This image was taken from a patient with crusted scabies.)

The predominant adverse effects of permethrin usage are dermal irritation, characterized by pruritus, edema, and erythema, which may manifest during scabies infestation and exhibit transient exacerbation after permethrin therapy. In addition, some may have a little sensation of burning or stinging.[102] In treating scabies, it is recommended to provide permethrin 5% cream to the entire body, starting from the neck and moving downward. This application should be on for 8 to 14 hours, after which it should be washed off. It is recommended that this application be repeated 1 week later.[103]

Data have indicated the equivalent efficacy of 1% topical ivermectin in similar cases of scabies. Concurrent administration of oral ivermectin and topical ivermectin in patients plagued with crusted scabies has been established as an appropriate course of treatment. The recommended 1% ivermectin cream dose is a once-daily application for two consecutive days. If symptoms persist after the initial treatment, a second course may be administered 1 week later.[104]

Intravenous ivermectin, a regimen that is indicated in a variety of severe parasitic infections, has also been used in cases of severe scabies.[105] Ivermectin works by paralyzing the scabies mite through interference with specific neurotransmitter receptors associated with the parasite's motor system.[106] One trial established a 100% cure rate in all three of the aforementioned drugs (oral/topical ivermectin and topical permethrin) after 3 weeks of application.[107]

Novel treatment options are currently being developed to address drug-resistant scabies mites. In fact, clinical ivermectin and permethrin resistance has already

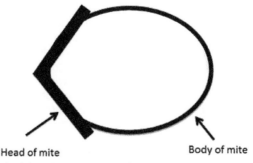

Head of mite   Body of mite

Fig. 4. Correlation of "delta-wing" sign to scabies mite.

been reported.[108,109] Scabies mite digestive proteases and complement inhibitors (for the evasion of host defense) have been identified to serve as potential drug targets.[110]

In 2022, the Journal of the American Academy of Dermatology published an article regarding the efficiency of 0.9% spinosad in the treatment of scabies. This topical medication primarily attacks the parasite's nervous system, destroying only the motile stages. Owing to the lack of ovicidal activities, they require further treatments to be effective. The number of applications depends on the severity of the disease.[111]

In this article, efficacy assessments supported 0.9% spinosad's potential to eliminate scabies in terms of both observed decreases in related symptoms and microscopically determined mite eradication. In addition, 0.9% spinosad was well tolerated and did not cause any safety concerns.[112] This is a brand new therapeutic option for drug-resistant scabies.

Clinicians must make special considerations when treating the elderly population for scabies. Clinicians should advise against hot showers before the application of topical treatment to avoid potential toxicity facilitated by extra absorbent skin. Normally, topical/oral ivermectin and topical permethrin are associated with only mild side effects that subside without further medical attention. Adverse effects of ivermectin may include mild headache, anorexia, asthenia, myalgia, and arthralgia, whereas side effects of permethrin may appear as a mild burning sensation at the point of application.[107]

One study aiming to assess the safety and efficacy of the most prominent scabies treatment included patients between the ages of 5 and 80 years.[107] However, the elderly demographic generally represents a subset of patients that is uniquely susceptible to the toxic effects of drugs. Monitored properly; however, elderly patients may be treated for scabies in concert with the recommended drug regimen without adverse events.

Clinicians must also address an elderly patient's living conditions to ensure the longevity of relief from scabies. In fact, reinfestations commonly occur when patients return to their home environments. Particularly in cases of crusted scabies, clinicians must advise the complete sanitization of potential fomites, including bedding, clothing, and furniture. It is recommended to machine wash bedding and clothing at temperatures of 50°C for a minimum of 10 minutes to improve the odds of completely eradicating the scabies mite and its eggs. Mite transmission typically occurs in squalid conditions. Often, cognitively impaired elderly patients neglect appropriate hygiene and general cleanliness practices. Clinicians should counsel patients about the importance of cleanliness in the avoidance of scabies and other pruritic diseases.

Section Summary Points

1. Scabies is common in the elderly population, particularly in patients who have dementia or other forms of cognitive impairment, immunologic or hematologic conditions, nutritional deficiencies, and infectious diseases.
2. The ease of skin-to-skin transmission, especially in residential institutions, prompts special attention to the disease in the elderly demographic.
3. The implications of scabies extend beyond severe widespread pruritus. Clinicians should be cognizant of the possibility of secondary infections (group A streptococci and S aureus) and the effects of prolonged scabies infections on the quality of life.
4. High efficacy of treatment correlates directly with prompt recognition and treatment of scabies.
5. Early recognition and treatment of scabies in the elderly population diminishes the risk of the rapid spread of the easily transmissible mite.

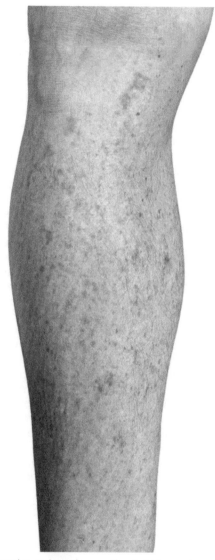

Fig. 5. Erythematous papules and patches on the right lower leg.

Case presentation

A 73-year-old Caucasian man reported significant pruritus over most of his body that began 4 weeks after COVID infection. Four weeks before the rash, the severe acute respiratory syndrome coronavirus-2 (SARS-CoV-2) antibody immunoglobulin G (IgG) was positive. Urticaria precedes the rash, which is followed by redness. There was no recent travel history, dietary changes, or new skin care products. Except for numerous brown and pink macules and papules 3 to 6 mm on the trunk and erythematous papules and patches on bilateral arms, legs, and trunk, the rest of the skin examination was within normal limits (**Fig. 5**).

Two 4-mm punch biopsies were done on two leg lesions. Initially, the patient was advised to switch to hypoallergenic detergent and skin care, avoid hot showers, and start a trial of oral hydroxyzine and topical triamcinolone. On both lesions, biopsies revealed spongiotic dermatitis with underlying inflammation. With triamcinolone, the patient observed a slight improvement. He claims that triamcinolone 0.1% cream provides some relief, reducing his pruritus score from 6 to 3 out of 10. The pruritus was more severe at night, primarily affecting the trunk and extremities. The patient's primary care practitioner also attempted to control his pruritus by prescribing Allegra, Zyrtec, Singulair, and Cimetidine daily; however, these medications did not provide any relief. Five months later, a daily naltrexone trial began to control his persistent pruritus. Laboratory orders were submitted during the same appointments to rule out an autoimmune condition. The erythrocyte sedimentation rate and C-reactive protein levels were within normal limits, and the antinuclear antibody test was negative. Naltrexone provided no alleviation. Because the patient had a history of hot tub use and the severity of rash on both thighs, a 2-week trial of doxycycline was attempted. Although doxycycline is an excellent treatment for bacterial folliculitis, the patient did not improve after completing the course. After 6 months of unsuccessful pharmacologic treatment, the patient began twice-weekly phototherapy. There was no improvement in symptoms 3 months following phototherapy. Because of the debilitating nature of this rash, a trial of therapy with Dupixent was discussed with the patient. The patient's insurance approved Dupixent; however, the patient could not afford the copay. Before paying the copay, the patient received free Dupixent samples. Six weeks after beginning Dupixent, the patient had a 50% reduction in pruritus. He had one flare in the previous 6 weeks. The provider explained to the patient that Dupixent typically takes 10 to 12 weeks to begin working, so the fact that he has already noticed improvement is promising. The patient's symptoms were resolved after 6 months of treatment with Dupixent.

The case report outlines the challenges of treating pruritus in a COVID-19-infected patient. This elderly patient developed pruritus 4 weeks after the COVID-19 infection, which persisted for months despite pharmacologic treatment. Hot showers and allergenic skin care products were avoided to reduce pruritus. Oral hydroxyzine and topical triamcinolone failed to treat. Spongiotic dermatitis with underlying inflammation was found in the biopsy, which may have caused pruritus to persist. Allegra, Zyrtec, Singulair, cimetidine, naltrexone, and doxycycline were tried, but none relieved the symptoms. Phototherapy twice a week also failed. Thus, Dupixent (dupilumab) was prescribed, which resolved symptoms in 10 weeks. This case suggests that Dupixent may be an effective remedy for COVID-19-related pruritus.

CLINICS CARE POINTS

- Persistent pruritus post COVID-19 infection can be a challenge to treat, and it may require multiple treatment strategies.
- Avoidance of hot showers and allergenic skin care products can be the first step in reducing pruritus.
- Pharmacological treatments like oral hydroxyzine and topical triamcinolone may not always be effective, indicating the need for alternative therapies.
- Spongiotic dermatitis with underlying inflammation, as found in skin biopsy, can contribute to persistent pruritus.
- A variety of treatments including Allegra, Zyrtec, Singulair, cimetidine, naltrexone, doxycycline, and phototherapy may be ineffective in some cases.

- Dupixent (dupilumab) could be a potential therapeutic option for COVID-19-related pruritus, as suggested by the resolution of symptoms in this case.

ACKNOWLEDGMENT

The authors would like to thank the TTUHSC Writing Center for their help editing and reviewing this article.

FUNDING

The authors have no funding sources to declare.

DISCLOSURE

Dr Bharat Panuganti and Dr Michelle Tarbox contribute equally to this article. Student doctor Shakira Meltan was responsible for the revision of this article. Dr Tarbox is a researcher for Castle Biosciences. Their products are not discussed in this article. The patient consent form was obtained.

REFERENCES

1. Yalcin B, Tamer E, Gur Toy G, et al. The prevalence of skin diseases in the elderly: analysis of 4099 geriatric patients. Int J Dermatol 2006;45:672–6.
2. Vespa J, Medina L, Armstrong D. Demographic Turning Points for the United States: Population Projections for 2020 to 2060 Population Estimates and Projections Current Population Reports.; 2020.
3. Ikoma A, Steinhoff M, Ständer S, et al. The neurobiology of itch. Nat Rev Neurosci 2006;7(7):535–47.
4. Stander S, Weisshaar E, Luger TA. Neurophysiological and neurochemical basis of modern pruritus treatment. Exp Dermatol 2008;17(3):161–9.
5. Mansfield AS, Nevala WK, Dronca RS, et al. Normal ageing is associated with an increase in Th2 cells, MCP-1 (CCL1) and RANTES (CCL5), with differences in sCD40L and PDGF-AA between sexes. Clin Exp Immunol 2012;170(2):186–93.
6. Bianchi J, Cameron J. Assessment of skin integrity in the elderly 1. Br J Community Nurs 2008;13(3):S26–8. S30–2.
7. Norman RA. Xerosis and pruritus in the elderly: recognition and management. Dermatol Ther 2003;16(3):254–9.
8. Pseudomonas dermatitis/folliculitis associated with pools and hot tubs-Colorado and Maine, 1999-2000. Can Commun Dis Rep 2001;27(3):24–8.
9. Boccanfuso SM, Cosmet L, Volpe AR, et al. Skin xerosis. Clinical report on the effect of a moisturizing soap bar. Cutis 1978;21(5):703–7.
10. Simpson E, Böhling A, Bielfeldt S, et al. Improvement of skin barrier function in atopic dermatitis patients with a new moisturizer containing a ceramide precursor. J Dermatolog Treat 2012;24(2):122–5.
11. Proksch E. Antilipemic drug-induced skin manifestations. Hautarzt 1995;46(2):76–80 [in German].
12. Tivoli YA, Rubenstein RM. Pruritus: an updated look at an old problem. J Clin Aesthet Dermatol 2009;2(7):30–6.
13. Summey BT Jr, Yosipovitch G. Pharmacologic advances in the systemic treatment of itch. Dermatol Ther 2005;18(4):328–32.

14. Yosipovitch G. Chronic pruritus: a paraneoplastic sign. Dermatol Ther 2010; 23(6):590–6.
15. Berger TG, Steinhoff M. Pruritus in elderly patients–eruptions of senescence. Semin Cutan Med Surg 2011;30(2):113–7.
16. Robinson-Bostom L, DiGiovanna JJ. Cutaneous manifestations of end-stage renal disease. J Am Acad Dermatol 2000;43(6):975–86 [quiz: 987–90].
17. McHutchison JG, Bacon BR. Chronic hepatitis C: an age wave of disease burden. Am J Manag Care 2005;11(Suppl 10):S286–95 [quiz: S307–11].
18. Cacoub P, Bourlie're M, Lubbe J, et al. Dermatological side effects of hepatitis C and its treatment: patient management in the era of direct-acting antivirals. J Hepatol 2012;56(2):455–63.
19. Kremer AE, Oude Elferink RP, Beuers U. Cholestatic pruritus: new insights into pathophysiology and current treatment. Hautarzt 2012;63(7):532–8 [in German].
20. Cohen KR, Frank J, Salbu RL, et al. Pruritus in the elderly: clinical approaches to the improvement of quality of life. P T 2012;37(4):227–39.
21. Kluger N, Raison-Peyron N, Rigole H, et al. Generalized pruritus revealing hereditary haemochromatosis. Acta Derm Venereol 2007;87(3):277.
22. Sliti N, Benmously R, Fenniche S, et al. Pruritus in the elderly: an epidemic clinical study (about 208 cases). Tunis Med 2011;89(4):347–9 [in French].
23. Carr TF, Saltoun CA. Chapter 21: urticaria and angioedema. Allergy Asthma Proc 2012;33(Suppl 1):S70–2.
24. Kimyai-Asadi A, Nousari HC, Kimyai-Asadi T, et al. Poststroke pruritus. Stroke 1999;30(3):692–3.
25. Cohen OS, Chapman J, Lee H, et al. Pruritus in familial Creutzfeldt-Jakob disease: a common symptom associated with central nervous system pathology. J Neurol 2011;258(1):89–95.
26. Laihinen A. Assessment of psychiatric and psychosocial factors disposing to chronic outcome of dermatoses. Acta Derm Venereol Suppl 1991;156:46–8.
27. Krishnan A, Koo J. Psyche, opioids, and itch: therapeutic consequences. Dermatol Ther 2005;18(4):314–22.
28. Koblenzer CS. Cutaneous manifestations of psychiatric disease that commonly present to the dermatologist—diagnosis and treatment. Int J Psychiatry Med 1992;22(1):47–63.
29. Kuritzky A, Mazeh D, Levi A. Headache in schizophrenic patients: a controlled study. Cephalalgia 1999;19(8):725–7.
30. Greenberger PA. Chapter 30: drug allergy. Allergy Asthma Proc 2012;33(Suppl 1):103–7.
31. Khandpur S, Verma P. Bullous pemphigoid. Indian J Dermatol Venereol Leprol 2011;77(4):450–5.
32. Kasteler JS, Callen JP. Scalp involvement in dermatomyositis. Often overlooked or misdiagnosed. JAMA 1994;272(24):1939–41.
33. Oaklander AL. Common neuropathic itch syndromes. Acta Derm Venereol 2012; 92(2):118–25.
34. Kostner L, Anzengruber F, Guillod C, et al. Allergic contact dermatitis. Immunol Allergy Clin North Am 2017;37(1):141–52.
35. Pearce JM. Meralgia paraesthetica (Bernhardt-Roth syndrome). J Neurol Neurosurg Psychiatry 2006;77(1):84.
36. Ivins GK. Meralgia paresthetica, the elusive diagnosis: clinical experience with14 adult patients. Ann Surg 2000;232(2):281–6.
37. Pérez-Pérez LC. General features and treatment of notalgia paresthetica. Skinmed 2011;9(6):353–9 [quiz: 359].

38. Yosipovitch G, Samuel LS. Neuropathic and psychogenic itch. Dermatol Ther 2008;21(1):32–41.
39. Ward JR, Bernhard JD. Willan's itch and other causes of pruritus in the elderly. Int J Dermatol 2005;44(4):267–73.
40. Moreau M, Seité S, Aguilar L, et al. Topical S. aureus - targeting endolysin significantly improves symptoms and QoL in individuals with atopic dermatitis. J Drugs Dermatol 2021;20(12):1323–8.
41. Papoiu AD, Valdes-Rodriguez R, Nattkemper LA, et al. A novel topical formulation containing strontium chloride significantly reduces the intensity and duration of cowhage-induced itch. Acta Derm Venereol 2013;93(5):520–6.
42. Savin JA. Diseases of the skin. The management of pruritus. Br Med J 1973; 4(5895):779–80.
43. Patel T, Yosipovitch G. The management of chronic pruritus in the elderly. Skin Therapy Lett 2010;15(8):5–9.
44. Ragamin A, Fieten KB, Tupker RA, et al. The effectiveness of antibacterial therapeutic clothing based on silver or chitosan as compared with non-antibacterial therapeutic clothing in patients with moderate to severe atopic dermatitis (ABC trial): study protocol for a pragmatic randomized controlled trial. Trials 2021; 22(1):902.
45. Fowler JF Jr, Fowler LM, Lorenz D. Effects of Merino wool on atopic dermatitis using clinical, quality of life, and Physiological outcome measures. Dermatitis 2019;30(3):198–206.
46. Ference JD, Last AR. Choosing topical corticosteroids. Am Fam Physician 2009; 79(2):135–40.
47. Rathi SK, D'Souza P. Rational and ethical use of topical corticosteroids based on safety and efficacy. Indian J Dermatol 2012;57(4):251–9.
48. du Vivier A, Stoughton RB. Tachyphylaxis to the action of topically applied corticosteroids. Arch Dermatol 1975;111(5):581–3.
49. Schnopp C. Topical steroids under wet-wrap dressings in atopic dermatitis a vehicle-controlled trial. Dermatology 2002;204(1):56–9.
50. Watson CP, Evans RJ, Watt VR. Post-herpetic neuralgia and topical capsaicin. Pain 1988;33(3):333–40.
51. Stander S, Luger T, Metze D. Treatment of prurigo nodularis with topical capsaicin. J Am Acad Dermatol 2001;44(3):471–8.
52. Goodless DR, Eaglstein WH. Brachioradial pruritus: treatment with topical capsaicin. J Am Acad Dermatol 1993;29(5 Pt 1):783–4.
53. Robbins BA. Brachioradial Pruritus. StatPearls - NCBI Bookshelf. Published September 12, 2022. https://www.ncbi.nlm.nih.gov/books/NBK459321/.
54. Siepmann D, Luger TA, Stander S. Antipruritic effect of cyclosporine microemulsion in prurigo nodularis: results of a case series. J Dtsch Dermatol Ges 2008; 6(11):941–6.
55. Sekine R. Anti pruritic effects of topical crotamiton, capsaicin, and a corticosteroid on pruritogen-induced scratching behavior. Exp Dermatol 2012;21(3): 201–4.
56. Yosipovitch G, Maibach HI, Rowbotham MC. Effect of EMLA pre-treatment on capsaicin-induced burning and hyperalgesia. Acta Derm Venereol 1999;79(2): 118–21.
57. Elmariah SB, Lerner EA. Topical therapies for pruritus. Semin Cutan Med Surg 2011;30(2):118–26.
58. Kusin S, Lank PM. Pediatric Overdoses. In: Adams JG, editor. Emergency medicine. 2nd edition. Philadelphia, PA: W.B. Saunders; 2013. p. 1343–50.e1.

59. Gupta S, Singh MM, Prabhu S, et al. Allergic contact dermatitis with exfoliation secondary to calamine/diphenhydramine lotion in a 9 year old girl. J Clin Diagn Res 2007;1(3):147–50.

60. Cassano N. Chronic pruritus in the absence of specific skin disease: an update on pathophysiology, diagnosis, and therapy. Am J Clin Dermatol 2010;11(6): 399–411.

61. Steinhoff M, Cevikbas F, Ikoma A, et al. Pruritus: management algorithms and experimental therapies. Semin Cutan Med Surg 2011;30(2):127–37.

62. Terg R. Efficacy and safety of oral naltrexone treatment for pruritus of cholestasis, a crossover, double blind, placebo-controlled study. J Hepatol 2002; 37(6):717–22.

63. Di Leo E. Cyclosporin-A efficacy in chronic idiopathic urticaria. Int J Immunopathol Pharmacol 2011;24(1):195–200.

64. Dehesa L. The use of cyclosporine in dermatology. J Drugs Dermatol 2012; 11(8):979–87.

65. Rezzani R. Cyclosporine A and adverse effects on organs: histochemical studies. Prog Histochem Cytochem 2004;39(2):85–128.

66. Ereshefsky L, Riesenman C, Lam YW. Antidepressant drug interactions and the cytochrome P450 system. The role of cytochrome P450 2D6. Clin Pharmacokinet 1995;29(Suppl 1):10–8 [discussion: 18–9].

67. Gupta MA, Guptat AK. The use of antidepressant drugs in dermatology. J Eur Acad Dermatol Venereol 2001;15(6):512–8.

68. Pour-Reza-Gholi F. Low-dose doxepin for treatment of pruritus in patients on hemodialysis. Iran J Kidney Dis 2007;1(1):34–7.

69. Drake LA, Fallon JD, Sober A. Relief of pruritus in patients with atopic dermatitis after treatment with topical doxepin cream. The Doxepin Study Group. J Am Acad Dermatol 1994;31(4):613–6.

70. Savin JA. Effects of trimeprazine and trimipramine on nocturnal scratching in patients with atopic eczema. Arch Dermatol 1979;115(3):313–5.

71. Goncalves F. Thalidomide for the control of severe paraneoplastic pruritus associated with Hodgkin's disease. Am J Hosp Palliat Care 2010;27(7):486–7.

72. Chen M, Doherty SD, Hsu S. Innovative uses of thalidomide. Dermatol Clin 2010; 28(3):577–86.

73. Wu JJ. Thalidomide: dermatological indications, mechanisms of action and side-effects. Br J Dermatol 2005;153(2):254–73.

74. Thalidomide: MedlinePlus Drug Information. Medlineplus.gov. Published December 2019. https://medlineplus.gov/druginfo/meds/a699032.html.

75. Blauvelt A, de Bruin-Weller M, Gooderham M, et al. Long-term management of moderate-to-severe atopic dermatitis with dupilumab and concomitant topical corticosteroids (LIBERTY AD CHRONOS): a 1-year, randomised, double-blinded, placebo-controlled, phase 3 trial. Lancet 2017;389(10086):2287–303.

76. Pousti BT, Valdes-Rodriguez R. Use of dupilumab in severe, multifactorial, chronic itch for geriatric patients. Cutis 2022;110(6):E31–2.

77. Weiser P, Brewer A. Dupixent side effects: what you should know. Medical News Today 2022. Available at: https://www.medicalnewstoday.com/articles/drugs-dupixent-side-effects#more-common-side-effects. Accessed March 14, 2023.

78. Han Y, Woo YR, Cho SH, et al. Itch and Janus kinase inhibitors. Acta Derm Venereol 2023;103:adv00869.

79. Seckin D, Demircay Z, Akin O. Generalized pruritus treated with narrowband UVB. Int J Dermatol 2007;46(4):367–70.

80. Rivard J, Lim HW. Ultraviolet phototherapy for pruritus. Dermatol Ther 2005; 18(4):344–54.
81. Zhang H, Yang Y, Cui J, et al. Gaining a comprehensive understanding of pruritus. Indian J Dermatol Venereol Leprol 2012;78(5):532–44.
82. Reiter M. Statin therapy has no significant effect on skin tissue cholesterol: results from a prospective randomized trial. Clin Chem 2005;51(1):252–4.
83. Ramsing D. Effect of systemic treatment with cholesterol-lowering drugs on the skin barrier function in humans. Acta Derm Venereol 1995;75(3):198–201.
84. Brazzelli V. Effects of systemic treatment with statins on skin barrier function and stratum corneum water-holding capacity. Dermatology 1996;192(3):214–6.
85. Neukam K. Supplementation of flaxseed oil diminishes skin sensitivity and improves skin barrier function and condition. Skin Pharmacol Physiol 2011;24(2): 67–74.
86. Rumble RH, Morgan K. Longitudinal trends in prescribing for elderly patients: two surveys four years apart. Br J Gen Pract 1994;44(389):571–5.
87. Alim N, Patel JY. Rapid oral desensitization to furosemide. Ann Allergy Asthma Immunol 2009;103(6):538.
88. White-Chu EF, Reddy M. Dry skin in the elderly: complexities of a common problem. Clin Dermatol 2011;29(1):37–42.
89. Upadhayai JB, Nangia AK, Mukhija RD, et al. Cutaneous reactions due to antihypertensive drugs. Indian J Dermatol Venereol Leprol 2006;51(3):189–91.
90. Thestrup-Pedersen K. Adverse reactions in the skin from anti-hypertensive drugs. Dan Med Bull 1987;34(Suppl 1):3–5.
91. Scheinfeld N. Controlling scabies in institutional settings: a review of medications, treatment models, and implementation. Am J Clin Dermatol 2004; 5(1):31–7.
92. Walton SF, Currie BJ. Problems in diagnosing scabies, a global disease in human and animal populations. Clin Microbiol Rev 2007;20(2):268–79.
93. Luk JHK, Chan HHL, Yeung NSL, et al. Scabies in the elderly: a revisit. Hong Kong Pract 2002;24:426–34.
94. Alexander JO. Arthropods and human skin. Heidelberg, Germany: Springer-Verlag; 1984. p. 422.
95. Burkhart CG, Burkhart CN, Burkhart KM. An epidemiologic and therapeutic reassessment of scabies. Cutis 2000;65(4):233–40.
96. Hengge UR. Scabies: a ubiquitous neglected skin disease. Lancet Infect Dis 2006;6(12):769–79.
97. Feldmeier H. Diagnosis of parasitic diseases. In: Maibach H, Gorouhi F, editors. Evidence- based Dermatology. 2nd edition. Shelton, CT: PMPH-USA; 2010.
98. Falk ES, Eide TJ. Histologic and clinical findings in human scabies. Int J Dermatol 1981;20(9):600–5.
99. Wu M, Hu S, Hsu C. Use of non- contact dermatoscopy in the diagnosis of scabies. Dermatol Sinica 2008;26(2):112–4.
100. Walter B. Comparison of dermoscopy, skin scraping, and the adhesive tape test for the diagnosis of scabies in a resource-poor setting. Arch Dermatol 2011; 147(4):468–73.
101. Palicka P. Laboratory diagnosis of scabies. J Hyg Epidemiol Microbiol Immunol 1980;24(1):63–70.
102. Nanda J, Juergens AL. Permethrin. PubMed. Published 2020. https://www.ncbi.nlm.nih.gov/books/NBK553150/.
103. Fawcett RS. Ivermectin use in scabies. Am Fam Physician 2003;68(6):1089–92.

104. Goldust M, Rezaee E, Raghifar R, et al. Treatment of scabies: the topical iver-mectin vs. permethrin 2.5% cream. Annals of Parasitology 2013;59(2):79–84.
105. Meinking TL. The treatment of scabies with ivermectin. N Engl J Med 1995; 333(1):26–30.
106. Dourmishev AL, Dourmishev LA, Schwartz RA. Ivermectin: pharmacology and application in dermatology. Int J Dermatol 2005;44(12):981–8.
107. Chhaiya SB. Comparative efficacy and safety of topical permethrin, topical iver-mectin, and oral ivermectin in patients of uncomplicated scabies. Indian J Der-matol Venereol Leprol 2012;78(5):605–10.
108. Currie BJ. First documentation of in vivo and in vitro ivermectin resistance in *Sar-coptes scabiei*. Clin Infect Dis 2004;39(1):e8–12.
109. Walton SF, Myerscough MR, Currie BJ. Studies in vitro on the relative efficacy of current acaricides for *Sarcoptes scabiei* var. hominis. Trans R Soc Trop Med Hyg 2000;94(1):92–6.
110. Fischer K. Scabies: important clinical consequences explained by new molec-ular studies. Adv Parasitol 2012;79:339–73.
111. Fernando DD, Fischer K. Spinosad topical suspension (0.9%): a new topical treatment for scabies. Expert Review of Anti-infective Therapy.
112. Seiler JC, Keech RC, Aker JL, et al. Spinosad at 0.9% in the treatment of scabies: efficacy results from 2 multicenter, randomized, double-blind, vehicle-controlled studies. J Am Acad Dermatol 2022;86(1):97–103.

Bacterial Skin and Soft Tissue Infections in Older Adults

Eamonn Maher, MD[a],*, Anya Anokhin, MD[b]

KEYWORDS

- Skin infection • Aging • Cellulitis • Fasciitis • Epidermis • Soft tissue • Surgical site
- Pressure ulcer

KEY POINTS

- Bacterial skin infections are the most common outpatient dermatologic diagnoses presenting to emergency department and to primary care provider.
- Skin and soft tissue infections are a persistent threat to the health of the aging population.
- The elderly population is at a higher risk of contracting bacterial infections due to weakened immune systems and comorbidities.

INTRODUCTION

Bacterial skin infections are the most common outpatient dermatologic diagnoses presenting to emergency department and to primary care providers. Skin and soft tissue infections (SSTIs) are a persistent threat to the health of the aging population. SSTIs are a common complication of hospitalization, occurring in 2% to 5% of all patients undergoing surgery in the United States and accounting for around 10% of overall hospital admissions.[1,2]

Humans are colonized by complex communities of microorganisms that are part of a beneficial resident microbiota.[3] In commensal relationships, the microbe and host benefit without causing harm to the other. This interaction is fundamentally important to human biology. Human skin and mucosa are colonized at birth, typically by travel through the birth canal, and have a lifelong codependent relationship with indigenous microbiota.[4] The capacity of invasive microorganisms to cause disease in healthy hosts is a result of fundamental biologic differences in their virulence factors from those of opportunistic and commensal species that rarely cause disease.

[a] Department of Dermatology, University of Minnesota, Phillips-Wangensteen Building, 516 Delaware Street SE, Suite 1-400, Minneapolis, MN 55455, USA; [b] University of Missouri, Phillips-Wangensteen Building, 516 Delaware Street SE, Suite 1-400, Minneapolis, MN 55455, USA
* Corresponding author.
E-mail address: maher297@umn.edu

Clin Geriatr Med 40 (2024) 117–130
https://doi.org/10.1016/j.cger.2023.09.006
0749-0690/24/© 2023 Elsevier Inc. All rights reserved.
geriatric.theclinics.com

RELEVANT SKIN BIOLOGY AND ECOLOGY

The epidermis is both an active and passive barrier to infection. The structurally intact epidermis is composed of tightly linked epithelial cells covered by tightly packed layers of keratin.[5,6] The stratum corneum, the epidermal top layer, is composed of terminally differentiated cells called corneocytes, which have lost their nuclei. In between the corneocytes in the stratum corneum are lipids that have been secreted by cells lower down in the epidermis. These corneocytes and intercellular lipids create what has been described as a "brick and mortar complex."[7] The mortar, composed of intercellular lipids, decreases transepidermal water loss and inhibits colonization and invasion by pathogenic organisms. Additionally, the skin produces a variety of unique defensive molecules called antimicrobial peptides that target microbial membranes.[8–11]

The combination of corneocytes and extracellular lipids create a hydrophobic matrix. The lipids that make up the "mortar" are secreted from lamellar bodies within keratinocytes in the spinous layer. The skin flora partially hydrolyzes the triglycerides, liberating fatty acids. The breakdown of these lipids and fatty acids creates an acidic environment, which is toxic to most pathogenic bacteria.[12] The so-called acid mantle (pH 5–6) and the normal skin flora both act to form a prohibitive environment for invading microbes. For instance, *Staphylococcus aureus* grows optimally at a pH of 6.5 to 7.[13] The flora of normal and altered skin has a bearing on understanding the causative organism in SSTIs. There is a varied ecology of microbe communities that colonize human skin (listed in **Table 1**). These communities vary in their composition across different body areas because the environment differs with respect to things such as moisture, sebum, and UV exposure. Alterations in this flora can enable the invasion of pathogenic bacteria.

Superficial skin infections that develop on healthy, seemingly intact, skin are referred to as primary infections. The portal of entry is often unknown or there is evidence of minor trauma. Secondary infections develop from skin lesions, wounds, surgical sites, burns, and maceration. These infections tend to be polymicrobial (**Box 1**).

CELLULITIS

Cellulitis and erysipelas (discussed later) are bacterial skin infections of the deep and superficial dermis, respectively. Cellulitis is a bacterial skin infection involving the deeper dermis and subcutaneous tissues. The skin of elderly patients is often afflicted with conditions that are associated with skin fragility, such as edema and skin tears

Table 1 Normal skin flora	
Organism	**Location**
Staphylococcus saprophyticus *Staphylococcus epidermidis* *Micrococcus* spp *S aureus*	All sites
Aerobic *Corynebacterium*	Intertriginous areas, including the toe webs
Anaerobic *Corynebacterium*	Sebaceous and hair follicles
Acinetobacter spp	Axillae, perineum, and antecubital fossae
Yeast including *Pityrosporum* spp and *M furfur*	Sebaceous areas of skin (eg, scalp)

Data from Hartmann AA. The influence of various factors on the human resident skin flora. Semin Dermatol 1990;9(4):305-8; and Blume JE, Levine EG, Heyman WR. Bacterial diseases. In: Bolognia JL, Jorizzo JL, Rapini RP, editors. Dermatology. London: Mosby; 2003. p. 1117.

Box 1
Superficial skin infections

- Primary skin infections tend to be single organisms and arise from common skin flora.
- Secondary skin infections arise from preexisting lesions and are often polymicrobial.

---

that predispose them to cellulitis. By 70 years of age, about 70% of persons will have at least one skin problem, such as edema that puts them at an increased risk for cellulitis.[14] Other risk factors include venous insufficiency, saphenectomy, earlier history of cellulitis, and presence of ulcers (**Box 2**).[15,16]

When cellulitis presents, it is typically sudden in onset and presents as a rapidly spreading erythema, edema, pain, and tenderness. Systemic symptoms and signs may occur but are often mild, including fever, tachycardia, and leukocytosis.[17] As with other bacterial infections, cellulitis in the elderly can present with atypical symptoms. Fever may be absent.

Less commonly, lymphangitic streaks and regional lymphadenopathy occur in cellulitis. Blood cultures show positive results in 4% to 5% of cases[18,19] and are not recommended unless there is evident systemic toxicity. Cultures of aspirates or punch biopsy specimens have low yields and thus have no role in routine clinical practice.

The lower extremity is the most common site for cellulitis in the elderly. The most common pathogens are Group A beta-hemolytic *Streptococci* (GABHS) and *S aureus*. Most cases are caused by *Streptococcal* species.[20] However, since the 1960s, the prevalence of methicillin-resistant *Staphylococcus aureus* (MRSA) as skin contaminates has been increasing steadily. There has been a dramatic increase in *S aureus* and MRSA infections at all sites during the last 50 years. Nasal carriage of MRSA, a risk factor, is increasing as well.[21] MRSA organisms have different virulence factors, including exotoxins that predispose to increased rates of purulence and abscess formation.[22] Therefore, MRSA should be suspected if there is purulence or abscess formation. MRSA has complicated the recommendation for empiric therapy for cellulitis. Oral doxycycline, trimethoprim-sulfamethoxazole, or linezolid are oral options for empiric antibiotic treatment of MRSA.[23] Clindamycin is not recommended because of inducible resistance.

There are several anatomic variants of cellulitis (**Table 2**). An important pair is preseptal and septal cellulitis. Preseptal cellulitis is a superficial infection of the skin of the

---

Box 2
Risk factors for cellulitis in the elderly

- Venous insufficiency
- Lymphatic obstruction
- Saphenous venectomy
- Skin tears and other minor trauma
- Surgical wounds
- Macerated skin
- Preexisting skin lesions and dermatoses
- Skin fissures (ie, toe webs)

Table 2
Cellulitis variants organism predilection by site

Cellulitis Variant	Location	Organism (Most Common)
Orbital	Contents of orbit (spares Globe)	
Periorbital (Preseptal)	Face and periorbital	S aureus, Streptococcus pneumoniae, group A streptococci
Buccal cellulitis	Cheek	Haemophilus influenzae
Cellulitis complicating body piercing	Ear, nose, and umbilicus	S aureus, group A streptococci
After mastectomy (with axillary node dissection)	Ipsilateral upper extremity	Non–group A β-hemolytic streptococcus
After saphenous vein harvest for coronary artery	Ipsilateral leg	Group A or non–group A β-hemolytic streptococci
After radical pelvic surgery, radiation therapy	Vulva, inguinal areas, and legs	Group B and group G streptococci
Postoperative (early) wound infection	Varies, for example, abdomen, chest, and hip	Group A streptococci
Perianal cellulitis	Perineum	Group A streptococcus
Injection drug use	Extremities	S aureus, streptococci (groups A, C, F, G) wide variety of others including: Enterococcus faecalis, viridians streptococci, coagulase-negative staphylococci

Data from Schwartz MN. Cellulitis. N Engl J Med 2004;350:904-12; and Siddiqui AR. Chronic wound infection: facts and controversies. Clin Dermatol 2010;28(5):519-26.

eyelid and surrounding face involving tissue anterior to the orbital septum. It does not involve the orbit. Patients present with erythema, eyelid pain, and swelling. Preseptal (periorbital) cellulitis needs to be distinguished from septal (orbital) cellulitis, a much more serious entity that can lead to loss of vision and intracranial spread of infection.

Orbital cellulitis, because it involves structures deep to the orbital septum such as the intraocular muscles, classically presents with diplopia, proptosis, and pain with eye movement. However, early orbital cellulitis and periorbital cellulitis can be difficult to distinguish clinically and the best diagnostic test is a contrast computed tomography (CT).[24] Most cases of orbital cellulitis develop from earlier bacterial rhinosinusitis. Other sources are orbital trauma, dental infection, and dacryocystitis.[25] The presence or absence of these risk factors can be helpful for evaluating the pretest probability of preseptal versus septal cellulitis.

A distinctive form of lower extremity cellulitis can occur in patients whose saphenous veins have been harvested for coronary artery bypass surgery.[26] There can be an associated lymphangitis. In these patients, episodes of cellulitis can be recurrent. The area of cellulitis extends along the course of the saphenous venectomy. Patients present with edema, erythema, local tenderness, and at times systemic toxicity.

Similarly, cellulitis of the breast or arm distal to axillary node dissection due to disruption of the lymphatic system can occur.[27] Recurrence is not uncommon. Compressive lymphedema sleeves may decrease recurrences.

ERYSIPELAS

Erysipelas (St. Anthony's fire) and cellulitis are, at times, used interchangeably. The diagnosis of erysipelas is based on a distinctive clinical presentation of intense erythema with well-demarcated advancing raised margins and significant edema. It is often painful and indurated with a peau d'orange appearance. Fever is not uncommon. The infection primarily involves the dermis and superficial lymphatics. Bullous erysipelas is a complication observed in about 5% of cases.[28] Recurrent bouts of lower extremity erysipelas can be difficult to treat. Episodes of infection involve the lymphatic system causing scarring and lymphedema. Between 20% and 30% of cases of lower extremity erysipelas and cellulitis recur,[29] sometimes at frequent intervals. Some studies have shown a benefit for prophylactic penicillin with respect to reducing recurrences.[30] Rarely, the infection extends more deeply and produces subcutaneous abscess and necrotizing fasciitis. At one time the face was the most frequent location but now the lower extremity is the most common (80%). When involving the face, the most commonly involved areas are the bridge of the nose and cheeks. It is a disease of the very young and older debilitated individuals, particularly those with lymphedema and venous stasis ulcers. Similar to cellulitis, most cases are due to GABHS and to a lesser degree *S aureus*, including MRSA (**Boxes 3** and **4**).

IMPETIGO

Streptococcal pyoderma, pyoderma, impetigo, and impetigo contagiosa are terms used synonymously to describe discrete purulent lesions that are primary infections of the skin in pediatrics. Adult infection is associated with contact with infected children. Predisposing factors include high humidity, poor hygiene, and minor skin trauma. *S aureus* and less commonly GABHS cause most cases of impetigo. This is particularly true for those with *S aureus* nasal or perianal carriage.

There are 2 forms of impetigo: nonbullous impetigo and bullous impetigo. The nonbullous form that develops in adults is described here.[31,32] The classic presentation is a single erythematous macule that rapidly becomes a pustule and then a crusted stuck-on honey-colored scale. The vesiculopustules are in the epidermis. Exudate from beneath the crust can be successfully cultured but is not necessary in most cases. The disease is benign and self-limiting. In stable hosts with limited disease, the scale is removed and the treatment is local with 2% mupirocin ointment without the need for systemic antibiotics.

ECTHYMA

Ecthyma is a deeper ulcerated form of nonbullous impetigo. Ecthyma lesions are found most frequently on the lower extremities in children and older adults, especially those with lymphedema and poor hygiene. Poor hygiene and trauma are the common contributing factors. The lesions begin as those of impetigo but penetrate through the

---

Box 3
Special treatment considerations in cellulitis and erysipelas

- Rule out more ominous causes of skin inflammation, such as necrotizing fasciitis and pyomyositis
- Edema-associated cellulitis is best treated by mobilizing edema fluid
- Know the rate of MRSA in your community

> **Box 4**
> **Complication of cellulitis in older patients**
>
> - Cellulitis of the lower extremities in older patients may be complicated by thrombophlebitis.
> - In patients with chronic-dependent edema, cellulitis may spread rapidly.
> - Infections of the upper lip and nose can result in spread of infection via the facial veins to the cavernous sinus.
>
> *Data from* Woo PC, Lum PM, Wong SS, et al. Cellulitis complicating lymphoedema. Eur J Clin Microbiol Infect Dis 2000;19:294-7.

epidermis and enlarge, often to 2 to 3 cm in diameter. The lesion is "punched out," has a purulent base, and a dried, often hemorrhagic crust. The lesions are usually few in number, and systemic symptoms are rare. The treatment is the same as for impetigo.

ERYTHRASMA

Erythrasma is a superficial localized infection of the stratum corneum. It is caused by *Corynebacterium minutissimum*, which favors moist occluded areas. The lesions are red well-defined patches covered with fine scale. In darkly pigmented individuals, erythema can be more difficult to appreciate, and the patches may seem more hyperpigmented. The organism can be grown from scrapings of the scale. Predisposing factors include advanced age, obesity, diabetes, and poor hygiene. The easiest way to make the diagnosis is to identify the characteristic coral red fluorescence under a Wood lamp. The coral red fluorescence is due to the production of coproporphyrinogen III by the bacteria.[33] Erythrasma can mimic tinea cruris and cellulitis. Treatment includes topical agents or oral erythromycin. Antimicrobial soaps can prevent future eruptions. There is little danger of institutional spread, and patients do not need to be isolated.

BACTERIAL FOLLICULITIS

Superficial bacterial folliculitis is a common skin infection located within hair follicles and the apocrine glands. The lesions consist of small erythematous papules often with a central pustule and a fine surrounding collar of desquamation.[34] Lesions in different stages of development (macules, papules, and papulopustules) are often present. If no pustules are present, this "collarette of scale" is a clue to the diagnosis. *S aureus* is the usual cause of folliculitis. *Pseudomonas aeruginosa* has been responsible for folliculitis acquired from swimming pools and hot tubs contaminated with large numbers of these organisms. Folliculitis preferentially involves the buttocks, hips, and axillae. The condition is typically self-resolving but topical or oral antibiotics that target *Pseudomonas*, such as gentamycin and fluoroquinolones, respectively, can be used.

Scarring develops only when a pustule progresses to furuncle formation. In immune-suppressed and human immunodeficiency virus patients, a myriad of atypical presentations can occur. In particular, herpes simplex virus (HSV) folliculitis (herpetic sycosis) occurs in men with recurrent facial HSV infection who shave with a razor. The herpetic lesions can disseminate in immunocompromised individuals.[35]

Candida may cause folliculitis, often presenting with pruritic satellite lesions surrounding areas of intertriginous candidiasis. This presentation is seen in diabetics and patients receiving prolonged antibiotic or corticosteroid therapy. The fungus *Malassezia furfur*, a common skin saprophyte, may also produce a folliculitis with pruritic erythematous papules typically distributed on the forehead, cheeks, upper shoulders, and chest.

FURUNCLES, CARBUNCLES, AND ABSCESSES

Folliculitis that extends into the subcutaneous tissue gives rise to furuncles. A furuncle or boil is a deep inflammatory nodule that develops from preceding folliculitis. A carbuncle is a larger lesion formed by coalescence of furuncles in the subcutaneous fat. *S aureus* is the most common isolate in infections of the extremities and trunk, whereas anaerobes are more common in the genital, perirectal, and inguinal regions.

A furuncle begins as a firm, tender, red nodule that soon becomes fluctuant. Spontaneous drainage of pus commonly occurs, and the lesion subsides. A carbuncle is a larger, deeper, indurated, more serious lesion, commonly located at the nape of the neck, on the back, or on the thighs. The results of a retrospective study published by the Centers for Disease Control and Prevention (CDC) of 361 patients in rural Alaska with SSTIs observed for 3.6 years reveal the breakdown of types of infection and sites.[36] The findings are shown in **Table 3**. *S aureus* is the principal isolate in infections of the extremities and trunk.

Furuncles occur on skin that contains hair follicles and is subject to friction, moisture, and occlusion. Predisposing factors include obesity, treatment with corticosteroids, immunosuppressive therapy, and diabetes. Fever is more common than in cellulitis. Some patients may manifest systemic toxicity and leukocytosis. As the lesions enlarge, they may drain externally along the course of multiple hair follicles. Bacteremia can occur and can cause endocarditis or metastatic foci.

Most furuncles are initially treated by the application of moist heat, which promotes localization and spontaneous drainage. Prompt surgical drainage with culture is indicated with enlarging or fluctuant lesions **Box 5**.

Data from the CDC reveals that 74% of furuncles and carbuncles are caused by CA-MRSA. Other causative organisms include nonresistant *Staphylococcus* spp and *Streptococcus* spp. It is extremely important to obtain culture of the purulent lesion to direct antibiotic treatment given the increase in CA-MRSA. Older texts quote resolution rates of lesions with drainage alone of 90%. Local hot compresses followed by drainage without antibiotics when there are no signs of cellulitis or systemic toxicity is accepted treatment. Few practitioners today would follow this conservative practice. Metastatic abscesses can occur during the course of bacteremia or endocarditis. They can be single, as in epidural abscess, or multiple and arise in subcutaneous tissue and other organs. These metastatic abscesses are tender and fluctuant. If

Table 3	
Breakdown 391 cases of skin and soft tissue infection in rural Alaska reported by CDC	
Type and Site of SSTI	**Percentage of Total Cases (%)**
Single furuncle (45.9% buttocks/low back/thigh)	62.9
Multiple furuncles (41.2% buttocks/low back/thigh)	21.7
Cellulitis (66% on extremities)	12.8
Folliculitis	1.0
Deep abscesses	1.5

From Stevens AM, Hennessy TW, Baggett HC, et al. Methicillin-resistant staphylococcus aureus carriage and risk factors for skin infections, Southwestern Alaska, USA. Emerg Infect Dis [serial on the Internet]. 2010;16(5):797-803. Available at: http://wwwnc.cdc.gov/eid/article/16/5/09-0851_article.htm.last. Accessed August 28, 2012.

Box 5
Treatment of furuncles, carbuncles, and abscesses

- Most lesions are caused by *Staphylococcus* spp and, increasingly, CA-MRSA.
- Drainage of pus is of primary importance.
- Culture of SSTIs is important in guiding antibiotic treatment.
- For recurrent boils, consider eradicating carriage state.[44]

Data from McBride DR. Furuncles and carbuncles. In: Rakel RE, Rakel DP, editors. Textbook of family medicine. 8th edition. Philadelphia: Saunders; 2011.

---

promptly identified and treated, the "seeding" process may be aborted before frank abscess formation occurs.

SURGICAL SITE INFECTION

The geriatric generalist may be required to follow postoperative patients, particularly in a postacute setting. Surgical site infections are common in spite of the administration of antimicrobial prophylaxis and optimal surgical technique.[37] Outcomes for the elderly surgical patient with a serious SSI is dismal with mortality at least 4 times greater than patients younger than 65 years of age.[38] The best evidence reveals 4 specific interventions to limit SSI: (1) appropriate, timed antimicrobial prophylaxis, (2) avoidance of hair removal, (3) glycemic control, and (4) maintaining postoperative normothermia. If hair removal is necessary, the use of clippers is preferred to shaving. The administration of antimicrobial prophylaxis increases the magnitude of the bacterial inoculum needed to produce infection.[39] The CDC has defined 3 levels of SSI: superficial incisional, deep incisional, and organ space SSI. Some degree of microbial surgical wound contamination is universal.[40] Pathogens are acquired from skin flora or from the operating room. The greatest risk period is from incision to closure. The time to first sign of infection varies with the virulence of the organism, the size of the inoculum, and host factors. There is a delay of 5 to as many as 20 days before there are clinical manifestations.

According to data collected by the National Nosocomial Infections Surveillance System, *S aureus* from the skin remains the most common SSI accounting for approximately 20% of the infections. Coagulase-negative staphylococci and *Enterococcus* spp make up another 30%. Surgeries of the abdomen and genitourinary tract will result in more gram-negative and anaerobic infections. Older and younger patient populations have the same SSI pathogen profiles.

If an SSI manifests in less than 5 days, unusual organisms must be suspected. Postoperative clostridial myonecrosis can have a fulminating course with hypotension and cardiovascular collapse. Cellulitis caused by GABHS can present as early as 6 hours postoperatively. Systemic signs of sepsis may be the initial sign of infection, often associated with bacteremia before incisional erythema is evident. A thin discharge may be expressed on compression of the wound margins. All incisional abscesses need drainage. It is imperative to distinguish uncomplicated superficial or deeper SSI from necrotizing soft tissue infection. Most often the patient has been discharged from the hospital. Emergent CT[27] or surgical referral (or both) is imperative.

INFECTION IN CHRONIC WOUNDS

A chronic wound (such as pressure ulcers and venous and arterial ulcers) is one where the normal healing process is stalled.[41,42] One of the principal reasons that an otherwise clean wound bed is not granulating or proceeding to closure is the presence of inflammation due to heavy bacterial burden. This finding is commonly erroneously labeled as "wound infection" without overt clinical signs of true infection. A true wound infection involves bacterial invasion of living tissue, not heavy growth of microbes obtained from swab culture of a wound base. There is a body of medical literature that labels a wound as "infected" if quantitative wound culture obtained at biopsy yields a microbial load of 10^6 or greater organisms per gram or milliliter of tissue.[43] This heavy bacterial load may lead to delayed healing and increased exudate but labeling the wound as infected without evidence of adjacent tissue invasion is misleading. In a recent review, Reddy and colleagues,[40] referring to wound infection, stated, "There were no studies identified that addressed the precision of symptoms, signs, or investigations in the diagnosis of chronic wounds."

All chronic wounds are polymicrobially colonized.[44] Large populations of bacteria that can produce toxins and proteolytic enzymes in a wound bed and disrupt orderly healing need to be eliminated by local measures. Biofilms that form on wound beds can delay healing and can be disrupted by cleansing. Increasing wound pain, surrounding cellulitis, and purulent exudate are reliable in distinguishing true superficial or deep wound infection[45] from bacterial colonization. True infections in chronic wounds are very uncommon, less than 1.4 wound infections per 1000 nursing home resident days in one study.[46]

Maintain a high index of suspicion when there is a necrotic wound bed. Wound infection is initiated from bacterial colonization of the wound base or tracts. Repeated debridement of necrotic tissue is the best preventative measure. Topical antimicrobials have a limited role. It is only when colonization is combined with other factors, such as decreased vascular supply, intrinsic virulence of specific bacteria, and host immune factors, that true infection occurs.[47] The microbiology of chronic wounds is complex, and it is difficult to discern which bacteria are culpable from simple swab cultures. Deep cultures or quantitative biopsies of wound tissue are necessary to determine organisms causing true infection. In some instances, it is appropriate to treat these wounds empirically with a combination of topical antiseptics and systemic antibiotics.[48]

In cellulitis complicating pressure ulcers, a broad range of microorganisms should be considered as potential pathogens. If this complication develops in a previously institutionalized patient, the known nosocomial pathogens should be considered when deciding on empiric antibiotic coverage. Clinically, it is important to distinguish liquefaction in wounds from purulence. Heavy necrotic wound burden alone can cause both odor and thick exudate. Silver sulfadiazine cream, when combined with exudate can produce a thick yellow exudate. These circumstances, in isolation, do not indicate infection in the surrounding viable skin and soft tissues.

NECROTIZING SKIN AND SOFT TISSUE INFECTIONS

Necrotizing skin and soft tissue infections (NSSTIs) are rare, rapidly progressive infections of the skin and deeper structures. They are characterized by necrosis of the skin, subcutaneous tissue, fascia, and at times skeletal muscle. The infection initially spreads along the superficial fascial planes, not the muscular aponeurosis. It starts superficially from skin or mucosa to involve and destroy deeper structures. NSSTIs can cause overwhelming sepsis if not recognized early.[49,50] Exact early categorization of bacterial infections of the soft tissues may be difficult.[51] The differences between a superficial SSTI and a classic gas gangrene infection are readily apparent. However, many times, the distinction between a superficial and deep infection is difficult. Because of the seriousness of necrotizing infections a high index of suspicion must be maintained.

The varied classification schemata of the necrotizing deep infections are based on the tissue level involved, suspected organisms, and/or clinical presentation. As a result, the nomenclature is very confusing. The NSSTIs are grouped into 3 categories.[52] Type I infections are polymicrobial and involve gram-negative and anaerobic organisms. Type II infections are single organism, most often *Streptococcus pyogenes*. Type III involve Clostridial species and are nicknamed "gas gangrene." This classification is not useful at the bedside. Some infections may involve multiple soft tissue elements, and several bacterial species may produce infections with similar or overlapping clinical presentations. This portion of the article discusses NSSTI as a single entity, called necrotizing fasciitis so as to distinguish it from the superficial, uncomplicated SSTI. Suspicion of necrotizing fasciitis requires emergent surgical consultation for exploratory incisional biopsy or aggressive debridement.

The initial lesion in an evolving NSSTI is a hot tender swollen area of cellulitis that rapidly spreads and does not respond to antibiotics. Skin color can change from red to violaceous in 24 hours and then to blister or necrotic eschar. The area can become anesthetic as dermal nerve endings are destroyed. A great deal of subcutaneous tissue destruction can occur before skin necrosis occurs. Patients rapidly become toxic with fever, chills, and delirium. Ten percent of the cases are due to GABHS, the remainder are polymicrobial. Polymicrobial NSSTIs are associated with the following:

- Surgical procedures involving the bowel or penetrating trauma
- Perianal abscess
- Heavily necrotic, pressure ulcers
- Spread from vulvovaginal infections or abscesses
- Intravenous drug injection sites
- Eroded urethral mucosa in catheterized patients (**Box 6**)

Prompt surgical intervention is diagnostic and therapeutic. Direct inspection by a surgeon is the best test. At the first suspicion of an NSTTI, a surgical consultation for an exploratory incisional biopsy to establish the diagnosis and to obtain tissue for culture is indicated. If no necrosis is found, no further debridement will be needed. The sensitivity of CT versus MRI is unclear. Waiting for imaging studies should not delay a surgical diagnosis.

Blood cultures show positive results in only 2% to 4% of patients with community-acquired cellulitis[53] and are not indicated or cost-effective. Blood cultures are more likely to be positive with cellulitis superimposed on lymphedema.[54] Blood cultures are definitively indicated in all case of suspected NSSTIs and in patients with systemic toxicity.

A detailed discussion of all the variant forms of NSSTI is beyond the scope of this article. Two well-known variants, Fournier gangrene and Clostridial myonecrosis will

---

Box 6
Sign to distinguish superficial from deep skin and soft tissue infection

- Failure to respond to initial antibiotic therapy
- Induration of the subcutaneous tissue beyond the superficial cellulitis
- Systemic toxicity
- Delirium
- Overlying bullous lesions
- Skin necrosis and/or ecchymoses

be mentioned briefly. The excellent review by File and Stevens[55] and others[56,57] are recommended for more detail.

FOURNIER GANGRENE

This NSSTI variant involves the scrotum, vulva, and perineum. The mean age of onset is 50 years. It is more common in men. Most patients have some predisposing disease such as diabetes. It can be insidious or explosive and rapidly progressive.[58] A urinary tract infection or infection of the perineum initiates the process and spreads along fascial planes. Many times Foley catheters are involved. It is a polymicrobial infection that if unchecked can spread widely from the perineal body into the abdominal wall.

CLOSTRIDIAL MYONECROSIS

If wound crepitus is noted, there is a wide differential diagnosis. The most urgent is clostridial myonecrosis (gas gangrene) because of the fulminating nature of the infection.[59] Treatment is emergent surgery. There are posttraumatic and spontaneous forms of gas gangrene. *Clostridium perfringens* is the most common Clostridial species found. *Clostridium septicum* and other species have been isolated. In some cases, clostridia are present in mixed culture.

SUMMARY

SSTIs in the elderly are common in all care settings.[60] The symptomatic older patient will often present first to the generalist. After careful history and skin surface examination, a distinction must be made between noninfectious inflammatory disorders and a superficial or deep infection. The deeper infections require a high index of suspicion and rapid referral to a surgical specialist for definitive diagnosis. Poor response in the first 24 hours of empiric therapy for a superficial infection should prompt reevaluation or referral to rule out deep infection.

Specific antibiotic treatment recommendations are always in flux and will vary based on the specific flora in each community. Most superficial SSTIs will respond to empiric treatment without culture data guidance. When indicated, blood cultures and carefully procured cultures of purulent exudate can refine antibiotic selection. Hospitals publish an "antibiogram" annually that delineates the antibiotic susceptibility of common bacterial isolates. The reader is referred to the useful references below to guide empiric antibiotic choices.

CLINICS CARE POINTS

- Necrotizing soft tissue infections are a surgical emergency, pain out of proportion to exam, woody induration, and crepitus can be clues to the diagnosis.

DISCLOSURE

No conflicts of interest for the authors.

REFERENCES

1. DiNubile MJ, Lipsky BA. Complicated infections of skin and skin structures: when the infection is more than skin deep. J Antimicrob Chemother 2004;53. https://doi.org/10.1093/jac/dkh202.

2. Hall MJ, Hall MJ, et al. National hospital discharge survey: 2007 summary. National health statistics reports 2010;29:1–24.
3. Relman DA, Falkow S. 1 – a molecular perspective of microbial pathogenicity. Mandell, Douglas, and Bennett's Principles and Practice of Infectious Diseases 2015;1–10. https://doi.org/10.1016/b978-1-4557-4801-3.00001-1. Published online January 1.
4. Dethlefsen L, McFall-Ngai MJ, Relman DA. An ecological and evolutionary perspective on human–microbe mutualism and disease. Nature 2007; 449(7164):811–8.
5. Fore-Pfliger J. The epidermal skin barrier: implications for the wound care practitioner, part I. Adv Skin Wound Care 2004;17(8):417–25.
6. Fore-Pfliger J. The epidermal skin barrier: implications for the wound care practitioner, part II. Adv Skin Wound Care 2004;17(8):417–25.
7. Fore J. A review of skin and the effects of aging on skin structure and function. Ostomy/Wound Manag 2006;52(9):24–35.
8. Hartmann AA. The influence of various factors on the human resident skin flora. Semin Dermatol 1990;9(4):305–8.
9. Fuchs E. Beauty is skin deep: the fascinating biology of the epidermis and its appendages. Harvey Lect 1998;94:47–77.
10. Zasloff M. Antimicrobial peptides of multicellular organisms. Nature 2002; 415(6870):389–95.
11. Kaźmierczak AK, Szewczyk EM. Bacteria forming a resident flora of the skin as a potential source of opportunistic infections. Pol J Microbiol 2004;53(4):249–55.
12. Role of lipids in the formation and maintenance of the cutaneous permeability barrier | Elsevier Enhanced Reader. doi:10.1016/j.bbalip.2013.11.007.
13. Iyer V, Raut J, Dasgupta A. Impact of pH on growth of Staphylococcus epidermidis and Staphylococcus aureus in vitro. J Med Microbiol 2021;70(9). https://doi.org/10.1099/jmm.0.001421.
14. Laube S, Farrell AM. Bacterial skin infections in the elderly: diagnosis and treatment. Drugs Aging 2002;19(5):331–42.
15. Dupuy A, Benchikhi H, Roujeau JC, et al. Risk factors for erysipelas of the leg (cellulitis): case-control study. BMJ 1999;318(7198):1591–4.
16. Björnsdóttir S, Gottfredsson M, Thorisdottir AS, et al. Risk factors for acute cellulitis of the lower limb: a prospective case-control study. Clin Infect Dis 2005; 41(10):1416–22.
17. Stevens DL, Bisno AL, Chambers HF, et al. Practice guidelines for the diagnosis and management of skin and soft-tissue infections. Clin Infect Dis 2005;41(10): 1373–406.
18. Swartz Mn, Swartz MN. Clinical practice. Cellulitis. N Engl J Med 2004;350(9): 904–12.
19. Perl B, Gottehrer NP, Raveh D, et al. Cost-effectiveness of blood cultures for adult patients with cellulitis. Clin Infect Dis 1999;29(6):1483–8.
20. Hirschmann JV, Raugi GJ. Lower limb cellulitis and its mimics: Part I. Lower limb cellulitis. J Am Acad Dermatol 2012;67(2). https://doi.org/10.1016/j.jaad.2012.03.024.
21. Baggett HC, Hennessy TW, Rudolph K, et al. Community-onset methicillin-resistant Staphylococcus aureus associated with antibiotic use and the cytotoxin panton-valentine leukocidin during a furunculosis outbreak in rural Alaska. JID (J Infect Dis) 2004;189(9):1565–73.
22. Daum RS, Robert S. Daum. skin and soft-tissue infections caused by methicillin-resistant staphylococcus aureus. N Engl J Med 2007;357(4):380–90.

23. Raff AB, Kroshinsky D. Cellulitis: a review. JAMA 2016;316(3):325–37.

24. Zacharias N, Velmahos GC, Salama A, et al. Diagnosis of necrotizing soft tissue infections by computed tomography. Arch Surg 2010;145(5):452–5.

25. Uzcátegui N, Warman R, Smith A, et al. Clinical practice guidelines for the management of orbital cellulitis. J Pediatr Ophthalmol Strabismus 1998;35(2):73–9, quiz 110-111.

26. Baddour LM, Bisno AL. Recurrent cellulitis after saphenous venectomy for coronary bypass surgery. Ann Intern Med 1982;97(4):493–6.

27. Simon MS, Cody RL. Cellulitis after axillary lymph node dissection for carcinoma of the breast. Am J Med 1992;93(5):543–8.

28. Guberman D, Gilead L, Zlotogorski A, et al. Bullous erysipelas: a retrospective study of 26 patients. J Am Acad Dermatol 1999;41(5):733–7.

29. McNamara DR, Tleyjeh IM, Berbari EF, et al. A predictive model of recurrent lower extremity cellulitis in a population-based cohort. JAMA Intern Med 2007;167(7): 709–15.

30. Thomas KS, Crook AM, Nunn AJ, et al. Penicillin to prevent recurrent leg cellulitis. N Engl J Med 2013;368(18):1695–703.

31. Darmstadt GL, Lane AT. Impetigo: an overview. Pediatr Dermatol 1994;11(4): 293–303.

32. Hirschmann JV. Impetigo: etiology and therapy. Curr Clin Top Infect Dis 2002;22: 42–51.

33. Masood M, Usatine RP, Heath CR. Erythrasma. Cutis 2022. https://doi.org/10. 12788/cutis.0662.

34. Levy AL, Simpson GL, Skinner RB. Medical pearl: circle of desquamation–a clue to the diagnosis of folliculitis and furunculosis caused by Staphylococcus aureus. J Am Acad Dermatol 2006;55(6):1079–80.

35. Campanelli A, Marazza G, Marazza G, et al. Fulminant herpetic sycosis: atypical presentation of primary herpetic infection. Dermatology 2004;208(3):284–6.

36. Stevens AM, Hennessy TW, Baggett HC, et al. Methicillin-resistant staphylococcus aureus carriage and risk factors for skin infections, southwestern Alaska, USA. Emerg Infect Dis 2010;16(5):797–803.

37. Mangram AJ, Horan TC, Pearson ML, et al. Guideline for prevention of surgical site infection, 1999. Centers for disease control and prevention (CDC) hospital infection control practices advisory committee. Am J Infect Control 1999;27(2): 97–132, quiz 133-134; discussion 96.

38. Lee J, Singletary R, Schmader KE, et al. Surgical site infection in the elderly following orthopaedic surgery. Risk factors and outcomes. J Bone Jt Surg Am Vol 2006;88(8):1705–12.

39. Houang ET, Ahmet Z. Intraoperative wound contamination during abdominal hysterectomy. J Hosp Infect 1991;19(3):181–9.

40. Wong E. Surgical site infection. 3rd edition. Philidelphia, PA: Lippincott, Williams, and Wilkins; 2004.

41. Reddy M, Gill SS, Wu W, et al. Does this patient have an infection of a chronic wound. JAMA 2012;307(6):605–11.

42. Mustoe TA, O'Shaughnessy KD, Kloeters O. Chronic wound pathogenesis and current treatment strategies: a unifying hypothesis. Plast Reconstr Surg 2006; 117. https://doi.org/10.1097/01.prs.0000225431.63010.1b.

43. Bendy RH, Nuccio PA, Wolfe E, et al. Relationship of quantitative wound bacterial counts to healing of decubiti: effect of topical gentamicin. Antimicrob Agents Chemother 1964;10:147–55.

44. Dow G, Browne A, Sibbald RG. Infection in chronic wounds: controversies in diagnosis and treatment. Ostomy Wound Manage 1999;45(8):23–7, 29-40; quiz 41-42.
45. Thomas DR. When is a chronic wound infected. J Am Med Dir Assoc 2012; 13(1):5–7.
46. Yoshikawa TT, Livesley NJ, et al. Infected pressure ulcers in elderly individuals. Clin Infect Dis 2002;35(11):1390–6.
47. Drinka PJ, Bonham PA, Crnich CJ. Swab culture of purulent skin infection to detect infection or colonization with antibiotic-resistant bacteria. J Am Med Dir Assoc 2012;13(1):75–9.
48. Siddiqui AR, Bernstein JM. Chronic wound infection: facts and controversies. Clin Dermatol 2010;28(5):519–26.
49. Harmonson JK, Tobar MY, Harkless LB. Necrotizing fasciitis. Clin Podiatr Med Surg 1996. Available at: https://www.semanticscholar.org/paper/Necrotizing-fasciitis.-Harmonson-Tobar/126907b3faf57c71b0e1274d34c2c24fbd96baed. Accessed March 5, 2023.
50. Miller LG, Perdreau-Remington F, Rieg G, et al. Necrotizing fasciitis caused by community-associated methicillin-resistant staphylococcus aureus in los angeles. N Engl J Med 2005;352(14):1445–53.
51. Seal DV. Necrotizing fasciitis. Curr Opin Infect Dis 2001;14(2):127–32.
52. Urschel JD. Necrotizing soft tissue infections. Postgrad Med J 1999;75(889): 645–9.
53. Hook EW, Hooton TM, Horton CA, et al. Microbiologic evaluation of cutaneous cellulitis in adults. JAMA Intern Med 1986;146(2):295–7.
54. Woo PCY, Lum PNL, Wong SSY, et al. Cellulitis complicating lymphoedema. Eur J Clin Microbiol Infect Dis 2000;19(4):294–7.
55. File T, Stevens DL. Necrotizing soft tissue infections. In: Tan JS, File T, Salata R, et al, editors. Expert guide to infectious diseases. 2nd edition. Philidelphia, PA: ACP Press; 2008. p. 643–62.
56. Fontes RA, Ogilvie CM, Miclau T. Necrotizing soft-tissue infections. J Am Acad Orthop Surg 2000;8(3):151–8.
57. Headley AJ, Headley AJ. Necrotizing soft tissue infections: a primary care review. Am Fam Physician 2003;68(2):323–8.
58. Eke N. Fournier's gangrene: a review of 1726 cases. Br J Surg 2000;87(6): 718–28.
59. McHenry CR, Piotrowski JJ, Petrinic D, et al. Determinants of mortality for necrotizing soft-tissue infections. Ann Surg 1995;221(5):558–65.
60. Anderson DJ, Kaye KS. Skin and soft tissue infections in older adults. Clin Geriatr Med 2007;23(3):595–613.

Cutaneous Fungal Infections in Older Adults

Saniya Shaikh, DO[a],*,[1], Aditya Nellore, MD[b],[1]

KEYWORDS

- Older adults • Dermatophytosis • Candidal cutaneous infection
- *Pityrosporum* infection

KEY POINTS

- The skin of older adults may be more prone to cutaneous fungal infections due to a history of long-term environmental exposures, as well as due to intrinsic metabolic and degenerative skin changes that occur over time.
- Dermatophytes, a type of mold, can invade and multiply within keratinized tissue to cause tinea pedis, tinea corporis, tinea unguium, and tinea capitis.
- *Candida albicans*, a yeast, can cause clinical infection of the skin, mucous membranes, and nails when the normal commensal balance of the skin is disturbed.
- Conditions such as seborrheic dermatitis, pityrosporum folliculitis, and tinea versicolor are caused by another yeast, *Pityrosporum ovale*.

INTRODUCTION

In 1900, the population of adults aged older than 65 years consisted only 4% of the population.[1] By 2050, that number is expected to increase to 22%.[2] The prevalence of dermatoses, specifically, cutaneous fungal infections, will increase accordingly. The skin of older adults is more susceptible to infection due to long-term exposure to ultraviolet light, smoking, and other environmental factors. Intrinsic degenerative and metabolic changes also occur, leading to thinning of the epidermis and damage with mild friction, creating a port of entry for microorganisms.[3]

Common cutaneous fungal infections can be divided into 3 broad causes.

1. The dermatophytes (a group of molds): tinea pedis, tinea corporis, tinea cruris, tinea unguium, and tinea capitis

Funding Source: None.

[a] Department of Dermatology, SSM Health SLU Care Physician Group Saint Louis University School of Medicine, 1225 S Grand Boulevard, Saint Louis, MO 63104, USA; [b] Department of Internal Medicine, St. Luke's Hospital, 232 S Woods Mill Road, Chesterfield, MO 63017, USA

[1] Co-first authors, both authors contributed equally to this article.

* Corresponding author.

E-mail address: saniya.shaikh@ssmhealth.com

https://doi.org/10.1016/j.cger.2023.09.008
0749-0690/24/© 2023 Elsevier Inc. All rights reserved.
geriatric.theclinics.com

2. *Candida* (a yeast species): candidiasis, perleche, intertrigo, erosio interdigitalis blastomycetica, vaginitis, balanitis, and chronic paronychia
3. *Pityrosporum* (another yeast species): seborrheic dermatitis, tinea versicolor, and pityrosporum folliculitis

These pathogens cause superficial fungal infections, meaning they are limited to the stratum corneum, hair, and nails in immunocompetent patients.

DERMATOPHYTOSIS

Dermatophytosis refers to superficial skin, hair, and nail infections caused by dermatophytes. Dermatophytes can invade and multiply within keratinized tissue. There are 3 main genera: *Microsporum*, *Trichophyton*, and *Epidermophyton*. *Trichophyton rubrum* is the most common cause of dermatophytosis worldwide.[4]

Tinea Pedis

Tinea pedis, or athlete's foot, is a dermatophyte infection that localizes to the interdigital spaces and sides of the feet. *T rubrum*, *Trichophyton mentagrophytes*, and *Epidermophyton floccosum* are the most common pathogens involved. They flourish in warm, moist environments such as within occlusive footwear, pools, saunas, and gyms.[4] Older adults may dismiss dry, scaly skin as part of the normal aging process, and therefore, may experience a delay in diagnosis.

There are 3 clinical variants of tinea pedis: (1) moccasin, (2) interdigital, and (3) inflammatory (vesiculobullous).

The moccasin type presents as pruritic scaliness and mild erythema of the entire plantar surface and sides of the foot, creating a moccasin outline (**Fig. 1**). The most common causative agent is *T rubrum*. Patients may also present with unilateral hand involvement (tinea manuum), known as two feet–1 hand syndrome.[5]

The interdigital type, caused by *T rubrum*, is the most common presentation of tinea pedis. It begins with scaling, erythema, and erosion of the interdigital skin of the feet. Coinfection can lead to a malodorous and pruritic overlying bacterial infection.[6]

The inflammatory (vesiculobullous) variant is most commonly caused by *T mentagrophytes* and presents as vesicles or bullae on the foot.[7]

The differential diagnosis for tinea pedis includes contact dermatitis, dyshidrotic eczema, pustular psoriasis, and rarely, an autoimmune bullous dermatosis. Tinea manuum, tinea unguium, and tinea cruris are often seen in conjunction as a result of autoinoculation. Thus, the hands, nails, and groin should also be examined.

For diagnosis, a no.15 blade is used to scrape dry superficial scales onto a glass slide, which can then be examined under a microscope with 20% potassium

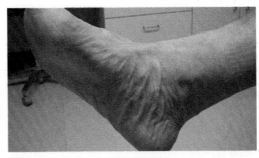

Fig. 1. Moccasin subtype of tinea pedis with scaliness on the plantar surface and sides of the foot.

hydroxide (KOH) or chlorazol black solution. Positive examination reveals long branching septate hyphae.

Treatment usually involves topical antifungals such as imidazoles (ie, ketoconazole, econazole) and allylamines (ie, terbinafine, butenafine) twice daily for 2 to 4 weeks.[3] Studies have shown no difference in efficacy between the 2 options.[8,9] If hyperkeratosis is present, keratolytics such as salicylic acid and lactic acid should be used to improve penetration of the antifungal agents. Oral therapy should be given to patients who have difficulty applying topicals to their feet. Pulse doses of 150 mg fluconazole once weekly for 2 to 6 weeks, 400 mg itraconazole daily for 7 days, and 250 mg terbinafine daily for 2 weeks have been shown to be effective.[10] Failure to treat the infection can lead to secondary bacterial infection such as cellulitis.[11,12] Patients should be taught preventative measures including wearing shower shoes in common bathrooms, completely drying feet after showering, and using a prophylactic antifungal powder or cream intermittently.

Tinea Corporis

Tinea corporis presents as a pruritic, scaly, annular, erythematous plaque on the trunk or extremities (**Fig. 2**). Spread through contact with contaminated shed skin cells, causative fungi thrive in warm and moist environments.[13] Thus, occlusive clothing that traps heat can predispose to infection.[14] The differential diagnosis is vast and includes nummular dermatitis, psoriasis, contact dermatitis, and pityriasis rosea.[5] Diagnosis is made through microscopic examination of scraped scale prepared with KOH.

Treatment is limited to topical antifungal agents unless the area of involvement is extensive or difficult to reach. Topical azoles and allylamines can be used for 2 to 4 weeks. The best oral option is terbinafine 250 mg daily for 1 to 2 weeks because it has the fewest interactions with other drugs.[15] Fluconazole (150–200 mg once weekly for 2–4 weeks) or itraconazole (200 mg daily for 7 days) can also be used for treatment.[16]

Tinea Cruris

Tinea cruris, or jock itch, presents as a red, scaly, annular plaque on the inguinal folds, perineum, and/or buttocks. It is often spread through clothes contaminated by other infected body parts while dressing. Sources of autoinoculation include tinea pedis, tinea manuum, and tinea unguium. Therefore, the hands, nails, and feet should be examined. Patients with these conditions should be encouraged to put on gloves or socks before dressing to prevent spread.[17] Notably, tinea cruris is more common in

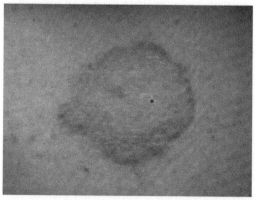

Fig. 2. Classic tinea corporis presents as an erythematous, scaly plaque with central clearing.

men than women because the external genital male anatomy predisposes to warmth and moisture. The differential diagnosis includes candida intertrigo, erythrasma, and inverse psoriasis. Tinea cruris can be distinguished from candidal infection because it spares the penis and scrotum. Treatment is similar to that of tinea corporis.[18]

Tinea Unguium

Tinea unguium is a type of onychomycosis in which there is a dermatophyte infection of the nail bed and plate.[19,20]

Generally, onychomycosis can be divided into 3 clinical types: (1) distal subungual, (2) proximal subungual, and (3) white superficial. The first 2 are most often caused by dermatophytes such as *T rubrum*, *T mentagrophytes*, *Trichophytonrichophyton tonsurans*, and *E floccosum*. The third, most commonly caused by *T mentagrophytes*, can also be caused by nondermatophyte molds such as *Aspergillus terreus*, *Fusarium oxysporum*, and *Acremonium potonii*.

Distal subungual onychomycosis is the most common form and leads to yellowing, thickening, subungual hyperkeratosis, and onycholysis of the toenails (**Fig. 3**). Secondary bacterial infection can occur, leading to additional green or black discoloration.[20]

Proximal subungual infection seems as a white nail with proximal subungual hyperkeratosis and onycholysis. This finding may be an indicator of an underlying immunosuppressed state.[20]

The nail in the white superficial type becomes crumbly and soft with a chalky white discoloration and rough dorsal surface.[20]

For diagnosis, a nail clipping can be submitted for fungal culture and/or microscopic examination. A separate clipping sample is submitted for each test. Submitting a nail clipping for histologic examination, when possible, tends to have a higher sensitivity (85%) compared with culture (32%).

There is a broad differential for onychodystrophy, including psoriasis, trauma, chronic eczematous dermatitis, and lichen planus.[4]

Treatment of onychomycosis is the same regardless of whether a dermatophyte or nondermatophyte is cultured. Terbinafine 250 mg daily for 12 weeks for toenails and the same dose for 6 weeks for fingernails is the treatment of choice. Terbinafine pulse therapy (500 mg daily for 1 week per month, 2 pulses for fingernails and 3 pulses for toenails), itraconazole pulse therapy (200 mg twice daily for 1 week per month, for 3 months), griseofulvin, and fluconazole can also be effective but have lower cure rates and more drug interactions.[21,22]

A yellow or white streak in the nail indicates a dermatophytoma, which is a walled off mass of fungus. Dermatophytomas should be removed surgically.[23] Superficial white

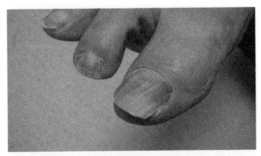

Fig. 3. Distal subungual onychomycosis characteristically presents with yellow, thick nails and onycholysis.

onychomycosis is localized to the dorsal nail surface and can be treated with topical azoles and ciclopirox 8% lacquer with occlusion.[24]

Due to the slow growth of toenails, resolution of onychomycosis can take 12 to 18 months, depending on how much of the nail is involved. Recurrence is common, with a 42% recurrence rate during a 1-year period, despite treatment with oral antifungals.[25]

Old shoes are a common source of reinfection. Therefore, patients should be advised to treat them with over-the-counter antifungal sprays or discard them altogether.

Tinea Capitis

Tinea capitis is a dermatophyte infection of the hair shaft, most commonly occurring in children. However, adults can also be affected, presenting with scalp scale and associated alopecia, pruritus, and/or posterior cervical lymphadenopathy. These symptoms may be mistaken for persistent dandruff or psoriasis, so precautionary testing in this setting is important.

Tinea capitis can be classified as endothrix or ectothrix depending on how the pathogen invades. In endothrix infections, it invades the hair shaft itself, often causing hairless patches with black dots (broken hair shafts). In ectothrix infections, the microorganisms cover the outside of the hair, resulting in scaly patches of alopecia known as gray patch tinea capitis (**Fig. 4**). The differential includes seborrheic dermatitis, eczematous dermatitis, or psoriasis. Severe inflammation can lead to kerion formation, which is a pustular eruption with scarring alopecia.

To prevent spread, anyone in close contact with a symptomatic patient should be treated with ketoconazole 2% shampoo. Fomites such as combs, hats, and hair accessories should also be disinfected or discarded. Some also advocate for the evaluation of home pets, who often serve as a persistent source of reinfection.

Diagnosis can be made with KOH examination, culture, or Wood lamp examination. *T tonsurans* is the most common cause of tinea capitis in the United States and does not fluoresce under a Wood lamp. However, the second most common cause, *Microsporum canis*, does fluoresce a characteristic yellow-green color.[4] Fungal cultures should be taken with a cotton swab swept over the scaly region. Broken hairs should also be included within the culture tube.

A dosage of 20 to 25 mg/kg daily of micronized griseofulvin for 6 to 8 weeks has historically been the gold standard treatment of tinea capitis caused by *Trichophyton* species.[5] However, multiple clinical trials have shown terbinafine to be just as effective with a shorter treatment duration (4 weeks).[26] Resolution can be achieved with either medication (**Table 1**).

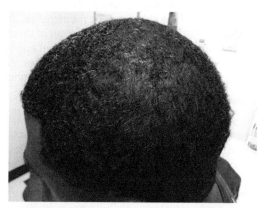

Fig. 4. Ectothrix tinea capitis classically causes scaly gray patches of alopecia.

Table 1 Treatment options for dermatophyte infections		
Disease	Systemic Treatment	Amount
Tinea pedis	Fluconazole Itraconazole Terbinafine	150 mg/wk × 2–6 wk 400 mg/d × 7 d 250 md/d × 2 wk
Tinea corporis/cruris	Terbinafine Fluconazole Itraconazole	250 mg/d × 1–2 wk 150–200 mg/wk × 2–4 wk 200 mg/d × 7 d
Tinea unguium	Terbinafine	250 mg/d × 12 wk (toenails) 250 mg/d × 12 wk (fingernails)
Tinea capitis	Griseofulvin Terbinafine	20–25 mg/kg/d × 6–8 wk 250 mg/d × 4 wk

KEY POINTS

- Dermatophytosis refers to superficial skin, hair, and nail infections caused by dermatophytes.
- These molds flourish in warm, moist environments and have the ability to invade keratinized tissue.
- Tinea pedis localizes to the feet and interdigital spaces. The infection is spread by walking barefoot on contaminated surfaces.
- Tinea corporis, or ringworm, presents as a pruritic, scaly, annular, erythematous plaque on the trunk or extremities.
- Tinea cruris, or jock itch, involves the inguinal folds, perineum, and/or buttocks. It presents as a red, scaly, annular plaque.
- Tinea unguium is a dermatophyte infection of the nail bed and plate. Resolution can often take 12 to 18 months.
- Tinea capitis is a dermatophyte infection of the hair shaft most commonly found in children. It can also be found in older adults but is often overlooked.

CANDIDAL CUTANEOUS INFECTIONS

Cutaneous candidiasis is most commonly caused by *Candida albicans*, a yeast that is part of the normal flora balance of the skin, mucous membranes, and nails of healthy humans. A disturbance of this balance can lead to infection of these sites, typically in either the very young or elderly. Note that chronic and recurrent episodes of candidiasis in older adults may indicate underlying conditions such as diabetes, malignancy, vitamin deficiency, or malnutrition. Appropriate workup and investigation should be performed.

Oral Candidiasis or Candidiasis (Thrush)

The oral cavity is the most common location for overgrowth of *Candida* species. Older adults are predisposed to this infection due to the frequent occurrence of dry mouth (xerostomia), along with the use of systemic, inhaled, or topical corticosteroids, broad-spectrum antibiotics, immunosuppressive drugs, and dentures.[27]

Gray-white plaques loosely adherent to the surface of the tongue, buccal mucosa, palate, and pharynx are clinically suspicious. These are easily removed with a tongue depressor to reveal a red, beefy, moist base.[28] Oral hairy leukoplakia and lichen planus may seem similarly, however, the plaques will be fixed. Acute oral candidiasis can sometimes present with a glossy, red tongue with atrophic papillae.[27] Diagnosis can be confirmed by performing a fungal culture on a swab of the mucosal surface.

An important first step in treatment is to address any predisposing factors, such as denture cleanliness and potential medication causes. Pharmacologic treatment of patients with mild disease includes clotrimazole troches (1–2 tablets 4–5 times daily up to 14 days) or nystatin solution. Patients requiring systemic treatment can be given fluconazole (200 mg on day 1, then 100–200 mg daily continued for 7–14 days).[29]

Denture Stomatitis

Denture stomatitis presents as a localized, sharply demarcated, erythematous, and edematous lesion in denture-occluded areas. Candida infection is the most common cause for denture stomatitis. Predisposing factors include poor denture care and wearing dentures for longer than 24 hours.[30] Prevention involves removing dentures before sleeping, confirming a proper fit to prevent any trauma to the region, and cleaning them properly.[31]

Perleche (Angular Cheilitis)

Angular cheilitis, often associated with denture stomatitis, presents with maceration, fissuring, and crusting at the angles of the mouth. It is often caused by candida infection although infection with *Staphylococcus aureus* may also be causative. Patients with this condition are often edentulous and collect saliva in the affected area. Treatment involves a combination of topical anticandidal creams and low-to-mid potency topical corticosteroids (eg, 2.5% hydrocortisone). As a preventative measure, vaseline can be applied to the corners of the mouth at bedtime.

Candidal Intertrigo

Candidal intertrigo refers to inflammation (rash) in various intertriginous areas of the body. Patients present with sharply demarcated, pruritic to painful, erythematous, macerated patches, which are often studded with satellite pustules or a thin peripheral collarette of scale. Predisposing factors include free-hanging, overlapping skin, obesity, diabetes, chronic bed rest, inadequate personal hygiene, and use of broad-spectrum antibiotics.[28]

Diagnosis can be confirmed by a fungal swab culture. Erythrasma, a *Corynebacterium* bacterial infection, can present similarly but is distinguished by a characteristic coral red fluorescence on Wood lamp examination.

Treatment of candidal intertrigo involves the use of topical antifungals such as ketoconazole cream or nystatin powder twice a day for 2 to 4 weeks.[4] Low-potency topical steroids such as 2.5% hydrocortisone cream can be added to decrease inflammation but should not be used as monotherapy. Towels or washcloths moistened with a dilute vinegar solution can be used once or twice daily for 10 to 15 minutes to enhance medication penetration and provide additional antimicrobial effect. In severe or extensive cases, a course of oral antifungals at the same dosage as for oral candidiasis is appropriate. To keep the area dry and prevent recurrences, daily use of antifungal powders such as nystatin or miconazole after treatment of active infection should be encouraged.

Interdigital Candida (Erosio Interdigitalis Blastomycetica)

Another variant of intertrigo is interdigital Candida, also known as erosio interdigitalis blastomycetica. It presents as an area of macerated white skin on an erythematous, painful base between the middle and ring fingers of the hand and/or the fourth interspace of the feet. Predisposing factors include diabetes and repetitive immersion of the hands in water. In the feet, this can be difficult to distinguish from tinea pedis without culture. Additionally, erythrasma should be considered and can be distinguished by Wood lamp examination. Treatment is similar to candidal intertrigo with the use of topical azoles and keeping the area clean and dry.[28]

Candidal Vulvovaginitis and Balanitis

The common term "yeast infection" refers to candidal vulvovaginitis, which occurs from an overgrowth of *Candida* in the vagina. Although easily treatable, older women may experience a delay in diagnosis due to less frequent gynecologic visits. Affected patients complain of severe pruritus, burning, and sometimes dyspareunia. Examination shows labial erythema and a white cottage cheese-like discharge.[32]

Predisposing factors include diabetes, use of broad-spectrum antibiotics, and long-term use of tamoxifen.[28] Tamoxifen has an antiestrogen effect on malignant breast cells but an estradiol agonist effect in the genital tract of postmenopausal women, facilitating *Candida* colonization.[33]

Uncircumcised older men who have intercourse with an affected woman are at risk for candidal balanitis, an inflammation of the glans. Symptoms include mild burning and pruritus. Examination shows glassy erythema, and occasionally small satellite pustules, on the inner aspect of the foreskin. Although the most common source of transmission is through intercourse with an infected partner, infectivity is measured at only 10%.[34]

Visualization of yeast in a smear of vaginal discharge treated with KOH, or a fungal culture, confirms the diagnosis in a female. In a male, the surface of a pustule can be prepared with KOH or cultured. The treatment of choice is a single dose of fluconazole 150 mg. Other options for women include the use of topical or suppository antifungals such as miconazole and clotrimazole.[35,36]

Candidal Paronychia

Paronychia is inflammation of the skin around the nail, known as the nail fold. Although *S aureus* is the most common cause of acute paronychia, *Candida albicans* is found in 40% to 90% of chronic (>6 weeks) or recurrent cases and is thought to represent secondary colonization.[37] Similar to interdigital candidiasis, candidal paronychia is more common in diabetics and patients who do wet work.

Paronychia presents as painful erythema and edema of the nail fold, leading to separation from the nail plate and eventual loss of the cuticle. Chronic inflammation can lead to nail changes such as onycholysis and yellow-green discoloration.

Addressing predisposing factors is essential in the treatment of candidal paronychia. Patients should be advised to minimize wet work and seek treatment of underlying diabetes if present. Pharmacologically speaking, topical steroids have been found to be more effective than systemic antifungals as have topical calcineurin inhibitors such as tacrolimus.[38–40] This may indicate that chronic paronychia is more an inflammatory disorder of the proximal nail than a fungal infection. Still, a topical antifungal (ciclopirox) could be considered as adjunctive therapy in refractory cases but may or may not provide additional efficacy.

KEY POINTS

- Cutaneous candidiasis is most commonly caused by *C albicans*, a yeast that is part of the normal flora balance of the skin, mucous membranes, and nails of healthy humans. When this balance is disturbed, infection of these sites can occur.

- Oral candidiasis seems as grayish-white plaques that are loosely adherent to the surface of the tongue, buccal mucosa, palate, and pharynx.
- Denture stomatitis presents as a localized, sharply demarcated, erythematous, edematous lesion in an area that is occluded by the dentures and is most often caused by candidal infection.
- Angular cheilitis can be associated with denture stomatitis and affects the oral commissures, presenting with maceration, fissuring, and crusting at the angles of the mouth. *Candida* is the most common causative agent.
- Candidal intertrigo refers to candidal infection in various intertriginous areas of the body.
- Candidal vulvovaginitis occurs when there is an increased growth of *Candida* in the vagina.
- Paronychia is inflammation of the nail fold that often occurs after repetitive wet work.

PITYROSPORUM INFECTIONS

The yeast *Pityrosporum ovale* (also known as *Malassezia furfur*), a lipophilic fungus, causes seborrheic dermatitis, pityrosporum folliculitis, and tinea (or pityriasis) versicolor. A normal skin commensal, disease manifests when its numbers increase past a certain threshold.

Seborrheic Dermatitis

Patients with seborrheic dermatitis often complain of a dry, scaly scalp (**Fig. 5**). Additionally, pink patches with greasy scale can occur in other areas rich in sebaceous glands, such as the eyebrows, external ear canals, paranasal folds, and forehead (**Fig. 6**).

Sebocyte turnover rate decreases with age, leading to an increased incidence of seborrheic dermatitis in older adults.[41] Diagnosis is made clinically based on the classic distribution and appearance of the lesions. Patients with scalp involvement can be treated with antifungal (ketoconazole 2% and ciclopirox 1%) and cytostatic (zinc pyrithione and selenium sulfide) shampoos.[42] If severe, addition of topical steroid solutions or gels can help with inflammation and pruritus. Mild topical steroids (hydrocortisone 2.5% cream) and topical antifungals (ketoconazole 2% cream) can be used for the involvement of other areas such as the ears, neck, face, and chest.[43] Topical steroids should be discontinued on resolution. However, continued intermittent use of topical antifungals can prevent recurrence.

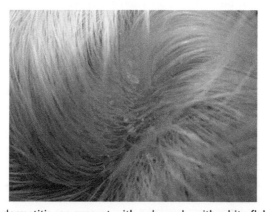

Fig. 5. Seborrheic dermatitis can present with a dry scalp with white flakes.

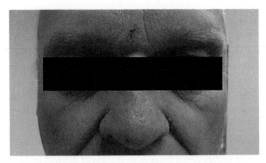

Fig. 6. Seborrheic dermatitis, seen as greasy scale on the eyebrows.

Pityrosporum Folliculitis

Pityrosporum folliculitis presents clinically with pruritic follicular papules and pustules, usually on the trunk. Although uncommon in older adults, it should be considered when patients complain of itching on the back. Predisposing factors include diabetes and use of corticosteroids or broad-spectrum antibiotics.[44] The diagnosis can be made clinically or by visualizing the *Pityrosporum* yeast on skin biopsy; it cannot be cultured with normal fungal culture medium. Response to therapy can also be used for diagnosis. Systemic treatment with itraconazole (200 mg daily for 1–3 weeks) or fluconazole (100–200 mg daily for 1–4 weeks or 300 mg weekly for 4–8 weeks) can be considered.[45] Topical therapy with selenium sulfide 2.5% or ketoconazole 2% shampoo can be used as adjunctive therapy. This condition is prone to relapse, so prophylactic treatment with selenium sulfide, econazole cream, or ketoconazole shampoo a few times weekly is beneficial even after treatment.[28]

Tinea Versicolor

Tinea, or pityriasis, versicolor is a common skin disorder that causes well-defined, slightly scaly, hypopigmented (most commonly) or hyperpigmented macules and patches (**Fig. 7**). Areas of change are more apparent in tanned individuals. The condition is more common in the summer months and in oily areas of the skin. The classic distribution involves the chest, back, neck, and face.

Diagnosis is confirmed by skin scraping and direct microscopy using KOH or chlorazol black. The classic "spaghetti and meatballs" appearance of the yeast with short hyphae and oval yeast forms confirms the diagnosis.

Tinea versicolor can be treated with selenium sulfide 2.5%, clotrimazole 1%, or ketoconazole 2% shampoo applied once daily for 2 to 4 weeks. Oral therapy with fluconazole 300 mg weekly for 2 weeks or itraconazole 200 mg daily for 5 to 7 days can be given, especially to older adults who may not be able to apply topicals.[46–48] The condition often recurs, therefore weekly use of an antiyeast shampoo is recommended long-term. Patients should be informed that this condition is neither contagious nor related to hygiene and that the color change will resolve within a few weeks to months. See **Table 2** for treatment options for canididal and pityrosporum infections.

KEY POINTS

- The yeast *P ovale* (also known as *M furfur*) causes seborrheic dermatitis, pityrosporum folliculitis, and tinea (or pityriasis) versicolor.

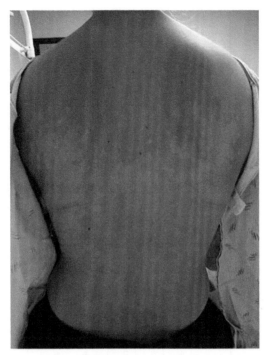

Fig. 7. Tinea versicolor presents as hypopigmented macules and patches on the back of this patient.

- Patients with seborrheic dermatitis have patches of greasy scale on the scalp, eyebrows, external ear canals, paranasal folds, and/or forehead. It can be treated with antifungal and cytostatic shampoos.
- Pityrosporum folliculitis presents clinically with pruritic follicular papules and pustules that usually involve the trunk. It can be treated systemically with the oral azole antifungals and topical antifungal shampoos.
- Tinea versicolor causes pigmentary changes in the skin that seem as hypopigmented or hyperpigmented patches in most individuals.

SPECIAL CONSIDERATIONS REGARDING SYSTEMIC ANTIFUNGAL TREATMENT

Systemic antifungal medications should be prescribed and used with caution due to interactions with other medications and potential side effects.

- All systemic azole antifungals can be hepatotoxic, so liver function tests should be checked before prescribing. Specifically, oral ketoconazole is discouraged from use because it can cause severe liver damage, adrenal gland issues, and harmful interactions with other medications.[49,50]
- Itraconazole can cause negative inotropic effects and should not be used in those with a history of congestive heart failure.[51]
- Itraconazole inhibits the cytochrome P3A4 enzyme, responsible for the metabolism of medications like H1 receptor antagonists, warfarin, and others, increasing the risk for medication-related side effects.[49,52]

Table 2
Treatment options for cutaneous candida and pityrosporum infections

Disease	Topical treatment	Systemic treatment
Oral candidiasis	Clotrimazole troches; 1–2 tablets 4–5/d × 14 d Nystatin solution; 4–6 mL 4/d × 7–14 d	Fluconazole 200 mg on day 1; 100–200 mg/d × 7–14 d
Candidal intertrigo	Ketoconazole cream or nystatin powder; twice daily × 2–4 wk	Fluconazole 200 mg on day 1; 100–200 mg/d × 7–14 d
Candidal vulvovaginitis and balanitis	Clotrimazole 1% cream; 5 g/d × 7–14 d Miconazole 2% cream; 5 g/d × 7 d	Fluconazole; 150 mg
Candidal paronychia	Medium-High potency topical steroid or topical calcineurin inhibitor ± topical ciclopirox solution	
Seborrheic dermatitis	Ketoconazole 2% cream and shampoo Zinc pyrithione or selenium sulfide shampoo Ciclopirox 1% shampoo	
Pityrosporum folliculitis	Selenium sulfide 2.5% or ketoconazole 2% shampoo (adjunctive therapy)	Itraconazole 200 mg/d × 1–3 wk Fluconazole; 100–200 mg/d × 1–4 wk or 300 mg/wk × 4–8 wk
Tinea versicolor	Selenium sulfide 2.5%, clotrimazole1%, or ketoconazole 2% shampoo once daily × 2–4 wk	Fluconazole; 300 mg/wk × 2 wk Itraconazole 200 mg/d × 5–7 d

- Fluconazole has fewer medication interactions because it is metabolized through the CYP 2C9 and 2C19 pathways, which are not commonly used for the metabolism of medications.
- Although griseofulvin is the mainstay therapy for tinea capitis, its liquid form has a poor compliance rate due to its bitter taste. Its side effect profile includes cytochrome P450 induction, photosensitivity, headache, and gastrointestinal upset.[28] Additionally, it must be taken with high-fat foods for optimal absorption.
- Terbinafine inhibits the CYP 2D6 system and can affect the metabolism of beta-blockers and tricyclic antidepressants.[5]

SUMMARY

As the patient population aged older than 65 years increases, it becomes more important to recognize and treat skin conditions seen in this age group. When determining treatment choice, it is important to consider different physiologic characteristics faced by older adults, their often lengthy medication lists (warfarin, metformin, hydrochlorothiazide, clopidogrel, and so forth), and their social living conditions. These patients should be prescribed simple regimens with a low risk of drug interactions. Treating skin conditions in older adults can lead to a significant increase in quality of life. Additionally, some fungal infections may become a port of entry for more serious infections, such as bacterial cellulitis, which can have significant morbidity and mortality in this patient population.

CLINICS CARE POINT

- Fungal infections tend to affect the hair, skin, and nails of older adults.

- Proper diagnosis requires an understanding of the clinical features unique to the various diseases discussed in this article. Once diagnosed, treatment of these infections is generally similar (topical ± oral antifungal medications).

ACKNOWLEDGMENTS

Reena S. Varade, MD; Nicole M. Burkemper, MD.

CONFLICT OF INTEREST OR DISCLOSURE

The authors have no conflict of interest to declare.

REFERENCES

1. Johnson ML. Aging of the United States population: the dermatologic implications. Clin Geriatr Med 1989;5:41–51.
2. US Census Bureau. Age and sex. Washington, DC: US Department of Commerce; 2020.
3. Wey SJ, Chen DY. Common cutaneous disorders in the elderly. Journal of Gerontology and Geriatrics 2010;1:36–41.
4. Sobera JO, Elewski BE. Fungal diseases. In: Bolognia JL, Jorizzo JL, Rapini RP, editors. Dermatology. 2nd edition. St Louis: Elsevier; 2008. p. 1135–63.
5. Schieke SM, Garg A. Superficial fungal infection. In: Fitzpatrick's dermatology in internal medicine. 8th edition. New York: McGraw-Hill; 2012. p. 1807–21.

6. Leyden JJ. Progression of interdigital infections from simplex to complex. J Am Acad Dermatol 1993;28:S7–11.
7. Neri I, Piraccini BM, Guareschi E, et al. Bullous tinea pedis in two children. Mycoses 2004;47:475–8.
8. Rotta I, Sanchez A, Goncalves PR, et al. Efficacy and safety of topical antifungals in the treatment of dermatomycosis: a systematic review. Br J Dermatol 2012;166: 927–33.
9. Parish LC, Parish JL, Routh HB, et al. A randomized, double-blind, vehicle-controlled efficacy and safety study of naftifine 2% cream in the treatment of tinea pedis. J Drugs Dermatol JDD 2011;10:1282–8.
10. Gupta AK, Cooper EA. Update in antifungal therapy of dermatophytosis. Mycopathologia 2008;166:353.
11. Dawber R, Bristow I, Turner W. Skin disorders. In: Dunitz M, editor. Text atlas of podiatric dermatology. Malden (MA): Blackwell Science; 2001. p. 31–76.
12. Strauss H, Spielfogel W. Foot disorders in the elderly. Clin Geriatr 2003;52:595–602.
13. Drake LA, Dinehart SM, Farmer ER, et al. Guidelines of care for superficial mycotic infections of the skin: tinea corporis, tinea cruris, tinea faciei, tinea manuum, and tinea pedis. J Am Acad Dermatol 1996;34:282–6.
14. Martin AG, Kobayashi GS. Superficial fungal infection: dermatophytosis, tinea nigra, piedra. In: Feedberg IM, Eisen AZ, Wolff K, et al, editors. Fitzpatrick's dermatology in general medicine. 5th edition. New York: McGraw-Hill; 1999. p. 2337–57.
15. Lesher JL. Oral therapy of common superficial fungal infections of the skin. J Am Acad Dermatol 1999;40:S31–4.
16. Elewski BE, Hughey LC, Sobera JO. Fungal diseases. In: Bolognia JL, Jorizzo JL, Schaffer JV, editors. Dermatology2, 3rd edition. London: Elsevier Limited; 2012. p. 1251.
17. Gupta AK, Chaudhry M, Elewski B. Tinea corporis, tinea cruris, tinea nigra, and piedra. Dermatol Clin 2003;21:395–400.
18. Loo DS. Cutaneous fungal infections in the elderly. Dermatol Clin 2004;22:33–50.
19. Elewski B, Charif MA. Presence of onychomycosis in patients attending a dermatology clinic in northeaster Ohio for other conditions. Arch Dermatol 1999;133: 1172–3.
20. Amsden G, Elewski B, Ghannoum M, et al. Managing onychomycosis: issues in diagnosis, treatment and economics. Am J Clin Dermatol 2000;1:19–26.
21. Cribier BJ, Bakshi R. Terbinafine in the treatment of onychomycosis: a review of its efficacy in high-risk populations and in patients with nondermatophyte infections. Br J Dermatol 2004;150:414–20.
22. Kreijkamp-Kaspers S, Hawke K, Guo L, et al. Oral antifungal medication for toenail onychomycosis. Cochrane Database Syst Rev 2017 Jul 14;7(7):CD010031.
23. Burkhart CN, Burkhart CG, Gupta AK. Dermatophytoma: recalcitrance to treatment because of existence of fungal biofilm. J Am Acad Dermatol 2002;47:629–31.
24. Baran R, Kaoukhov A. Topical antifungal drugs for the treatment of onychomycosis: an overview of current strategies for monotherapy and combination therapy. J Eur Acad Dermatol Venereol 2005;19:21–9.
25. Heikkila A, Stubb S. Long-term results of patients with onychomycosis treated with itraconazole. Acta Derm Venereol 1997;77:70–1.
26. Alkeswani A, Cantrell W, Elewski B. Treatment of tinea capitis. Skin Appendage Disord 2019;5:201–10.
27. Turner MD, Ship JA. Dry mouth and its oral effects on the health of elderly people. J Am Dent Assoc 2007;138:15S–20S.

28. James WD, Berger T, Elston D. Diseases resulting from fungi and yeast: candidi-asis. In: James WD, Berger T, Elston D, editors. Andrews' diseases of the skin. 11th edition. Philadelphia: Saunders Elsevier; 2011. p. 297–9.
29. Martin ES, Elewski BE. Cutaneous fungal infections in the elderly. Clin Geriatr Med 2002;18:59–75.
30. Collins JJ, Stafford GD. A survey of denture hygiene in patients attending Cardiff dental hospital. Eur J Prosthodont Restor Dent 1994;3:67–71.
31. Kulak-Ozkan Y, Kazazoglu E, Arikan A. Oral hygiene habits, denture cleanliness, presence of yeasts and stomatitis in elderly people. J Oral Rehabil 2002;29:300–4.
32. Nathan L. Vulvovaginal disorders in the elderly woman. Clin Obstet Gynecol 1996;39:933–45.
33. Sobel JD, Chaim W, Leahman D. Recurrent vulvovaginal candidiasis associated with long-term tamoxifen treatment in postmenopausal women. Obstet Gynecol 1996;88:704–6.
34. English JC 3rd, Laws RA, Keough GC, et al. Dermatoses of the glans penis and prepuce. J Am Acad Dermatol 1997;37:1–24.
35. Peter GP, Carol AK, David RA, et al. Clinical practice guideline for the manage-ment of candidiasis: 2016 update by the infectious diseases society of America. Clin Infect Dis 2016;62(Issue 4):e1–50.
36. Workowski KA, Bachmann LH, Chan PA, et al. Sexually transmitted infections treat-ment guidelines, 2021. MMWR Recomm Rep (Morb Mortal Wkly Rep) 2021;70(No. RR-4):1–187.
37. Shafritz AB, Coppage JM. Acute and chronic paronychia of the hand. J Am Acad Orthop Surg 2014 Mar;22(3):165–74.
38. Tosti A, Piraccini BM, Ghetto E, et al. Topical steroids versus antifungals in the treatment of chronic parohychia: an open, randomized double-blind and double dummy study. J Am Acad Dermatol 2002;47:73–6.
39. Rigopoulos D, Gregoriou S, Belyayeva E, et al. Efficacy and safety of tacrolimus ointment 0.1% vs betamethasone17-valerate 0.1% in the treatment of chronic pa-ronychia: an unblinded randomized study. Br J Dermatol 2009;160:858–60.
40. Leggit JC. Acute and chronic paronychia. Am Fam Physician 2017 Jul 1;96(1):44–51.
41. Mastrolonardo M, Diaferio A, Vendemiale G, et al. Seborrheic dermatitis in the elderly: inferences on the possible role of disability and loss of self-sufficiency. Acta Derm Venereol 2004;84:285–7.
42. Faergemann J. Treatment of seborrheic dermatitis of the scalp with ketoconazole shampoo: a double-blind study. Acta Derm Venereol 1990;70:171–2.
43. Elewski BE, Abramovits W, Kempers S, et al. A novel foam formulation of ketoco-nazole 2% for the treatment of seborrheic dermatitis on multiple body regions. J Drugs Dermatol 2007;6:1001–8.
44. Gupta AK, Batra R, Bluhm R, et al. Skin diseases associated with Malassezia species. J Am Acad Dermatol 2004;51:785–98.
45. Hald M, Arendrup MC, Svejgaard EL, et al. Evidence-based Danish guidelines for the treatment of Malassezia-related skin diseases. Acta Derm Venereol 2015 Jan;95(1):12–9.
46. Gupta AK, Lane D, Paquet M. Systematic review of systemic treatments for tinea versicolor and evidence-based dosing regimen recommendations. J Cutan Med Surg 2014 Mar-Apr;18(2):79–90.
47. Gupta AK, Foley KA. Antifungal treatment for pityriasis versicolor. J Fungi (Basel) 2015 Mar 12;1(1):13–29.

48. Leung AK, Barankin B, Lam JM, et al. Tinea versicolor: an updated review. Drugs Context 2022 Nov 14;11:2022–9.
49. Wong-Beringer A, Kriengkauykiat J. Systemic antifungal therapy: new options, new challenges. Pharmacotherapy 2003;23:1441–62.
50. Center for Drug Evaluation and Research. FDA drug safety communication. U.S. Food and Drug Administration, FDA; 19 2016.
51. Ahmad SR, Singer SJ, Leissa BG. Congestive heart failure associated with itraconazole. Lancet 2001;357:766–1767.
52. Albengres E, Louet HL, Tillement JP. Systemic antifungal agents: drug interactions of clinical significance. Drug Saf 1998;18:83–97.

Diagnostic Methods and Management Strategies of Herpes Simplex and Herpes Zoster Infections

Sino Mehrmal, DO[a], Rafael Mojica, DO[b],
Aibing Mary Guo, MD, MS[a], Tricia A. Missall, MD, PhD[b],*

KEYWORDS

- Herpesvirus • Diagnosis • Complications • Immunosuppression • Treatment

KEY POINTS

- The distribution of herpes simplex and herpes zoster varies; however, the primary lesion is a vesicle on an erythematous base often preceded by sensory alterations.
- Always consider herpes zoster in the differential diagnosis when an elderly patient presents with dermatomal pain or altered mental status.
- Polymerase chain reaction assays are preferred for a rapid diagnosis with high sensitivity.
- Immediate treatment with antivirals is recommended for herpes simplex and herpes zoster. Early antiviral intervention can decrease the incidence of postherpetic neuralgia.

INTRODUCTION

Herpesviruses are medium-sized double-stranded DNA viruses. Of more than 80 herpesviruses identified, only 9 human herpesviruses have been found to cause infection in humans. These include herpes simplex viruses 1 and 2 (HSV-1 and HSV-2), varicella-zoster virus (VZV), human cyto-megalovirus (HCMV), Epstein–Barr virus (EBV), and human herpesvirus (HHV-6A, HHV-6B, HHV-7, HHV-8). HSV-1, HSV-2, and VZV can be problematic given their characteristic neurotropism which is the ability to invade via fusion of its plasma membrane and reside within neural tissue. HSV and VZV primarily infect mucocutaneous surfaces and remain latent in the dorsal root ganglia for a host's entire life. Reactivation causes either asymptomatic shedding of virus or clinical manifestation of vesicular lesions.[1–3]

[a] Department of Dermatology, Saint Louis University School of Medicine, 1225 South Grand Boulevard, Saint Louis, MO 63104, USA; [b] Department of Dermatology, University of Florida College of Medicine, 4037 Northwest 86th Terrace, Gainesville, FL 32606, USA
* Corresponding author. Department of Dermatology, 4th floor, 4037 NW 86th Terrace, Gainesville, FL 32606.
E-mail address: triciamissall@dermatology.med.ufl.edu

Clin Geriatr Med 40 (2024) 147–175
https://doi.org/10.1016/j.cger.2023.09.003
0749-0690/24/© 2023 Elsevier Inc. All rights reserved.

The clinical presentation is influenced by the portal of entry, the immune status of the host, and whether the infection is primary or recurrent.[1] Affecting 60% to 95% of adults, herpesvirus-associated infections include gingivostomatitis, orofacial and genital herpes, and primary varicella and herpes zoster. Symptomatology, treatment, and potential complications vary based on primary and recurrent infections as well as the patient's immune status.

OROFACIAL HERPES SIMPLEX AND GENITAL HERPES
Primary Herpetic Gingivostomatitis

Orolabial herpes infection is essentially caused by HSV-1 infection, although HSV-2 infection can occur (**Figs. 1–3**). Most initial orolabial infections are subclinical and, therefore, go unrecognized. Latest data from the National Health and Nutrition Examination survey showed that during 2015 to 2016, the prevalence of HSV-1 was 47.8% and of HSV-2 was 11.9% among those aged 14 to 49.[2]

A small proportion of newly infected patients develop primary herpetic gingivostomatitis (PHGS). Classically, PHGS begins as transient perioral vesicles that quickly rupture, producing painful superficial ulcerations. The perioral vesiculo-ulcerative lesions are often preceded by a sensation of burning or paresthesia at the site of inoculation. Initial primary infections often occur within 1 to 26 days after inoculation and can last for 10 to 14 days. Although most orolabial infections are asymptomatic, they can be preceded by a prodrome of fever, chills, fatigue, muscle aches, and cervical and submandibular lymphadenopathy.[3-5]

Recurrent Herpes

Recurrent herpes labialis (RHL) affects up to one-third of the American population and typically presents at the vermillion border of the lip in 90% of cases. Recurrence may occur on eyelids, cheeks, perioral skin, nasal mucosa, or oral mucosa. If it recurs intraorally, it mostly recurs on keratinized mucosa, such as on the hard palate, gingiva, and occasionally dorsum of the tongue. Conditions associated with oral ulcers include orolabial herpes infection, aphthous ulcers, herpangina, hand-foot-mouth disease, lichen planus, drug-induced ulcers (with drugs like beta-blockers, antimetabolites, and alkylating agents, among others), erythema multiforme, pemphigus vulgaris, and Behcet's Disease (**Table 1**). For RHL specifically, papules on an erythematous base progress to vesicles and within 72 to 96 hours become ulcerated and crusted before healing.

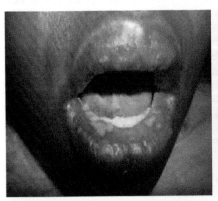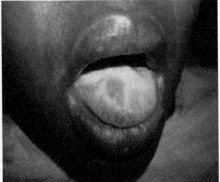

Fig. 1. Primary herpetic gingivostomatitis with coalescing grouped erosions with scalloped borders. The diagnosis was confirmed by viral culture.

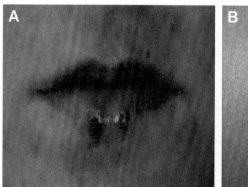
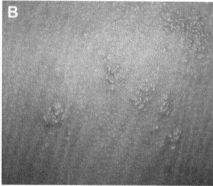

Fig. 2. (*A*) Recurrent herpetic labialis. (*B*) Recurrent cutaneous herpes.

About 60% of people experience a prodrome of tingling, itching, and burning within 24 hours of skin lesions. Overall, symptoms and duration are milder and shorter than primary infections.[3] Common triggers are illness, surgery, sun exposure, trauma, emotional stress, and menses. At least one-half of all immunocompetent individuals who experience an episode of HSV infection will have a recurrent episode in their lifetime.[4]

Genital Herpes Simplex Virus Infection

HSV-2 is the most common strain in genital herpes (**Fig. 4**); however, the percentage due to HSV-1 infection is increasing in developed countries.[7] This may be due to the fact that among people 14 to 19 years of age, the seroprevalence of HSV-1 has decreased by 30% over the past 30 years; thus, an increasing proportion of adolescents lack protective HSV-1 antibodies when they become sexually active.[8] Independent risk factors for HSV-2 seropositivity include female sex, older age, lifetime number of sexual partners, lower education or income level, cocaine use, and black or Hispanic race.[9] Approximately half of patients with symptomatic genital lesions report headache, fever, malaise, dysuria, or tender inguinal lymphadenopathy. However, most patients with initial genital herpes do not have conspicuous lesions and systemic symptoms.[8] Atypical presentations include edema, crusts, fissures, erythematous patches, or transient irritation, and back pain without genital lesions.

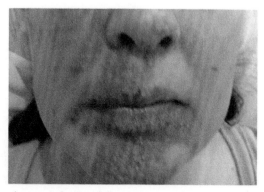

Fig. 3. Recrudescent herpes infection following a neurosurgical procedure.

Table 1
Differential diagnosis of oral ulcers

Orolabial herpes infection	Keratinized mucosa (hard palate, gingiva)
Aphthous ulcers	No vesicles, nonkeratinized, and moveable mucosa
Herpangina	Acute, multiple ulcers, posterior oral cavity, mild systemic symptoms, more common in children
Hand-food-mouth disease	Anterior oral cavity, hand, and foot lesions
Lichen planus[a]	Wickham striae[b], other skin or genital mucosal lesions
Drug induced	Beta-blockers, mycophenolate, anticholinergic bronchodilators, clopidogrel, nonsteroidal anti-inflammatory drugs, captopril, antimetabolites, taxanes, alkylating agents, vinca alkaloids
Erythema multiforme[a]	Often spared gingiva, widespread, irregular ulcers, blood-crusted lips, with or without targetoid skin lesions
Pemphigus vulgaris[a]	Posterior oral cavity and gingival ulcers
Behcet's disease	Uveitis, genital ulcers, acneiform lesions, pseudofolliculitis, erythema nodosum-like lesions, arthritis

[a] Biopsy is needed to confirm the diagnosis.
[b] Wickham striae are pathognomonic for lichen planus and appear as white reticulated patches on the buccal mucosa.
Data from Refs.[5,6]

Potential complications are urinary retention, aseptic meningitis, pharyngitis, and psychological morbidity.[10] The differential diagnosis for genital ulcers includes genital HSV in addition to other infectious and inflammatory causes (**Table 2**).

Transmission of Orofacial Herpes and Genital Herpes

Transmission of orofacial, intraoral, and genital herpes occurs by direct contact between mucous membranes, respiratory droplets, or impaired skin with mucosal secretions or ulcerative lesions of a person with active primary or recurrent infection. Clinicians often misuse the term "recurrence." Viral reactivation that results in asymptomatic viral shedding is considered a recurrence, whereas viral reactivation that produces clinical disease or symptoms is termed "recrudescence."[15]

Symptomatic lesions are more infectious because they contain higher virus titers; however, asymptomatic shedding is the predominant mode of transmission. Studies have shown that only approximately 20% to 50% of people with HSV-2 serology

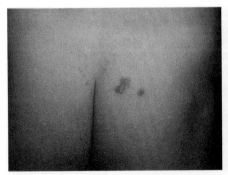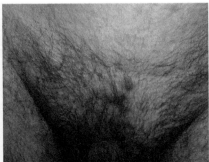

Fig. 4. Primary genital herpes caused by HSV-2.

Table 2	
Differential diagnosis of genital ulcers	
Differential Diagnosis	**Clinical Features**
Infectious causes	
Syphilis	Painless chancre with nontender LAD
Chancroid	Painful ulcer and LAD
Lymphogranuloma venereum	Painless ulcer, lymphadenitis
Donovanosis	Painless ulcerations, no LAD
Scabies	Excoriated red papules, burrows
Candida	Shallow, bright red
Cutaneous Crohn disease	Genital edema, linear "knife-like" ulceration, abdominal symptoms
Behcet's disease	Painful oral ulcers, uveitis, pathergy, arthralgias, gastrointestinal symptoms
Contact dermatitis	Complex topical products (ie, scented feminine hygiene products)
Reactive arthritis	Arthritis, uveitis, urethritis, cervicitis, buccal, mucosal and glans penile ulcers
Lichen planus	Inner aspect labia majora or glans penis
Pemphigus vulgaris	Oral ulcers and flaccid bullae/erosions on skin
Pyoderma gangrenosum	Painful ulcers with purpuric borders and undermined margins
Erythema multiforme	Herpes simplex virus, *Mycoplasma* associated, drug-induced

Abbreviation: LAD, lymphadenopathy
Data from Refs.[11–14]

are aware that they are infected.[16] Asymptomatic or unrecognized viral shedding is responsible for transmission of more than half of primary cases.[17]

Asymptomatic shedding varies by location, subtype, and primary or recurrent status. High-risk periods of asymptomatic shedding for genital herpes occur most commonly in the first 3 months after primary infection, during the prodrome, and the week following a symptomatic recurrence.[18–20] Infections that are primary, HSV-2 positive, and located to the perineum have a longer duration of shedding.[21,22] Having symptomatic genital herpes does not increase the risk of subclinical shedding compared with patients who are seropositive without a history of clinically evident disease.[22,23]

Anticipatory Guidance for Patients Regarding Herpes Simplex Virus-1 and Herpes Simplex Virus-2 Transmission

Patients with recrudescent genital herpes should be counseled to practice safe sex behaviors, including abstinence during outbreaks, and using condoms in all sexual encounters. Asymptomatic seropositive patients pose a greater challenge. However, when educated on the signs and symptoms of genital herpes, many "asymptomatic" patients begin to recognize clinical symptoms. Although asymptomatic seropositive patients experience less viral shedding than symptomatic seropositive patients, they can still transmit genital herpes in an unpredictable manner. Daily antiviral suppressive therapy has been shown to decrease HSV recrudescence, viral shedding, and transmission in serodiscordant sexual partners.[24]

Should everyone be screened for HSV-1 and HSV-2 with a blood test? This is a controversial public health question. Many clinicians fear the psychosocial consequences of mass serotesting and labeling millions of people with an incurable disease in addition to significant burdens to the health care system. Mass screening may be associated with severe anxiety to patients, increased psychological counseling, more costs related to testing, and an increase in suppressive therapy regimens related to increased diagnoses. Serologic testing may also be associated with a high rate of false-positive test results.[25] Patients with HSV have also expressed concerns related to personalized stigma, disclosure concerns, negative self-image, and concern with public attitudes.[25] The latest US Preventive Services Task Force (USPSTF) in 2016 recommend against routine serologic screening for genital HSV infections in asymptomatic adolescents and adults, including those who are pregnant.[26]

It is generally considered appropriate to initiate suppressive therapy for serodiscordant couples in which 1 partner is seropositive and the other is not and for patients who have psychological distress to their diagnosis.

HERPES SIMPLEX VIRUS INFECTION IN THE IMMUNOCOMPROMISED PATIENT

Patients who are immunocompromised (ie, those who are human immunodeficiency virus [HIV] positive, have undergone bone marrow or solid organ transplants, or are dependent on hemodialysis) have a heightened risk of acquiring opportunistic infections. Additionally, they may exhibit atypical symptoms of common infections like herpesvirus infections. While the clinical manifestations of HSV-1 and HSV-2 infections are similar between those with normal and compromised immune systems, the latter group may present variations in symptomatology. Infections in the immunocompromised patient group are more frequent, symptomatic, progressive, poorly responsive to therapy, associated with longer duration of shedding, involve multiple sites, and are at higher risk for viremic dissemination. Intraoral lesions are more extensive, surrounded by white elevated border and involve both keratinized and nonkeratinized mucosa. Genital HSV-1 and HSV-2 can be more atypical, such as painful verrucous nodules and persistent ulcers. Cutaneous HSV infection lesions have presented with ulceration of "knife-like" skin fissures in the abdominal, infra-abdominal, and inframammary skin folds, the interlabial and the gluteal cleft, and the inguinal crease.[5,27]

ECZEMA HERPETICUM

Eczema herpeticum (EH) describes herpes-infected dermatitis. Atopic dermatitis (AD) is the most common dermatitis implicated in EH with about 3% of patients developing this complication over their lifetime, but herpes simplex can secondarily infect many other chronic dermatoses. Other dermatoses that can be affected are pemphigus foliaceus, mycosis fungoides, ichthyosis vulgaris, Hailey–Hailey disease, irritant contact dermatitis, pityriasis rubra pilaris, and burns. Hematological abnormalities with a report of EH include cutaneous T-cell lymphoma and Sézary disease.[28] Classically, patients present with disseminated widespread monomorphic vesicles accompanied by fever, malaise, and lymphadenopathy. The vesicles crust over and heal by 6 weeks in most cases. However, often the presentation is more subtle, fissured disseminated plaques, flaring atopic dermatitis with punched out erosions, and a component of periorbital involvement with blepharitis can all indicate an occult herpes infection. The head, neck, and trunk are the most affected sites.

The use of topical corticosteroids has not been shown to increase the risk of EH. Topical calcineurin inhibitors may predispose a patient who is at increased risk and are contraindicated in acute EH. Antiviral therapy should be set up as soon as EH is suspected as EH can potentially be fatal with a mortality rate of 10% to 75% in its severe form.[29] Clinicians must maintain a high index of suspicion for herpes infection when a patient with chronic dermatosis presents with a flaring dermatosis or widespread monomorphic vesicles within the chronic dermatosis. All patients should be questioned about recent herpes outbreaks.

HERPES SIMPLEX ENCEPHALITIS

Herpes simplex encephalitis (HSE) has an incidence of 1 to 3 per million.[30] There is a bimodal age distribution affecting patients younger than 20 and older than 50 with a peak between 60 and 64. More than 90% of HSE in immunocompetent patients are HSV-1 related. Only 1.6% to 6.5% of HSE cases are HSV-2 related and typically occur in immunosuppressed patients.[30,31] HSE is the most frequent cause of sporadic necrotizing encephalitis in adults. Worldwide it accounts for 5% to 10% of all cases of encephalitis.[32]

HSE is generally not considered a sign of immunocompromise except in cases of bone marrow transplantation and acquired immunodeficiency syndrome (AIDS).[33,34] There are a number of reports of HSE following neurosurgery (eg, cervical spine laminectomy, acoustic neuroma resection).[35,36] Recent studies have elucidated *toll-like receptor*-(TLR 3) interferon pathways resulting in increased susceptibility to HSE. Both animal models and humans also indicate that cytolytic viral replication and immune-mediated responses (including cytotoxic T lymphocytes and immune mechanisms mediated by TLR 2) contribute to the pathology of HSV.[37]

Patients in the following settings should have cerebrospinal fluid (CSF) examination for HSV: patients presenting with fever, headache, and malaise for several days with progression to behavioral changes, seizures, focal neurologic signs, or cognitive difficulties, especially in patients with neuroimaging alterations (particularly in the medial temporal lobes, insular cortex, and orbital frontal lobes).[34] Central nervous system (CNS) manifestations might occur before the skin eruptions.[38] A personal history or an exposure history of "cold sores" or genital herpes should be elicited. In patients with AIDS, HSE may present with personality and behavioral changes but without fever or headache.[39]

The current gold standard confirmatory test for HSE is polymerase chain reaction (PCR) to detect HSV DNA in the CSF, whose sensitivity is approximately 96% with a specificity of 99% in experienced laboratories. Analysis on CSF frequently demonstrates WBC count of 100 to 200 cells/mm^3 with mild to moderately elevated CSF protein levels ($\sim$100 mg/dL) and normal glucose.[32] Diagnosis of HSE can be difficult, viral DNA by PCR can be negative initially. CSF cell count is normal in 5% to 10% of patients, computed tomography (CT) results are normal in the first week of illness in up to 33% of patients and MRI can be normal in up to 10% of patients.

ANTI-N-METHYL-D-ASPARTATE RECEPTOR ANTIBODY ENCEPHALITIS

Autoimmune encephalitis or anti-N-methyl-d-aspartate (NMDA) receptor (NMDAR) antibody encephalitis is a newly described cause of encephalitis within the last decade. It is critically important to distinguish this disease entity from HSE as therapeutic approaches are very different. Anti-NMDAR immunoglobulin (Ig)G serology in the blood and CSF coupled by symptoms of choreoathetosis, memory, behavioral changes, and seizures in the setting of previously diagnosed HSV encephalitis can aid in this distinction. The optimal management of autoimmune encephalitis is still unclear. Key questions, such as whether intravenous immunoglobulin is beneficial as a first-line therapy, remain to be clarified by randomized controlled trials. In contrast, intravenous acyclovir for HSE is a life-saving treatment and has reduced mortality from above 70% to around 10% to 20%.[32,37]

Varicella-zoster virusVaricella-zoster virus (VZV) produces 2 clinically distinct diseases. Primary infection with VZV causes varicella or "chickenpox," a vesicular rash most seen in young children. Unlike HSV-1 and HSV-2, primary VZV infection has a systemic phase of viremia. Inhalation of infectious particles colonizes respiratory lymphoid tissue and then spread systemically to the dermis via cutaneous vasculature.[40] This neurotropic virus later becomes latent, primarily in neurons in peripheral autonomic ganglia throughout the entire neuroaxis including dorsal root ganglia (DRG), cranial nerve ganglia such as the trigeminal ganglia (TG), and autonomic ganglia including those in the enteric nervous system. Reactivation of VZV infection results in herpes zoster or "shingles" which occurs up to decades following primary inoculation, presenting as a painful dermatomal vesicular rash. Unlike HSV, VZV tends to reactivate with increasing age and people older than 60 years are 8 to 10 times more likely to develop herpes zoster. VZV cell-mediated immunity declines with age despite unchanged or increased antibody titers. Reactivation of VZV may also cause a wide variety of neurologic syndromes, the most significant of which is a vasculitis, which is treated with corticosteroids and the antiviral drug acyclovir. Other VZV reactivation complications include encephalitis, segmental motor weakness and myelopathy, cranial neuropathies, and Guillain–Barré syndrome in which the viral reactivation occurs in the absence of the characteristic dermatomal distributed vesicular rash of herpes zoster.[41–44]

Primary Varicella

Primary varicella (VZV) or "chickenpox" is predominantly a disease of childhood. The incidence has dramatically decreased since the advent of the childhood vaccine in 1995. Although uncommon, adults can contract primary varicella. A seronegative adult can contract primary varicella from a person with varicella by inhalation of respiratory secretions, contact with skin lesions, or from mucocutaneous contact with someone with herpes zoster. Patients who are susceptible and exposed to VZV should be placed under airborne and contact precautions (**Table 3**).[45] According to the Centers for Disease Control and Prevention, an immunocompetent patient is considered contagious 2 days before the onset of a rash until about 5 days after rash onset and all lesions are dry and crusted.[46] Immunocompromised patients may be contagious for a longer period. Psychosocial needs must be balanced with infection control in long-term care facilities because of psychosocial risks associated with restriction.[46]

Primary varicella infection in adults or in an immunocompromised patient may be more severe. The conjunctiva and the upper respiratory tract mucosa are the most common portals of entry. The virus undergoes a primary viremia between days 4

Table 3 Isolation guidelines for varicella		
	Immunocompetent	**Immunocompromised**
Localized herpes zoster	Standard precautions Completely cover lesions	Standard precautions + airborne (until disseminated herpes zoster is ruled out)
Disseminated herpes zoster	Standard precautions + airborne contact	Standard precautions + airborne contact

and 6 in the regional lymph nodes, and then travels to the liver and spleen before hematogenous spread to other organs (eg, lungs, CNS, and skin).[47]

In addition to a low-grade fever and malaise, patients can develop a pruritic rash that evolves through several stages. Erythematous macules and papules present early in the disease course on the scalp and face. Within 12 to 24 hours, the rash may progress to the characteristic vesicles on an erythematous base and then ultimately pustules and crusted scabs.[44] Patients may exhibit lesions in various stages of healing, develop new lesions every few days, and display centripetal rash spread (ie, from the face to the trunk and extremities).[44] Adult primary varicella resembles the childhood type, but can have larger and an increased number of lesions as well as prolonged fever, and other constitutional symptoms. Primary varicella in immunocompromised patients may be more severe and even fatal.[44,48]

The most common cutaneous complication is bacterial superinfection secondary to *Staphylococcus aureus* or *Streptococcus pyogenes,* which can contribute to scarring.[48] Cases of staphylococcal and streptococcal toxic shock and severe soft tissue infections such as varicella-associated necrotizing fasciitis have been reported. Beta hemolytic streptococcal necrotizing fasciitis requires early, aggressive surgical debridement and targeted antibiotics.[49]

Adults and immunocompromised patients have a higher risk of developing complications from chickenpox compared to healthy children (eg, pneumonitis and neurologic sequelae). The mortality rate of adult varicella pneumonia ranges between 10% and 30% and up to 50% in those requiring mechanical ventilation.[50] The most common neurologic symptoms of primary VZV include acute cerebellitis and stroke (especially in childhood).[51] Other neurologic symptoms include myelitits, meningitis, and acute demyelinating radiculoneuropathy. Most cases with neurologic sequelae occur a week following rash onset, but symptoms may also develop without a rash.[51] Presenting symptoms may include the abrupt or gradual onset of fever, headache, vomiting, lethargy, seizures, meningismus, and coma.[51] CSF evaluation sometimes shows a low-grade lymphocytosis and elevated protein.[52] Fortunately, the cerebellar ataxias are self-limited and most patients recover within 1 to 3 weeks without permanent deficits.

Varicella encephalitis is the most serious CNS complication with mortality ranging from 5% to 10% and up to 80% in immunocompromised patients.[53] Other rare systemic complications of primary varicella in adults include myocarditis, glomerulonephritis, appendicitis, pancreatitis, hepatitis, Henoch–Schonlein vasculitis, orchitis, arthritis, optic neuritis, keratitis, and iritis.[54]

Herpes Zoster (Shingles)

Herpes zoster typically affects people older than 60 years secondary to decreased VZV-specific cell-mediated immunity (**Figs. 5** and **6**). Risk factors include chemotherapy, immunosuppressive agents (eg, prednisone used in transplant recipients and treatments for autoimmune disorders), biologics, and HIV/AIDS. It can be the first manifestation of HIV.[55]

Classic herpes zoster is characterized by an acute onset, sharp radicular pain, and the eruption of grouped vesicles on an erythematous base distributed in up to 3 dermatomes. Cutaneous lesions tend to respect the midline, which is a helpful feature to differentiate from HSV infection. Lesions on the chest (thoracic dermatomes) are the most common, followed by the face (trigeminal dermatome).[41]

Pain is often accompanied with pruritus, decreased sensation, and allodynia within the affected dermatome(s). In more than 90% of cases, pain precedes the skin eruption by days to a week.[56] It is easy to misdiagnose the pain as myocardial infarction,

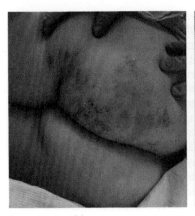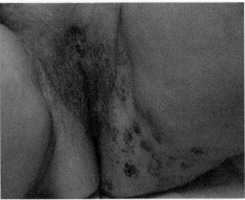

Fig. 5. Perineal herpes zoster.

pleurisy, cholecystitis, appendicitis, duodenal ulcer, ovarian cyst, herniated intervertebral disc, thrombophlebitis, or even biliary or renal colic. Zoster sine herpete describes a zoster-like neuropathic pain in a dermatomal distribution without an accompanying rash.[57] Reported cases noted rising titers of VZV-specific antibody

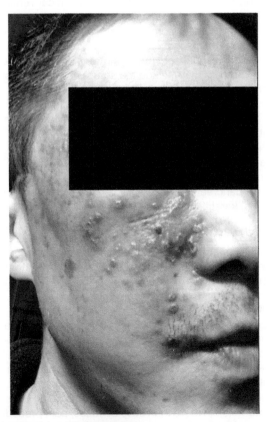

Fig. 6. Herpes zoster involving V2 dermatome.

in the serum and CSF as well as VZV DNA detected in the CSF and peripheral blood mononuclear cells by PCR.[41] Disseminated VZV is clinically like disseminated HSV and immunocompromised patients are at a significantly higher risk. Dissemination is defined as 20 or more individual vesicles distributed beyond the primary and adjacent dermatomes. Multisystem organ involvement (eg, lung, liver, and CNS) follows cutaneous dissemination in about 10% of high-risk patients.[58] Like primary varicella, the pain and extent of skin involvement in herpes zoster is more severe in the elderly and immunocompromised.

Neurologic Complications of Herpes Zoster

Possible neurologic sequelae of VZV reactivation are protean and include postherpetic neuralgia (PHN), cranial neuropathies, vasculopathy, myelitis, necrotizing retinitis, and zoster sine herpete. These complications can present as transient ischemic attacks, ischemic or hemorrhagic stroke, aneurysm, contralateral hemiparesis, bowel or bladder incontinence, chest pain, and blindness (**Box 1**).

PHN is the most common cause of morbidity in patients older than 60 years. It is defined as pain that persists for months to years after resolution of the herpes zoster cutaneous eruption.[62] There is a disproportionate frequency of PHN in patients older than 60 years (67%) compared to the number of herpes zoster cases (38%) in this age group.[63] The frequency and severity of PHN increases with age. About 20% of people aged 60 to 65 who have had acute herpes zoster developed PHN, compared to over 30% of people aged 80 or older. Cranial neuropathies and vasculopathy-associated neurologic symptoms can occur weeks after acute zoster.[41]

VZV infection of large or small cerebral arteries may cause an occlusive or inflammatory VZV vasculopathy with varied clinical presentations. When affecting the first division of the trigeminal nerve, the patient can experience delayed contralateral hemplegia days to weeks following herpes zoster. There is often no rash at the time of neurologic symptoms (headache, fever, mental status changes, and focal deficits). PCR can detect viral DNA in the CSF and MRI T2-weighted images may reveal focal enhancement at involved sites.[71–73] Viral invasion of vessels can produce cerebral aneurysms, hemorrhage, myelitis, and retinal necrosis. Although uncommon, when CNS sequelae are present, immunocompetent patients tend to develop large-vessel granulomatous arteritis, whereas immunocompromised patients are more apt to develop small-vessel encephalitis.[41]

Box 1 Neurologic complications	
CNS Location	**Clinical Presentation Including Neurologic Signs and Symptoms**
Oculomotor (CNIII) > Trochlear (CNIV) > Abducens (CNVI)	Ophthalmoplegia, optic neuritis, or both[59–61]
Trigeminal (CNV) Ophthalmic division	Keratitis, vesicles on nasal tip (Hutchinson sign), blindness
Maxillary and mandibular divisions	Osteonecrosis and spontaneous exfoliation of teeth[64,65]
Facial (CNVII)	Unilateral facial muscle weakness, rash of ipsilateral external ear, anterior two-thirds tongue, or hard palate (Ramsay Hunt syndrome))[41,66]
Cervical spine	Arm weakness >>> diaphragmatic paralysis[67–69]
Lumbosacral spine	Leg weakness >>> bladder, bowel dysfunction[70]

Herpes Zoster in Human Immunodeficiency Virus/Acquired Immunodeficiency Syndrome

Herpes Zoster (HZ) is an HIV-associated opportunistic infection. HIV infected populations have a 3-fold to 20-fold higher risk of contracting HZ than HIV-seronegative individuals.[74] The presence of VZV antibodies shows past exposure to chickenpox or vaccination, but in HIV-infected individuals, it is the low CD4 count and lack of antiretroviral therapy (ART) use, not VZV antibody levels, that better predict future shingles outbreaks.[75] Even though the introduction of ART has improved the survival of those living with HIV, the incidence of HZ among HIV cohorts remains higher than that of the general population.[74]

Clinically, patients with HIV may develop zoster in more than 1 dermatome. Cutaneous lesions can be atypical, such as hyperkeratotic, ulcerative with a black eschar, chronic in nature, and lacking a dermatomal distribution.[76,77] Certain severe complications are almost exclusively seen in HIV/AIDS or patients with impaired cell-mediated immunity. Chronic VZV encephalitis can occur months after a herpes zoster outbreak and present subacutely with headache, fever, mental status changes, seizures, and focal neurologic defects, as well as visual field cuts. The underlying pathology is a VZV-induced small-vessel vasculitis and demyelination. MRI is the best modality to investigate this type of acute encephalitis. There are anecdotal reports that high-dose intravenous acyclovir may be of benefit and adjunctive treatment with steroids remains a matter of debate; however, the clinical course is often progressive and results in death. A progressive and potentially fatal myelitis is also a possibility in the immunocompromised subset. Studies have shown a mortality rate between 4% and 25%. Factors associated with poor outcomes include mechanical ventilation and older age.[76,78] Overall, HIV patients with zoster show increased neurologic (eg, aseptic meningitis, radiculitis, and myelitis) and ophthalmologic complications, particularly peripheral outer retinal necrosis.

LABORATORY DIAGNOSIS OF HERPES SIMPLEX VIRUS AND VARICELLA-ZOSTER VIRUS

Several factors contribute to the ability to isolate herpes simplex and herpes zoster. Host factors, as well as selecting the appropriate test and executing the proper collection, transport, and storage of the specimen, are important. Lesions from immunosuppressed patients have a higher virus load than those from immunocompetent patients. Regardless of the host, an early vesicle has the highest viral yield compared with healed crusted lesions. Similarly, it is easier to detect virus in a primary infection compared with a secondary infection (primary infections have higher titers of virus). Each test has its own advantages and disadvantages. Combining 2 or more methods can increase sensitivity of detection.[79]

There are numerous laboratory tests available to identify herpetic infections. They can be categorized into 5 main methods: morphologic, immunologic, serologic, virologic, and molecular.[80,81] Physicians confirm their diagnosis using diverse laboratory techniques such as Tzanck smear, HSV culture, direct immunofluorescence (IF), or PCR. When it comes to diagnosis, molecular biological techniques are preferentially chosen because of their ease of use, reliability, and high sensitivity. Indeed, PCR is positive in 100% of cases when performed on early lesions, and positivity rates remain higher than 80% on later lesions as well (over 30 days).[82]

Viral culture is considered the gold standard diagnostic modality. Other diagnostic tests are often compared with viral culture when evaluating sensitivity and specificity. Rapid viral culture is available for HSV and VZV, which shortened the time for isolation to 4 days.[82] With newer PCR protocols (eg, real-time, nested) that take approximately 1 day to process, it has been proposed that PCR replace viral culture as the gold standard diagnostic test.[83]

Morphologic: Tzanck Smear and Tissue Biopsy

Tzanck smear is a common in-office procedure that is rapid and inexpensive but performer dependent. A fresh vesicle is more likely to result in a positive Tzanck smear than a pustule or crusted ulcer.[84–86] The base of a vesicle is scraped and then the cellular contents are mounted on a slide and stained with Giemsa, Wright, or Papanico laou. A positive smear demonstrates multinucleated giant cell formation, margination of nuclear chromatin, and molding of the nuclei by light microscopy. Tzanck smear cannot differentiate between HSV and VZV, and it requires an experienced interpreter.

A punch or shave skin biopsy from the edge of a lesion is positive if it displays characteristic viral cytopathic effect, such as ballooned or multinucleated keratinocytes with nuclear molding and margination of chromatin. Necrotic hair follicles can be a clue to adjacent herpetic infection as well. The sensitivity and specificity of a lesional skin biopsy are similar to a lesional Tzanck smear.[87] Like a Tzanck smear, a skin biopsy with routine staining cannot delineate HSV-1 from HSV-2 or VZV without immunohistochemical staining. Histologic examination is a reasonable choice to confirm HSV in an old, atypical lesion and to exclude other disease processes with similar clinical features.[81]

Immunomorphologic: Immunofluorescence and Immunoperoxidase Staining

Immunomorphologic techniques are used to identify viral antigens. Direct immunofluorescence uses direct application of viral antigen-specific fluorescein-tagged antibodies to a specimen. This method is rapid, sensitive, and specific and can be done on frozen or formalin-fixed paraffin-embedded sections. It can distinguish between HSV-1, HSV-2, and VZV. Immunoperoxidase technique is not as sensitive but is more specific. It can be performed on fixed or fresh tissue.[88] For VZV, immunofluorescence is more sensitive than viral culture or Tzanck smear. Combining viral antigen methods with viral culture can more rapidly detect HSV or VZV than biopsy, as it may take time for cytopathic effect to evolve.

Serologic Tests

Serologic tests are used to detect previous infection with HSV-1 or HSV-2 when a viral culture is not feasible, or the clinical presentation is unclear. Serologic tests use specific viral proteins, purified or recombinant.[89] These tests use serum to detect the presence of antibodies against HSV 1 and HSV-2. Due to the limited timeframe for the treatment of HSV, these tests must be obtained within the period of acute illness and 3 to 4 weeks later.

By the time a primary infection is established using this method, it is not clinically helpful, as the patient is outside the effective treatment window but provides information to guide future treatment. Fewer than 5% of patients with recurrent HSV infection will have a significant rise in antibody level.[90] Although antibody titers can fluctuate, these fluctuations do not reliably predict recurrent episodes or asymptomatic viral shedding.[91,92] There are certain circumstances in which serologic testing makes sense. The presence of old lesions and inadequate transport of specimens (and therefore compromised quality of specimen) are instances in which a serologic test may help. Serology is also valuable in screening pregnant women who may require acyclovir prophylaxis for HSV-2.

The diagnosis of genital herpes causes significant psychological distress. Despite a characteristic clinical history (eg, prodromal symptoms, recurrent crusted papules), a negative culture or indeterminate examination is a source of frustration for a patient. In this instance, establishing seropositivity to HSV-2 by serology can provide the patient with objective confirmation of genital herpes. Conversely, the absence of seropositivity can exclude the diagnosis of genital herpes.[93] Serologic diagnosis of HSV-2 should ideally be performed only if patients and providers are aware of the test's high sensitivity but low specificity.[94] In a study by Munday and colleagues, serologic testing contributed to diagnosis in 79% of cases of recurrent genital ulcerations.[95] Seropositivity of HSV-1 is more difficult to interpret. Historically, HSV-1 was considered restricted to orolabial infections; however, there is an increased prevalence of HSV-1 genital infection. A seropositive HSV-1 result cannot delineate an orolabial from a genital infection with certainty.[93]

Serologic tests are either type specific (differentiates HSV-1 from HSV-2) or non–type specific. Non–type-specific serologic modalities include complement fixation tests, direct hemagglutination, fluorescent antibody to membrane antigen, and enzyme-linked immunosorbent assay (ELISA). Complement fixation test has been the most used and is considered the standard serologic test for HSV identification but is less sensitive than other serologic tests. Western blot is considered the epidemiologic gold standard, but it is expensive, labor intensive, and performed at research centers only. Although historically ELISA tests were not the most reliable, newer assays in the past 10 years have improved significantly. Recombinant ELISA assays have excellent sensitivity and specificity. The sensitivity and specificity of the recombinant assay for HSV-1 immunoglobulin G (IgG) were 93.1% to 98.0% and 99.3% to 100.0%, respectively, whereas the sensitivity and specificity of the novel assays for HSV-2 IgG are 100.0% and 94.6% to 97.6%. respectively.[96]

Type-specific tests are neutralization tests, protein-specific assays, and Western blot (immunoblot) analysis. Type-specific tests are more challenging, as both HSV-1 and HSV-2 share many immunogenic antigens. Preexisting HSV-1 seropositivity impairs the sensitivity of HSV-2 serologic response. Seropositivity to HSV-2 can be blunted by the presence of type-common antigens recognized in earlier HSV-1 infections.[93] Western blot is best used for this clinical scenario. Identification of the type of HSV provides clinically helpful prognostic information to the patient, as type 1 versus type 2 exhibits different rates of shedding, recurrence, and transmission. Newer techniques such as the testing of dried blood samples (DBS) allow for a noninvasive sample collection and longer shelf life.[89] Currently, standardized testing protocols for DBS are being developed for review and approval by regulatory agencies.[97]

Virologic & Molecular

While viral cultures are considered to be the gold standard for diagnosing HSV and VZV, viral PCR tests allow for a more sensitive and rapid diagnosis.[98,99] By day 4 of a recurrent lesion outbreak, it is unlikely to obtain positive cultures from an ulcer or crusted lesion and the sensitivity of a positive viral culture is about 50% for genital ulcers.[21] HSV grows faster than VZV and therefore more than 50% of inoculations are positive within 24 to 48 hours and more than 90% are positive within 3 to 4 days. However, VZV takes 7 days to 2 weeks to process by traditional viral culture. New culture techniques (shell vial technique and blind passage) provide a rapid and more sensitive method, which takes only 4 days and increases the rate of VZV isolation from tissue.[100]

Tips for obtaining viral culture and viral PCR.

- Identify a new vesicle if possible.

- Unroof intact vesicle with a sharp (eg, 11 blade or 25-gauge) needle and be aware that vesicle fluid may splash. Vigorously scrape base of ulcer, as this increases likelihood of obtaining specimens with live virus.[80]
- If lesions are crusted, remove necrotic debris with sterile saline before scraping base for culture.[80,101]
- Use viral culture medium (should be refrigerated until use) and a plastic applicator with a Dacron (or rayon) tip. If viral media is not available, the culture swab should be kept moist with non-bacteriostatic sterile saline.
- If transport time is longer than 8 hours, the swabs should be removed after swirling in the medium.
- A wood applicator with cotton tip should never be used, as they may harbor substances that kill the virus.
- Specimen should be refrigerated at 4°C until inoculation.

PCR is a very sensitive molecular technique to isolate viral DNA. It can distinguish HSV-1 from HSV-2 and VZV. It can detect occult HSV, atypical presentations of HSV, and zoster sine herpete. PCR is the test of choice for VZV, as it is more rapid, highly sensitive, and specific (compared to culture).[81] A classic clinical presentation of herpes zoster may not necessitate laboratory testing; however, if the eruption is more than 3 day old or atypical, it may be prudent to proceed with PCR testing.

DIAGNOSIS OF NEUROLOGIC MANIFESTATIONS
Herpes Simplex Encephalopathy

The sensitivity and specificity for CSF PCR HSV-1 DNA are 98% and 94%, respectively, compared with histology on brain biopsy.[80] The most fruitful window to obtain a positive CSF PCR in HSE is between 2 and 10 days after the onset of illness.[102] CT scanning can be normal in the first 4 to 6 days of illness. MRI is more sensitive than CT, demonstrating high-signal-intensity lesions on T2-weighted, diffusion-weighted, and fluid-attenuated inversion recovery images earlier in the course.[103,104]

Zoster Encephalopathy

Detecting VZV DNA by PCR and VZV IgM and IgG antibodies to VZV in the CSF are confirmatory. Antibodies in the CSF alone without amplification of VZV DNA are supportive in the appropriate clinical setting. Serum antibodies are not relevant because most adults have persistent antibodies to VZV in their serum.[105]

WOLF POSTHERPETIC ISOTOPIC RESPONSE

Immunity-dependent disorders can occur in a zoster-affected dermatome, or after an HSV or varicella infection (**Box 2**). This phenomenon is called Wolf's postherpetic isotopic response (PHIR). An altered secretary immunopeptide milieu is hypothesized to be the cause of PHIR. Zoster-affected sensory neurons may display dysfunctional neuropeptide release, affecting local immune responses.[107]

MANAGEMENT OF HERPES SIMPLEX VIRUS AND VARICELLA-ZOSTER VIRUS

The immune status of the patient, comorbidities, the type of infection (primary vs recurrent), and the extent of the infection (dermatomal vs disseminated) all influence the management of herpes viral infection (**Tables 4** and **5**). Nucleoside analogs that inhibit viral DNA synthesis are the main-stay of herpes viral infections. Acyclovir, valacyclovir, and famciclovir are all in this class of medication, but vary based on dosing schedule and bioavailability. Acyclovir has poor bioavailability (10% to 20% compared

---

Box 2
Skin diseases with predilection for previously VZV-infected dermatomes

Granulomatous reactions
   Granuloma annulare
   Sarcoidosis

Malignant tumors
   Breast cancer
   Basal cell carcinoma
   Squamous cell carcinoma
   Angiosarcoma
   Kaposi sarcoma
   Metastases from cutaneous or visceral malignancies

Inflammatory reactions
   Lichen planus
   Lichen sclerosus et atrophicus
   Graft-versus-host disease
   Drug rash
   IgA linear dermatosis
   Psoriasis

Infections (bacterial, fungal, viral)

Acneiform lesions

Rosacea

Pseudolymphoma

Mucinosis

Data from Wolf R, Brenner S, Ruocco V, et al. Isotopic Response. Int J Dermatol 1995;34(5):341-8.[106]

---

to its prodrug, valacyclovir).[115] Oral valacyclovir can achieve a similar plasma level as intravenous (IV) acyclovir. IV acyclovir is contraindicated in renal disease given its association with crystalline nephropathy.[116] Famciclovir has been shown to be superior to valacyclovir in reducing herpes zoster pain.[117] The benefit of antiviral therapy is most effective when initiated within the first 72 hours of disease onset. The number of recurrences of HSV each year helps guide the decision to initiate suppressive therapy. Chronic suppressive treatment may be indicated in patients who experience 6 or

Table 4
Adverse effects of antiviral therapies

Medication	Side Effects
Acyclovir	Nausea, vomiting, rarely headaches and diarrhea in long-term use—PO Phlebitis, reversible crystalline nephropathy—IV
Valacyclovir	Headache—PO Thrombotic microangiopathy in patients with long-term HIV
Famciclovir	Headache, nausea, vomiting
Foscarnet	Renal toxicity, electrolyte imbalances (hypocalcemia), nausea, vomting, anemia, penile ulcers
Cidofovir	Highly nephrotoxic - IV

Abbreviations: IV, intravenous; PO, oral.
Data from Refs.[5,108,109]

Table 5
Treatment schedules

	Acyclovir	Valacyclovir	Famciclovir
Herpes labialis			
Recurrent	400 mg 5 times/d for 5 d	2 g q 12 h for 1 d PO	1500 mg × 1 dose
Chronic suppression	400 mg BID-TID	500 mg daily PO or 1 g daily PO	500 mg BID PO
Immunosuppressed	400 mg TID 5–10 d	1 g BID for 5–10 d PO	
Genital HSV			
Primary	200 mg 5 times/d or 400 mg TID for 7–10 d PO	1 g BID for 7–10 d PO	250 mg TID for 5–10 d PO
Recurrent	200 mg 5 times/d for 5–10 d or 400 mg TID for 5 d or 800 mg TID for 2 d PO or 800 mg TID for 5 d PO	0.5 g BID for 3 d or 1 g qd for 5 d PO	1 g BID for 1 d or 500 mg for 1 d then 250 mg BID for 2 d then 125 mg BID for 5 d PO
Immunosuppressed	400 mg TID for 5–10 d	1 g BID for 5–10 d	500 mg BID for 5–10 d
Chronic suppression	400 mg BID PO	1 g daily or 500 mg daily	250 mg BID
Immunosuppressed	400–800 mg BID or TID PO	500 mg BID PO	500 mg BID
Cutaneous HSV			
Primary			
Recurrent in HIV	400 mg TID for 5–10 d PO	1 g BID for 5–10 d	500 mg BID
Chronic suppression in HIV	400–800 mg BID or TID PO	500 mg BID PO	500 mg BID
Varicella			
Primary	10 mg/kg IV q8 h or 20 mg/kg (1 g max) TID × 5 d PO		
Immunosuppressed	VZIG within 72 h[a]		
Herpes zoster			
Primary	5–10 mg/kg body weight TID for 7 d IV or 800 mg 5 times/d for 7 d PO	100 mg TID for 7 d PO	500 mg TID for 7 d PO
Disseminated	10–15 mg/kg IV q 8 h × 7 d or 500 mg/m^2 IV q 8 h × 7 d		

(continued on next page)

Table 5
(continued)

	Acyclovir	Valacyclovir	Famciclovir
Eczema herpeticum			
Mild[29,109,110]	Children: 3–60 mg/kg TID Adults: 400 mg TID	Children: 20 mg/kg/day Adults: 500 mg TID	
Severe[111]	Acyclovir IV 5–10 mg/kg q 8 h		

Abbreviations: bid, twice a day; HSV, herpes simplex virus; IV, intravenous; PO, oral; q, every; tid, 3 times a day; VZIG, varicella zoster immunoglobulin.

[a] In immunocompromised seronegative patients, VZIG if administered within the first 72 h can prevent dissemination.

Data from Refs.[29,108–114]

more recurrences of HSV a year, have severe pain or disfigurement, difficulty swallowing, or a protracted disease course.[108]

Topical antivirals are an additional treatment modality (**Table 6**). Randomized placebo-controlled clinical studies assessing acyclovir topical treatments (creams vs ointments, 5% vs 10%) show mixed outcomes. Most evidence shows topical acyclovir ointment is not effective in treating recurrent herpes labialis because of poor penetration. Five percent acyclovir cream can reduce the duration of lesions if applied during the prodromal stage, but does not reduce pain.[112] 1% penciclovir cream can decrease duration of the lesions and pain if applied every 2 hours after the onset of prodromal symptom.[118] Topical docosanol (10%) can reduce healing time of recurrent herpes labialis when applied 5 times a day for 10 days.[119,120] Foscarnet cream (3%), when used on pre-vesicular lesions, reduces HSV shedding, lesion size, and duration, as well as prevents the development of vesicles. However, it requires compounding and is expensive and should be reserved for acyclovir-resistant HSV infections.[121] Topical therapies may be an option for patients with renal insufficiency.

ACYCLOVIR RESISTANCE

Acyclovir resistance occurs in the immunocompromised population, whereas it is quite rare in immunocompetent patients. Bone marrow transplant recipients have a higher incidence than patients with HIV. Its prevalence is 4.1% to 7.1% in immunocompromised patients.[122] Docosanol cream and topical foscarnet do not exert antiviral effects by way of thymidine kinase and therefore are still viable options in

Table 6
Topical treatments for recurrent herpes labialis

Recurrent herpes labialis	Acyclovir Ointment[a]	Penciclovir[a]	Docosanol	Foscarnet
	Every 3 h for 7 d 0.5-in. ribbon/4 in.² Acyclovir/hydrocortisone 5%/1% cream 5 times/d for 5 d	Every 2 h for 4 d	5 times/d until healed	Every 2 h for 5 d

[a] In adults older than 18 y.

Data from Brady RC, Bernstein DI. Treatment of herpes simplex virus infections. Antiviral Res 2004;61:73–81.[112,113]

acyclovir- resistant infections. Cidofovir, although currently approved by the Food and Drug Administration (FDA) only for CMV retinitis in patients with AIDS, is used in acyclovir-resistant cases of herpes simplex infections. It must be administered intravenously with probenecid and aggressive hydration, as it is nephrotoxic. Cidofovir gel (1.0%) once daily for 5 days has been a useful therapy for acyclovir-resistant genital and perianal HSV in patients with AIDS; it produces statistically significant reduction in viral shedding, lesion size, and pain.[123] Foscarnet has also been used at 40 mg/kg IV every 8 to 12 hours for 2 to 3 weeks until all lesions are healed.

A new class of antiherpetic drugs which includes amenamevir and pritelivir are non-nucleoside, antiviral drug called "helicase-primase inhibitors" that block an essential enzyme complex for replication of viral genomic DNA.[124] Amenamevir has also demonstrated efficacy against acyclovir-resistant HSV isolates. Amenamevir was approved in Japan as once-daily treatment for 7 days for herpes zoster in July 2017.[125] Other novel agents such as the polyphenol mangiferin has recently been investigated in Brazil as an alternative treatment for acyclovir-resistant HSV strains.[126]

POSTHERPETIC NEURALGIA
Is it Preventable?

Prevention of PHN with oral antiviral drugs has not been shown to be effective after 6 months of treatment; nor has been the use of systemic steroids. Systemic steroids do not decrease the incidence of PHN; however, in conjunction with antivirals, it can reduce the acute pain of herpes zoster.[127–130] Acyclovir and valacyclovir have shown similar reductions in time to skin healing in herpes zoster, but valacyclovir has shown a 34% faster resolution of zoster-associated pain compared with acyclovir.[131] The addition of gabapentin to valacyclovir within 72 h of rash onset does not provide significant additional relief from acute herpetic pain nor prevention of PHN. In fact, a 2019 randomized controlled trial found that patients taking gabapentin reported worse health-related quality of life and poorer sleep quality.[132] Prior Zoster vaccine live ZVL is 65% effective in preventing PHN in all age groups. No difference has been shown between immunosuppressed and immunocompetent groups.[133]

Topical Agents:
- Lidocaine: Use 5% patches, up to 3 patches simultaneously for a maximum of 12 hours within a 24-h period.
- Trolamine salicylate and *Aloe vera*: Apply directly to the painful area.
- Capsaicin: Apply a single 8% capsaicin patch over the non-crusted, uninjured area. Leave in place for 60 minutes.

Oral Medications:
- Gabapentin:
  - Start with 300 mg orally.
  - Can be increased up to a maximum of 3600 mg per day (divided into 3 doses).
  - Note: Gabapentin combined with morphine provides better pain relief than gabapentin alone.
- Pregabalin:
  - Initial dosage: 150 mg/day in divided doses.
  - Can be increased to a maximum of 300 mg/day within a week.
  - Dosage range: 150 to 300 mg daily (either 75-mg to 150-mg doses twice a day or 50-mg to 100-mg doses 3 times a day).
- Tricyclic Antidepressants:
  - Amitriptyline (Elavil): Start with 10 to 25 mg orally at bedtime. Can be increased to a maximum dosage of 150 to 200 mg/day.

- o Other options: nortriptyline, maprotiline, desipramine.
- Carbamazepine: 600 to 1200 mg daily.
- Controlled-release oxycodone: 10 to 40 mg orally every 12 hours.
- Controlled-release morphine sulfate: Can be combined with tricyclic antidepressants.
- Levetiracetam: Start with 500 mg orally daily. Dose can be titrated up by 500 mg weekly until a maximum dosage of 1500 mg twice daily is reached.
- Diazepam: 2 mg taken 3 times a day. This can supplement any of the aforementionede therapies.

Treatment with analgesics, antivirals, and a 3-day to 5-day course of prednisone 60 mg daily is recommended in immunocompetent patients 50 years or older and is essential when treating ophthalmic-distribution zoster

VACCINATION

In 1995, a live-attenuated vaccine for varicella became available for children. The introduction of a universal vaccination in the United States has led to a dramatic reduction in the varicella incidence, its associated complications, hospitalizations, and fatality rate.[134] A combination measles, mumps, rubella, and varicella vaccine (MMRV) was licensed in the United States in 2005 for healthy children aged 12 months to 12 years.[135] In mega-analysis studies, the MMRV vaccine demonstrated well-tolerated safety profiles. However, it is worth noting that some children who received the MMRV vaccine may have an increased risk of fever and febrile seizure 6 to 12 days after the first vaccine dose when the peak in replication of the live-attenuated measles virus occurs.[136,137]

In 2021, the Advisory Committee on Immunization Practices recommended the recombinant zoster vaccine (RZV), 2-dose, subunit vaccine containing recombinant glycoprotein E in combination with a novel adjuvant (AS01$_B$), in adults aged $\geq$18 years who are or will be at increased risk for herpes zoster because of immunodeficiency or immunosuppression caused by known disease or therapy.[138] The Shingrix (recombinant zoster vaccine), FDA approved in 2017, is now the preferred vaccine, over Zostavax (zoster vaccine live), a shingles vaccine in use since 2006. The vaccine consists of 2 doses (0.5 mL each), administered intramuscularly, 2 to 6 months apart.[139] The protective efficacy of the vaccine lasts for at least 4 years and is well preserved in adults aged $\geq$ 70 year.[138,140,141] It is recommended to delay vaccination until after pregnancy. Vaccine may be given regardless of breastfeeding status.[142] In a 2016 randomized, placebo-controlled phase trial, RZV showed a good safety profile. Overall incidences of potential immune-mediated diseases, serious adverse events, and deaths were similar in the vaccine and placebo groups.[143]

Prophylactic genital herpes vaccine has been showing promising results in the prevention of HSV-2 in guinea pig models. More studies are underway to assess its safety and efficacy for prevention of HSV-2.[144]

SUMMARY

Herpes simplex and herpes zoster infections are incredibly common. Because of the neurotropic nature of these viruses, infection is lifelong. Recognition of early signs of infection is necessary to implement effective treatment and prevent complications. Various laboratory tests exist to confirm infection; however, outcomes depend on the stage of the lesion and proper collection technique. Immunosuppressed populations require special attention, as herpes infections may appear atypical and severe.

This group is at higher risk for disseminated disease. Immunocompetent adults older than 60 should get vaccinated for VZV, as neurologic sequelae can be serious.

CLINICS CARE POINTS

- **Orofacial herpes:** While most initial orolabial herpes infections are subclinical and often unrecognized, recurrent herpes labialis can be preceded by a prodrome of tingling, itching, and burning, with common triggers including illness, sun exposure, and emotional stress.

- **Post herpetic neuralgia:** While systemic steroids don't reduce the incidence of postherpetic neuralgia (PHN), they can lessen the acute pain of herpes zoster when used alongside antivirals.

- **Vaccination:** Be aware of the potential for an increased risk of fever and febrile seizure in some children 6 to 12 days after the first dose of the MMRV vaccine.

- **Herpes simplex encephalitis:** When evaluating patients with fever, headache, behavioral changes, seizures, or focal neurologic symptoms, especially with neuroimaging alterations in the medial temporal lobes, consider cerebrospinal fluid examination for HSV as herpes simplex encephalitis may be present, even if initial tests like PCR are negative.

- **Primary Varicella:** Adults and immunocompromised individuals contracting primary varicella are at a higher risk for severe manifestations and complications, including pneumonia and neurologic sequelae.

- **Herpes Zoster (Shingles):** Due to its prodromal pain, herpes zoster can be misdiagnosed as other conditions such as myocardial infarction or pleurisy; clinicians should be alert to differentiate based on symptomatology and the possibility of subsequent rash appearance.

- **Neurologic complications of herpes zoster:** Neurologic complications of herpes zoster can range from postherpetic neuralgia, which is more prevalent in older patients, to cranial neuropathies and vasculopathy, and may manifest even weeks after the acute zoster outbreak without any visible rash.

- **Herpes Zoster in Human Immunodeficiency Virus:** HIV-infected individuals with a low CD4 count and no antiretroviral therapy are at a heightened risk for future herpes zoster outbreaks, irrespective of their VZV antibody levels.

- **Laboratory diagnosis of HSC and VSV virus:** For optimal viral yield in diagnosis, target early vesicles over healed crusted lesions. Proper specimen collection, transport, and storage are crucial. Newer vesicles in immunosuppressed patients tend to have a higher viral load. While viral culture has been the gold standard for diagnosis, PCR offers higher sensitivity, especially for atypical presentations or older lesions. PCR can accurately differentiate between HSV-1, HSV-2, and VZV, and remains highly sensitive even on lesions over 30 days old.

- **Management of Herpes Simplex Virus and Varicella-Zoster Virus:** The efficacy of antiviral therapy is maximized when initiated within the first 72 hours of disease onset. While topical acyclovir ointment has limited effectiveness for recurrent herpes labialis due to poor penetration, 1% penciclovir cream can decrease the duration of lesions and associated pain when applied frequently after the onset of prodromal symptoms.

- **Acyclovir Resistance:** Acyclovir resistance is more common in the immunocompromised population, with bone marrow transplant recipients having a higher incidence than patients with HIV. Docosanol cream and topical foscarnet remain effective treatments for acyclovir-resistant infections as they don't act via thymidine kinase. Novel antiviral agents, like amenamevir and pritelivir, from the "helicase-primase inhibitors" class, offer potential treatments for acyclovir-resistant HSV, with amenamevir already demonstrating efficacy against resistant strains.

- **Genital Herpes Simplex Virus Infection:** Not all patients with initial genital herpes present with overt lesions; consider atypical presentations such as edema, fissures, or back pain without genital manifestations. Differential diagnosis for genital ulcers extends beyond HSV and should encompass other infectious and inflammatory causes.

- **Transmission of orofacial herpes and genital herpes:** Daily antiviral suppressive therapy can decrease HSV recrudescence, viral shedding, and transmission to serodiscordant partners. Routine serologic screening for genital HSV in asymptomatic individuals is not recommended due to potential psychosocial consequences, healthcare burdens, and high rates of false-positive results.

- **HSV infection in Immunocompromised patients:** Immunocompromise d patients such as those with HIV or post-transplant, may exhibit atypical and more severe manifestations of HSV infections, requiring vigilant monitoring and prompt therapeutic intervention.

- **Eczema herpeticum:** Clinicians must maintain a high index of suspicion eczema herpeticum in patients with chronic dermatosis, especially when presenting with flared conditions or widespread monomorphic vesicles and initiate antiviral therapy promptly due to its potentially fatal nature.

DISCLOSURE

The authors have no relevant disclosures.

REFERENCES

1. Simmons A. Clinical manifestations and treatment considerations of herpes simplex virus infection. J Infect Dis 2002;186(Suppl 1). https://doi.org/10.1086/342967.
2. McQuillan G, Kruszon-Moran D, Flagg EW, et al. Prevalence of herpes simplex virus type 1 and type 2 in persons aged 14-49: United States, 2015-2016. NCHS Data Brief 2018;(304):1–8.
3. Lynch DP. Oral viral infections. Clin Dermatol 2000;18(5):619–28.
4. Evans CM, Kudesia G, McKendrick M. Management of herpesvirus infections. Int J Antimicrob Agents 2013;42(2):119–28.
5. Fatahzadeh M, Schwartz RA. Human herpes simplex virus infections: epidemiology, pathogenesis, symptomatology, diagnosis, and management. J Am Acad Dermatol 2007;57(5):737–63.
6. Muñoz-Corcuera M, Esparza-Gómez G, González-Moles MA, et al. Oral ulcers: clinical aspects. A tool for dermatologists. Part II. Chronic ulcers. Clin Exp Dermatol 2009;34(4):456–61.
7. Gupta R, Warren T, Wald A. Genital herpes. Lancet 2007;370(9605):2127–37.
8. Gnann JW, Whitley RJ. Genital herpes. N Engl J Med 2016;375(7):666–74.
9. Brown TJ, Yen-Moore A, Tyring SK. An overview of sexually transmitted diseases. Part I. J Am Acad Dermatol 1999;41(4):511–32.
10. Corey L. Genital herpes simplex virus infections: clinical manifestations, course, and complications. Ann Intern Med 1983;98(6):958.
11. Edwards L, Lynch PJ. Genital dermatology atlas and manual. Philadelphia: LWW; 2017.
12. Keogan MT. Clinical Immunology Review Series: an approach to the patient with recurrent orogenital ulceration, including Behçet's syndrome. Clin Exp Immunol 2009;156(1):1–11.
13. Edwards L, Lynch PJ. Genital dermatology manual. Philadelphia: LWW; 2022.
14. Maliyar K, Mufti A, Syed M, et al. Genital ulcer disease: a review of pathogenesis and clinical features. J Cutan Med Surg 2019;23(6):624–34.
15. Wolff MH, Schmitt J, Rahaus M, et al. Clinical and subclinical reactivation of genital herpes virus. Intervirology 2002;45(1):20–3.

16. Koutsky LA, Ashley RL, Holmes KK, et al. The frequency of unrecognized type 2 herpes simplex virus infection among women. Implications for the control of genital herpes. Sex Transm Dis 1990;17(2):90–4.

17. Mertz GJ, Coombs RW, Ashley R, et al. Transmission of genital herpes in couples with one symptomatic and one asymptomatic partner: a prospective study. J Infect Dis 1988;157(6):1169–77.

18. Whitley RJ. Neonatal herpes simplex virus infections. J Med Virol 1993;Suppl 1(1 S):13–21.

19. Wald A, Zeh J, Selke S, et al. Reactivation of genital herpes simplex virus type 2 infection in asymptomatic seropositive persons. N Engl J Med 2000;342(12): 844–50.

20. Barton SE, Munday PE, Patel RJ. Asymptomatic shedding of herpes simplex virus from the genital tract: uncertainty and its consequences for patient management. The Herpes Simplex Virus Advisory Panel. Int J STD AIDS 1996;7(4): 229–32.

21. Lafferty WE, Coombs RW, Benedetti J, et al. Recurrences after oral and genital herpes simplex virus infection. Influence of site of infection and viral type. N Engl J Med 1987;316(23):1444–9.

22. Mertz GJ, Schmidt O, Jourden JL, et al. Frequency of acquisition of first-episode genital infection with herpes simplex virus from symptomatic and asymptomatic source contacts. Sex Transm Dis 1985;12(1):33–9.

23. Wald A, Zeh J, Selke S, et al. Virologic characteristics of subclinical and symptomatic genital herpes infections. N Engl J Med 1995;333(12):770–5.

24. Corey L, Wald A, Patel R, et al. Once-daily valacyclovir to reduce the risk of transmission of genital herpes. N Engl J Med 2004;350(1):11–20.

25. Wang K, Merin A, Rendina HJ, et al. Genital herpes stigma: toward the Measurement and Validation of a highly prevalent yet hidden public health problem. Stigma Health 2018;3(1):27.

26. Bibbins-Domingo K, Grossman DC, Curry SJ, et al. Serologic screening for genital herpes infection: US preventive Services Task Force Recommendation Statement. JAMA 2016;316(23):2525–30.

27. Cohen PR. The "Knife-Cut sign" Revisited: a distinctive presentation of linear erosive herpes simplex virus infection in immunocompromised patients. J Clin Aesthet Dermatol 2015;8(10):38–42.

28. Traidl S, Roesner L, Zeitvogel J, et al. Eczema herpeticum in atopic dermatitis. Allergy 2021;76(10):3017–27.

29. Wollenberg A. Viral infections in atopic dermatitis Pathogenic aspects and clinical management. J Allergy Clin Immunol 2003;112(4):667–74.

30. Whitney RJ. Varicella-zoster virus infections. In: Galasso GJ, editor. Antiviral agents and viral diseases of man. New York: Raven Press; 1990. p. 235.

31. Aurelius E, Johansson B, Sköldenberg B, et al. Encephalitis in immunocompetent patients due to herpes simplex virus type 1 or 2 as determined by type-specific polymerase chain reaction and antibody assays of cerebrospinal fluid. J Med Virol 1993;39(3):179–86.

32. Ellul M, Solomon T. Acute encephalitis - diagnosis and management. Clin Med 2018;18(2):155–9.

33. Kennedy PGE. Viral encephalitis: causes, differential diagnosis, and management. J Neurol Neurosurg Psychiatry 2004;75(90001):10i–115i.

34. Darville JM, Ley BE, Roome AP, et al. Acyclovir-resistant herpes simplex virus infections in a bone marrow transplant population. Bone Marrow Transplant 1998;22(6):587–9.

35. Jalloh I, Guilfoyle MR, Lloyd SKW, et al. Reactivation and centripetal spread of herpes simplex virus complicating acoustic neuroma resection. Surg Neurol 2009;72(5):502–4.

36. Raper DMS, Wong A, McCormick PC, et al. Herpes simplex encephalitis following spinal ependymoma resection: case report and literature review. J Neuro Oncol 2011;103(3):771–6.

37. Gnann JW, Whitley RJ. Herpes simplex encephalitis: an Update. Curr Infect Dis Rep 2017;19(3):13.

38. Álvarez de Eulate-Beramendi S, Santirso-Rodríguez D, Piña-Batista KM, et al. Herpes simplex virus type 1 encephalitis after meningioma resection. Neurologia 2015;30(7):455–7.

39. Grover D, Newsholme W, Brink N, et al. Herpes simplex virus infection of the central nervous system in human immunodeficiency virus-type 1-infected patients. Int J STD AIDS 2004;15(9):597–600.

40. Kinchington PR, Leger AJS, Guedon JMG, et al. Herpes simplex virus and varicella zoster virus, the house guests who never leave. Herpesviridae 2012;3(1):5.

41. Gilden DH, Kleinschmidt-DeMasters BK, LaGuardia JJ, et al. Neurologic complications of the reactivation of varicella–zoster virus. N Engl J Med 2000;342(9):635–45.

42. Burke BL, Steele RW, Beard OW, et al. Immune responses to varicella-zoster in the aged. Arch Intern Med 1982;142(2):291–3.

43. Gershon AA, Steinberg SP. Antibody responses to varicella-zoster virus and the role of antibody in host Defense. Am J Med Sci 1981;282(1):12–7.

44. Kennedy P, Gershon A. Clinical features of varicella-zoster virus infection. Viruses 2018;10(11):609.

45. Kim SH, Park SH, Choi SM, et al. Implementation of hospital Policy for Healthcare Workers and patients exposed to varicella-zoster virus. J Korean Med Sci 2018;33(36). https://doi.org/10.3346/JKMS.2018.33.E252.

46. Siegel JD, Rhinehart E, Jackson M, et al. 2007 Guideline for isolation precautions: preventing transmission of infectious agents in health care settings. Am J Infect Control 2007;35(10):S65.

47. Freer G, Pistello M. Varicella-zoster virus infection: natural history, clinical manifestations, immunity and current and future vaccination strategies. New Microbiol 2018;41(2):95–105. Available at: https://pubmed.ncbi.nlm.nih.gov/29498740/. Accessed January 14, 2023.

48. Aebi C, Ahmed A, Ramilo O. Bacterial complications of primary varicella in children. Clin Infect Dis 1996;23(4):698–705.

49. Clark P, Davidson D, Letts M, et al. Necrotizing fasciitis secondary to chickenpox infection in children. Can J Surg 2003;46(1):9. Available at: http://pmc/articles/PMC3211661/. Accessed January 14, 2023.

50. John KG, John TJ, Taljaard JJ, et al. The outcome of severe varicella pneumonia with respiratory failure admitted to the intensive care unit for mechanical ventilation. Eur Respir J 2018;52(1). https://doi.org/10.1183/13993003.00407-2018.

51. Amlie-Lefond C, Jubelt B. Neurologic manifestations of varicella zoster virus infections. Curr Neurol Neurosci Rep 2009;9(6):430–4.

52. Nagel MA, Cohrs RJ, Mahalingam R, et al. The varicella zoster virus vasculopathies: clinical, CSF, imaging, and virologic features. Neurology 2008;70(11):853.

53. Kodadhala V, Dessalegn M, Barned S, et al. 578. Crit Care Med 2019;47:269.

54. Gilden DH, Cohrs RJ, Mahalingam R. Clinical and molecular pathogenesis of varicella virus infection. Viral Immunol 2003;16(3):243–58.

55. Zachariah S, Sullivan A, Donato A. Shingles: a harbinger of chronic HIV infection. J Community Hosp Intern Med Perspect 2021;11(6):871.
56. Patil A, Goldust M, Wollina U. Herpes zoster: a review of clinical manifestations and management. Viruses 2022;14(2). https://doi.org/10.3390/V14020192.
57. Zhou J, Li J, Ma L, et al. Zoster sine herpete: a review. Korean J Pain 2020; 33(3):208.
58. McCrary ML, Severson J, Tyring SK. Varicella zoster virus. J Am Acad Dermatol 1999;41(1):1–16.
59. Carroll WM, Mastaglia FL. Optic neuropathy and ophthalmoplegia in herpes zoster oticus. Neurology 1979;29(5):726–9.
60. Sanjay S, Chan EWE, Gopal L, et al. Complete unilateral ophthalmoplegia in herpes zoster ophthalmicus. J Neuro Ophthalmol 2009;29(4):325–37.
61. Karmon Y, Gadoth N. Delayed oculomotor nerve palsy after bilateral cervical zoster in an immunocompetent patient. Neurology 2005;65(1):170.
62. Mallick-Searle T, Snodgrass B, Brant JM. Postherpetic neuralgia: epidemiology, pathophysiology, and pain management pharmacology. J Multidiscip Healthc 2016;9:447.
63. Klompas M, Kulldorff M, Vilk Y, et al. Herpes zoster and postherpetic neuralgia Surveillance using Structured Electronic data. Mayo Clin Proc 2011;86(12): 1146.
64. Manz HJ, Canter HG, Melton J. Trigeminal herpes zoster causing mandibular osteonecrosis and spontaneous tooth exfoliation. South Med J 1986;79(8): 1026–8.
65. Schwartz O, Kvorning SA. Tooth exfoliation, osteonecrosis of the jaw and neuralgia following herpes zoster of the trigeminal nerve. Int J Oral Surg 1982;11(6): 364–71.
66. Asnis D, Micic L, Giaccio D. Ramsay Hunt syndrome presenting as a cranial polyneuropathy. Cutis 1996;57(6):421–4.
67. Thomas JE, Howard FM. Segmental zoster paresis—a disease profile. Neurology 1972;22(5):459.
68. Ö Yoleri, Ölmez N, Öztura I, et al. Segmental zoster paresis of the upper extremity: a case report. Arch Phys Med Rehabil 2005;86(7):1492–4.
69. Kawajiri S, Tani M, Noda K, et al. Segmental zoster paresis of limbs: report of three cases and review of literature. Neurol 2007;13(5):313–7.
70. Stowasser M, Cameron J, Oliver WA. Diaphragmatic paralysis following cervical herpes zoster. Med J Aust 1990;153(9):555–6.
71. Nau R, Lantsch M, Stiefel M, et al. Varicella zoster virus-associated focal vasculitis without herpes zoster: recovery after treatment with acyclovir. Neurology 1998;51(3):914–5.
72. Gilden DH, Lipton HL, Wolf JS, et al. Two patients with unusual forms of varicella-zoster virus vasculopathy. N Engl J Med 2002;347(19):1500–3.
73. Fukumoto S, Kinjo M, Hokamura K, et al. Subarachnoid hemorrhage and granulomatous angiitis of the basilar artery: demonstration of the varicella-zoster-virus in the basilar artery lesions. Stroke 1986;17(5):1024–8.
74. Ku HC, Tsai YT, Konara-Mudiyanselage SP, et al. Incidence of herpes zoster in HIV-infected patients undergoing Antiretroviral therapy: a Systematic review and Meta-analysis. J Clin Med 2021;10(11):2300.
75. Pomerantz HS, Xu X, White J, et al. Association between quantitative varicella-zoster virus antibody levels and zoster reactivation in HIV-infected persons. AIDS Res Ther 2018;15(1):25.

76. Gilson IH, Barnett JH, Conant MA, et al. Disseminated ecthymatous herpes varicella-zoster virus infection in patients with acquired immunodeficiency syndrome. J Am Acad Dermatol 1989;20(4):637–42.

77. VAUGHAN JONES SA, McGIBBON DH, BRADBEER CS. Chronic verrucous varicella-zoster infection in a patient with AIDS. Clin Exp Dermatol 1994;19(4):327–9.

78. Mirouse A, Sonneville R, Razazi K, et al. Neurologic outcome of VZV encephalitis one year after ICU admission: a multicenter cohort study. Ann Intensive Care 2022;12(1):32.

79. Schiffer JT, Corey L. New concepts in understanding genital herpes. Curr Infect Dis Rep 2009;11(6):457–64.

80. Cohen PR. Tests for detecting herpes simplex virus and varicella-zoster virus infections. Dermatol Clin 1994;12(1):51–68.

81. Eisen D. The clinical characteristics of intraoral herpes simplex virus infection in 52 immunocompetent patients. Oral Surg Oral Med Oral Pathol Oral Radiol Endod 1998;86(4):432–7.

82. Damour A, Garcia M, Seneschal J, et al. Eczema herpeticum: clinical and Pathophysiological aspects. Clin Rev Allergy Immunol 2020;59(1):1–18.

83. LeGoff J, Péré H, Bélec L. Diagnosis of genital herpes simplex virus infection in the clinical laboratory. Virol J 2014;11(1):83.

84. BROWN ST, JAFFE HW, ZAIDI A, et al. Sensitivity and specificity of diagnostic tests for genital infection with herpesvirus hominis. Sex Transm Dis 1979;6(1):10–3.

85. Solomon AR, Rasmussen JE, Varani J, et al. The Tzanck smear in the diagnosis of cutaneous herpes simplex. JAMA 1984;251(5):633–5.

86. Johnston C. Diagnosis and management of genital herpes: Key questions and review of the evidence for the 2021 centers for disease control and prevention sexually transmitted infections treatment guidelines. Clin Infect Dis 2022;74(Supplement_2):S134–43.

87. Solomon AR. New diagnostic tests for herpes simplex and varicella zoster infections. J Am Acad Dermatol 1988;18(1 Pt 2):218–21.

88. Sheibani K, Tubbs RR. Enzyme immunohistochemistry: technical aspects. Semin Diagn Pathol 1984;1(4):235–50.

89. García-Cisneros S, Sánchez-Alemán MÁ, Conde-Glez CJ, et al. Performance of ELISA and Western blot to detect antibodies against HSV-2 using dried blood spots. J Infect Public Health 2019;12(2):224–8.

90. Ashley RL. Genital herpes infections. Clin Lab Med 1989;9(3):405–20.

91. Reeves WC, Corey L, Adams HG, et al. Risk of recurrence after first episodes of genital herpes. N Engl J Med 1981;305(6):315–9.

92. CESARIO TC, POLAND JD, WULFF H, et al. Six years experience with herpes simplex virus in a CHILDREN'S HOME1. Am J Epidemiol 1969;90(5):416–22.

93. Goldman BD. Herpes serology for dermatologists. Arch Dermatol 2000;136(9). https://doi.org/10.1001/archderm.136.9.1158.

94. Feltner C, Grodensky C, Ebel C, et al. Serologic screening for genital herpes. JAMA 2016;316(23):2531.

95. Munday PE, Vuddamalay J, Slomka MJ, et al. Role of type specific herpes simplex virus serology in the diagnosis and management of genital herpes. Sex Transm Infect 1998;74(3):175–8.

96. Sauerbrei A, Wutzler P. Novel recombinant ELISA assays for determination of type-specific IgG antibodies against HSV-1 and HSV-2. J Virol Methods 2007;144(1–2):138–42.

97. Hobbs MM, Mwanyumba SW, Luseno WK, et al. Evaluation of herpes simplex virus type 2 serological tests for Use with dried blood spots in Kenya. Sex Transm Dis 2017;44(2):101–3.

98. Gitman MR, Ferguson D, Landry ML. Comparison of Simplexa HSV 1 & 2 PCR with culture, immunofluorescence, and laboratory-developed TaqMan PCR for detection of herpes simplex virus in swab specimens. J Clin Microbiol 2013; 51(11):3765.

99. Dominguez SR, Pretty K, Hengartner R, et al. Comparison of herpes simplex virus PCR with culture for virus detection in Multisource surface swab specimens from Neonates. J Clin Microbiol 2018;56(10). https://doi.org/10.1128/JCM. 00632-18.

100. Weinberg A, Clark JC, Schneider SA, et al. Improved detection of varicella zoster infection with a spin amplification shell vial technique and blind passage. Clin Diagn Virol 1996;5(1):61–5.

101. Erlich KS. Laboratory diagnosis of herpesvirus infections. Clin Lab Med 1987; 7(4):759–76.

102. Davis LE, Tyler KL. Molecular diagnosis of CNS viral infections. J Neurol Neurosurg Psychiatry 2005;76(1):10.

103. Dutt MK, Johnston IDA. Computed tomography and EEG in herpes simplex encephalitis. Their value in diagnosis and prognosis. Arch Neurol 1982;39(2): 99–102.

104. Steiner I. Herpes simplex virus encephalitis: new infection or reactivation? Curr Opin Neurol 2011;24(3):268–74.

105. Gilden DH, Bennett JL, Kleinschmidt-Demasters BK, et al. The value of cerebrospinal fluid antiviral antibody in the diagnosis of neurologic disease produced by varicella zoster virus. J Neurol Sci 1998;159(2):140–4.

106. Wolf R, Brenner S, Ruocco V, et al. Isotopic response. Int J Dermatol 1995;34(5): 341–8.

107. Wolf R, Wolf D, Ruocco E, et al. Wolf's isotopic response. Clin Dermatol 2011; 29(2):237–40.

108. Cernik C, Gallina K, Brodell RT. The treatment of herpes simplex infections: an evidence-based review. Arch Intern Med 2008;168(11):1137–44.

109. Sohail M, Khan FA, Shami HB, et al. Management of eczema herpeticum in a Burn Unit. J Pak Med Assoc 2016;66(11):1357–61.

110. Luca NJC, Lara-Corrales I, Pope E. Eczema herpeticum in children: clinical features and factors predictive of hospitalization. J Pediatr 2012;161(4):671–5.

111. Zhuang K, Wu Q, Ran X, et al. Oral treatment with valacyclovir for HSV-2-associated eczema herpeticum in a 9-month-old infant: a case report. Medicine 2016;95(29):e4284.

112. Woo S bin, Challacombe SJ. Management of recurrent oral herpes simplex infections. Oral Surg Oral Med Oral Pathol Oral Radiol Endod 2007;103(Suppl): S12.e1-18. https://doi.org/10.1016/J.TRIPLEO.2006.11.004.

113. Brady RC, Bernstein DI. Treatment of herpes simplex virus infections. Antiviral Res 2004;61(2):73–81.

114. Lilie HM, Wassilew SW. The role of antivirals in the management of neuropathic pain in the older patient with herpes zoster. Drugs Aging 2003;20(8):561–70.

115. Bomgaars L, Thompson P, Berg S, et al. Valacyclovir and acyclovir Pharmacokinetics in immunocompromised children. Pediatr Blood Cancer 2008; 51(4):504.

116. Koshy E, Mengting L, Kumar H, et al. Epidemiology, treatment and prevention of herpes zoster: a comprehensive review. Indian J Dermatol Venereol Leprol 2018;84(3):251.

117. Ono F, Yasumoto S, Furumura M, et al. Comparison between famciclovir and valacyclovir for acute pain in adult Japanese immunocompetent patients with herpes zoster. J Dermatol 2012;39(11):902–8.

118. Spruance SL, Rea TL, Thoming C, et al. Penciclovir cream for the treatment of herpes simplex labialis: a randomized, multicenter, double-blind, placebo-controlled trial. JAMA 1997;277(17):1374–9.

119. Habbema L, de Boulle K, Roders GA, et al. n-Docosanol 10% cream in the treatment of recurrent herpes labialis: a randomised, double-blind, placebo-controlled study. Acta Derm Venereol 1996;76(6):479–81.

120. Sacks SL, Thisted RA, Jones TM, et al. Clinical efficacy of topical docosanol 10% cream for herpes simplex labialis: a multicenter, randomized, placebo-controlled trial. J Am Acad Dermatol 2001;45(2):222–30.

121. Lawee D, Rosenthal D, Aoki FY, et al. Efficacy and safety of foscarnet for recurrent orolabial herpes: a multicentre randomized double-blind study. CMAJ (Can Med Assoc J): Canadian Medical Association Journal 1988;138(4):329. Available at: http://pmc/articles/PMC1267623/?report=abstract. Accessed January 14, 2023.

122. Bacon TH, Levin MJ, Leary JJ, et al. Herpes simplex virus resistance to acyclovir and penciclovir after two decades of antiviral therapy. Clin Microbiol Rev 2003; 16(1):114–28.

123. Lalezari J, Schacker T, Feinberg J, et al. A randomized, double-blind, placebo-controlled trial of Cidofovir gel for the treatment of acyclovir-Unresponsive mucocutaneous herpes simplex virus infection in patients with AIDS. J Infect Dis 1997;176(4):892–8.

124. Shiraki K, Yasumoto S, Toyama N, et al. Amenamevir, a helicase-primase inhibitor, for the optimal treatment of herpes zoster. Viruses 2021;13(8):1547.

125. Kawashima M, Imafuku S, Fujio K, et al. Single-dose, patient-initiated amenamevir therapy for recurrent genital herpes: a phase 3, randomized, double-blind, placebo-controlled study. Open Forum Infect Dis 2022;9(10). https://doi.org/10.1093/ofid/ofac494.

126. Rechenchoski DZ, Agostinho KF, Faccin-Galhardi LC, et al. Mangiferin: a promising natural xanthone from Mangifera indica for the control of acyclovir – resistant herpes simplex virus 1 infection. Bioorg Med Chem 2020;28(4):115304.

127. Whitley RJ. Acyclovir with and without prednisone for the treatment of herpes zoster. Ann Intern Med 1996;125(5):376.

128. KECZKES K, BASHEER AM. Do corticosteroids prevent post-herpetic neuralgia? Br J Dermatol 1980;102(5):551–5.

129. Eaglstein WH, Katz R, Brown JA. The effects of early corticosteroid therapy on the skin eruption and pain of herpes zoster. JAMA 1970;211(10):1681–3.

130. Kost RG, Straus SE. Postherpetic neuralgia — pathogenesis, treatment, and prevention. N Engl J Med 1996;335(1):32–42.

131. Beutner KR, Friedman DJ, Forszpaniak C, et al. Valaciclovir compared with acyclovir for improved therapy for herpes zoster in immunocompetent adults. Antimicrob Agents Chemother 1995;39(7):1546–53.

132. Bulilete O, Leiva A, Rullán M, et al. Efficacy of gabapentin for the prevention of postherpetic neuralgia in patients with acute herpes zoster: a double blind, randomized controlled trial. PLoS One 2019;14(6):e0217335.

133. Klein NP, Bartlett J, Fireman B, et al. Long-term effectiveness of zoster vaccine live for postherpetic neuralgia prevention. Vaccine 2019;37(36):5422-7.
134. Holmes SJ. Review of recommendations of the Advisory Committee on Immunization practices, centers for disease control and prevention, on varicella vaccine. JID (J Infect Dis) 1996;174(Supplement 3):S342-4.
135. Marin M, Broder KR, Temte JL, et al. Use of combination measles, mumps, rubella, and varicella vaccine: recommendations of the Advisory Committee on Immunization Practices (ACIP). MMWR Recomm Rep (Morb Mortal Wkly Rep) 2010;59(RR-3):1-12.
136. MacDonald SE, Dover DC, Simmonds KA, et al. Risk of febrile seizures after first dose of measles–mumps–rubella–varicella vaccine: a population-based cohort study. Can Med Assoc J 2014;186(11):824-9.
137. Ma SJ, Li X, Xiong YQ, et al. Combination measles-mumps-rubella-varicella vaccine in healthy children. Medicine 2015;94(44):e1721.
138. Food and Drug Administration. Shingrix [package insert]. US Department of Health and Human Services, Food and Drug Administration.; 2021.
139. Dooling KL, Guo A, Patel M, et al. Recommendations of the Advisory Committee on Immunization practices for Use of herpes zoster vaccines. MMWR Morb Mortal Wkly Rep 2018;67(3):103-8.
140. McKay SL, Guo A, Pergam SA, et al. Herpes zoster risk in immunocompromised adults in the United States: a Systematic review. Clin Infect Dis 2020;71(7): e125-34.
141. Yun H, Yang S, Chen L, et al. Risk of herpes zoster in autoimmune and inflammatory diseases: Implications for vaccination. Arthritis Rheumatol 2016;68(9): 2328-37.
142. Syed YY. Recombinant zoster vaccine (Shingrix®): a review in herpes zoster. Drugs Aging 2018;35(12):1031-40.
143. Cunningham AL, Lal H, Kovac M, et al. Efficacy of the herpes zoster subunit vaccine in adults 70 Years of age or older. N Engl J Med 2016;375(11):1019-32.
144. Bernstein DI, Pullum DA, Cardin RD, et al. The HSV-1 live attenuated VC2 vaccine provides protection against HSV-2 genital infection in the Guinea pig model of genital herpes. Vaccine 2019;37(1):61-8.

Paraneoplastic Dermatoses and Cutaneous Metastases

Andrea Murina, MD*, Ashley Allen, MD

KEYWORDS

- Paraneoplastic • Metastasis • Cutaneous • Malignancy

KEY POINTS

- Cutaneous paraneoplastic syndromes require recognition in order to perform a targeted workup for associated solid tumors or hematologic malignancies.
- Cutaneous metastases are most commonly from breast and lung carcinomas and can present as nodules, vascular lesions, eczematous dermatitis, or inflammatory lesions.
- The most common histologic presentation of cutaneous metastasis is that of a dermal-based or subcutaneous-based nodule with sparing of the epidermis. Determination of origin of tumor requires immunohistochemistry and clinical correlation.

PARANEOPLASTIC SYNDROMES
Introduction

Paraneoplastic syndromes are skin manifestations that occur in association with internal malignancies. Their presentations are highly varied, so knowledge of their clinical features aids in the diagnosis of the associated malignancy. Certain paraneoplastic syndromes are associated with a stronger likelihood of specific internal malignancies, whereas others have weaker or less-specific associations. The first section will discuss paraneoplastic syndromes associated with solid tumors, and the second section will discuss syndromes associated with hematologic disease.

CLINICAL VARIANTS: PARANEOPLASTIC SYNDROMES ASSOCIATED WITH SOLID TUMORS
Acrokeratosis Paraneoplastica

Acrokeratosis paraneoplastica is the appearance of acral hyperkeratotic plaques with associated paronychia and onychodystrophy. The histology of the eruption resembles psoriasis with acanthosis, orthokeratosis, and hyperkeratosis. It occurs in men aged older than 40 years and is most associated with malignances of the upper gastrointestinal tract. If the skin signs are clinically suspicious, a lymph node examination, otolaryngology consult, chest x-ray, and upper endoscopy are indicated.[1]

Department of Dermatology, Tulane University School of Medicine, 1430 Tulane Avenue #8036, New Orleans, LA 70112, USA
* Corresponding author.
E-mail address: amurina@tulane.edu

Clin Geriatr Med 40 (2024) 177–195
https://doi.org/10.1016/j.cger.2023.09.005
0749-0690/24/© 2023 Elsevier Inc. All rights reserved.

Antilaminin Mucous Membrane Pemphigoid

The antilaminin subtype of mucous membrane pemphigoid (MMP) is the pemphigoid type with the strongest association with malignancy. In pooled reports, 25% of patients with serum antibodies against laminin 332 have been associated with solid cancers of the lung, breast, prostate, tongue, uterus, and bladder.[2] Patients with MMP are diagnosed by direct immunofluorescence (DIF) microscopy showing linear deposits of immunoglobulins at the basement membrane zone. For the antilaminin subtype, indirect immunofluorescence (IIF) on salt split skin will show immunoglobulin G (IgG) and C3 on the dermal side of the blister. Patients with negative collagen VII, bulllous pemphigoid antigen (BPAG) 1 and 2 serum antibodies should undergo testing for antilaminin MMP. Either an enzyme-linked immunosorbent assay or IIF microscopy can be used to detect antilaminin antibodies.[3] Because the range of associations is wide, patients should start with age-appropriate cancer screening followed by history or symptom-guided testing.

Erythema Gyratum Repens

Erythema gyratum repens is characterized by serpiginous plaques with a wood-grain appearance that spreads centrifugally on the trunk. In a review of 83 cases presented in the literature, 70% presented with a concomitant malignancy, with bronchial cancer being the most common. There was also an association with drugs including azathioprine and interferon-alfa.[4]

Tylosis with Esophageal Cancer

Tylosis with esophageal cancer is a genetic syndrome characterized by focal thickening of the skin of the hands and feet and a high risk of developing squamous cell carcinoma of the esophagus. The syndrome is inherited in an autosomal dominant fashion with children of 7 to 8 years of age presenting with the disease. The risk of cancer is very high and surveillance with annual upper endoscopy is indicated.[5]

Hypertrichosis Lanuginosa Acquisita

Hypertrichosis lanuginosa acquisita is a rare form of facial hypertrichosis that presents with an increase in lanugo hairs, which are long, thin and unpigmented. These hairs are normally present in utero and shed in the first months after birth. The occurrence of lanugo hairs on the head and neck in an adult should prompt workup for possible adenocarcinoma of the lung or colon. Rarely, it has been associated with breast cancer, endometrial cancer, and lymphoma.[6] Screening with a blood count, chest x-ray, and colonoscopy are indicated if these findings occur.

Sign of Leser-Trelat

The sign of Leser-Trelat is a sudden eruption of seborrheic keratoses in association with malignancy of the gastrointestinal tract such as gastric or colon cancer. Hematologic malignancies have also been associated. The Leser-Trelat sign is controversial due to the overall high prevalence of seborrheic keratoses in the elderly, who are at the highest risk of malignancy.[7] Reports of coexisting malignant acanthosis nigricans and/or tripe palms helps to support a shared paraneoplastic correlation. Patients with who report an "eruptive onset" of seborrheic keratosis should be screened by endoscopy, colonoscopy, and blood count.

Malignant Acanthosis Nigricans and Tripe Palms

Malignant acanthosis nigricans and tripe palms are similar disorders of keratinization that lead to thick and velvety plaques on the face, neck, trunk, and palms. Acanthosis nigricans is a common skin condition that involves the folds but the malignant subtype is usually mucosal and more extensive. Tripe palms are a form of focal hyperkeratosis with enhancement of the epidermal ridges, which resembles the gastric lining of ruminant animals[8] (**Fig. 1**). Tripe palms can be associated with adenocarcinomas of the lung or gastrointestinal tract, whereas malignant acanthosis nigricans is more likely to be associated with gastrointestinal malignancies.

Necrolytic Migratory Erythema

Necrolytic migratory erythema (NME) is an eruption characterized by scaly, erosive, annular erythematous plaques that are intermittent in nature and affect the perioral and intertriginous regions of the body. Each episode evolves during 1 to 2 weeks and may leave scaling and hyperpigmentation.[9] Histology may show nonspecific features or superficial epithelial necrosis of the upper spinous layer with vacuolated keratinocytes. NME is part of the glucagonoma syndrome, associated with an alpha-cell pancreatic tumor (glucagonoma), and can be the presenting manifestation in most patients. Patients will also have high blood glucagon levels and either diabetes mellitus or glucose intolerance.[9] Half of patients may have metastatic disease at the time of presentation.

Superficial Migratory Thrombophlebitis

Thrombosis of a superficial vein can occur in different segments of a given vein over time, which is known as migratory thrombophlebitis. Thrombotic events of other types, such as deep vein thromboses or disseminated intravascular coagulopathy can precede malignancies; however, the original report of a paraneoplastic sign by

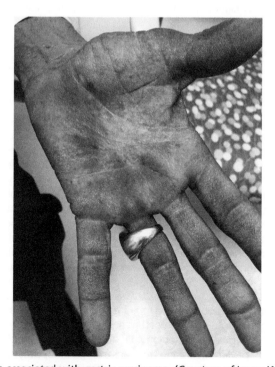

Fig. 1. Tripe palm associated with gastric carcinoma. (*Courtesy of* Laura Williams, MD.)

Trousseau included only superficial thrombophlebitis. Superficial migratory thrombophlebitis can be associated with pancreatic, brain, and lung malignancies.[10]

SUMMARY

Paraneoplastic syndromes can be exaggerated forms of skin lesions that are commonly seen in the dermatology clinic, such as malignant acanthosis nigricans or the sign of Leser-Trelat. Others can be confused with common inflammatory diseases such as palmoplantar psoriasis or keratoderma such as acrokeratosis neoplastica and tylosis with esophageal cancer. It is important to screen patients with any skin finding suspicious for paraneoplasia and select referrals based on the most common associated malignancies.

CLINICS CARE POINTS

- Acrokeratosis paraneoplastica in patients with hyperkeratotic plaques of the palms and associated nail dystrophy should have upper endoscopy for screening.
- The diagnosis of antilaminin MMP requires high clinical suspicion based on direct immunofluorescence microscopy and serum testing results.
- Erythema gyratum repens is associated with bronchial malignancy.
- Focal thickening of the acral skin of children or young adults should prompt evaluation for esophageal cancer screening.
- The presence of multiple lanugo facial hairs on an adult should prompt screening for an adenocarcinoma of the lung or colon.
- Malignant acanthosis nigricans, sign of Leser-Trelat and tripe palms are associated with gastrointestinal malignancy.
- NME is a part of the glucagonoma syndrome and presents as erythematous, eroded plaques in the intertriginous areas associated with metastatic pancreatic cancer.

CLINICAL VARIANTS: HEMATOLOGIC-ASSOCIATED CUTANEOUS SYNDROMES
Introduction

Monoclonal gammopathies and hematologic malignancies are associated with a wide range of cutaneous paraneoplastic syndromes (**Table 1**). Recognition of these syndromes is important to monitor for both new onset hematologic disease and recurrences. Hematologic malignancies can metastasize to the skin as leukemia/lymphoma cutis or plasmacytoma, which are diagnosed based on histology. Paraneoplastic syndromes, in contrast, do not reveal the underlying hematologic disorder on histopathology but instead must be recognized as cutaneous indicators. Complete blood counts, serum and urine electrophoresis, and immunofixation are generally the initial workup for these syndromes. Further studies in conjunction with specialists in hematology/oncology will aid in the specific diagnosis via bone marrow or lymph node biopsies.

Type I Cryoglobulinemia

Cryoglobulins are immunoglobulins or a mixture of immunoglobulins and complement components that precipitate from the serum and plasma. In type I cryoglobulinemia, the cryoglobulins are typically monoclonal IgG or immunglobulin M (IgM) and occur in the setting of a protein-secreting monoclonal gammopathy such as multiple myeloma, Waldenstrom macroglobulinemia, chronic lymphocytic leukemia, or

Table 1
Paraneoplastic syndromes associated with plasma cell disorders

Syndrome	Patterns	Association
Type I cryoglobulinemia	Digital ischemia Livedo reticularis Skin necrosis Raynaud phenomenon	Multiple myeloma MGUS CLL Waldenstrom macroglobulinemia
Necrobiotic xanthogranuloma	Periorbital papules and plaques	Multiple myeloma MGUS IgG-kappa subtype
DNPX	Symmetric xanthomas of the face, neck, and trunk	Monoclonal gammopathy Multiple myeloma
POEMS syndrome	Hyperpigmentation Glomeruloid hemangioma Acrocyanosis	Monoclonal gammopathy Lambda-subtype
Schnitzler syndrome	Urticarial papules and plaques	IgM-kappa monoclonal gammopathy
Scleromyxedema	Firm waxy red to skin-colored papules	IgG-lambda monoclonal gammopathy

Abbreviations: CLL, chronic lymphocytic leukemia; DNPX, diffuse normolipemic plane xanthoma; MGUS, monoclonal gammopathy of undetermined significance.

monoclonal gammopathy of undetermined significance (MGUS). The high viscosity of the circulating immunoglobulins leads to microthrombi in small size vessels which will appear in the skin as digital ischemia, livedo reticularis or skin necrosis (**Fig. 2**). Raynaud phenomenon is also a frequent sign as is peripheral neuropathy and arthritis.[11] Histopathology commonly shows noninflammatory thrombotic lesions. Treatment should focus on the hyperviscosity and the underlying malignancy.

Necrobiotic Xanthogranuloma

Necrobiotic xanthogranulomas (NXGs) are red-brown or yellow indurated plaques that typically occur in the periorbital area. Scarring and ulceration are very common. They are strongly associated with monoclonal gammopathy in 80% of patients, most commonly IgG-kappa. MGUS and multiple myeloma are the most common associated hematologic disorder but other hematologic diseases have been reported in association.[12] The mean time from the development of NXG to the development of a hematologic disorder is 2.4 years.[13] Histopathologic features include palisading granulomas with bands of necrobiosis. Patients should be screened with serum and urine electrophoresis and immunofixation. A bone marrow biopsy is warranted if there is concern for myeloma or leukemia.

Paraneoplatic Pemphigus

Paraneoplastic pemphigus (PNP) is a mucocutaneous blistering disease that is induced by a lymphoproliferative disorder. Its frequency may be decreasing due to an increased use of anti-CD20 monoclonal antibody therapy for non-Hodgkin lymphoma and chronic lymphocytic leukemia.[14] PNP produces an erosive stomatitis and polymorphous skin lesions. The most common associated disorders are non-Hodgkin lymphoma, chronic lymphocytic leukemia, and thymoma. Castleman disease is the most common associated disorder in children. The mucositis can involve the lips, tongue, nasopharynx, conjunctiva, and anogenital regions (**Fig. 3**). Pulmonary

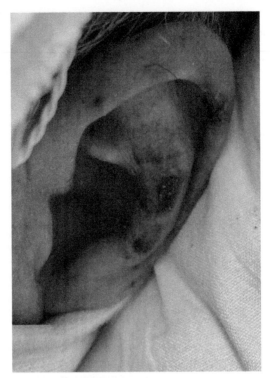

Fig. 2. Type I cryoglobulinemia showing purpuric and necrotic papules on the ear.

involvement can occur late in the course of disease as a restrictive bronchiolitis, or bronchilolitis obliterans. Workup should include skin biopsies for routine histology and DIF, which will show a suprabasal acantholysis with keratinocyte necrosis and lichenoid interface dermatitis with epidermal IgG or C3 intercellulary and at the basement membrane zone. IIF on rat bladder epithelium will help to differentiate PNP from pemphigus vulgaris.[15]

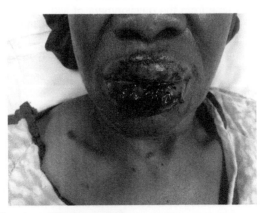

Fig. 3. Severe erosive stomatitis due to PNP.

Diffuse Normolipemic Plane Xanthoma

Plane xanthomas are thin yellow plaques that are commonly found on the eyelids, neck, trunk, shoulders, and axillae. One variant of plane xanthoma is a rare subtype of Langerhans-cell histiocytosis, known as diffuse normolipemic plane xanthoma (DNPX). DNPX is a symmetric eruption on the face, neck, and upper trunk in the absence of lipid abnormalities. This subtype has been associated with hematologic diseases including monoclonal gammopathy, multiple myeloma, leukemia, and other lymphoproliferative disorders.[16]

Polyneuropathy, Organomegaly, Endocrinopathy, M-protein, Skin changes Syndrome

POEMS is a syndrome of neurologic and endocrine symptoms that are associated with an underlying plasma cell neoplasm. The acronym indicates some of the main clinical features: polyneuropathy, organomegaly, endocrinopathy, M-protein, skin changes. Other important features are papilledema, extravascular volume overload, thrombocytosis, erythrocytosis, elevated vascular endothelial growth factor, increased risk of thrombosis, and abnormal pulmonary function tests. The skin changes include a variety of presentations including hyperpigmentation, hypertrichosis, glomerular hemangioma, acrocyanosis, and white nails. Sclerodermoid changes to the skin and facial lipoatrophy have also been reported. Bone marrow biopsy will show clonal plasma cells in the majority of cases, predominantly of the lambda subtype.[17] A Castleman's variant of POEMS syndrome lacks a monoclonal gammopathy.

Schnitzler Syndrome

Schnitzler syndrome is an acquired autoinflammatory disorder associated with a neutrophil-predominant urticaria and an IgM monoclonal gammopathy, predominantly the kappa subtype. Additional symptoms can include fever, lymphadenopathy, bone pain, arthralgia, headache, fatigue, and neuropathy.[18] Elevated c-reactive protein levels and leukocytosis are common. Treatment is with anti-IL-1-directed therapies.

Scleromyxedema

Scleromyxedema is a diffuse mucinosis that affects the skin of the hands, head, upper trunk, and thighs with firm waxy reddish to skin-colored papules (**Fig. 4**). Deep furrows of the face can lead to leonine facies and indurated plaques with central depression over the joints of the hands can seem as the "donut sign." Sclerodactyly, Raynaud syndrome, arthralgia, myopathy, and a polyarthritis can be associated. Neurologic symptoms such as carpal tunnel syndrome, neuropathy, and dermato-neuro syndrome, a flu-like prodrome with seizures and coma, can occur. A monoclonal spike is found in 90% of patients, usually of an IgG lambda subtype.[19]

Malignancy-Associated Sweet Syndrome

Sweet syndrome can be associated with an underlying hematologic malignancy such as myelodysplastic syndrome or acute myeloid leukemia. The diagnosis of malignancy-associated Sweet syndrome is the sentinel sign of newly diagnosed or recurrent malignancy. The characteristic tender erythematous plaques and nodules are the same as the classic (idiopathic) variant of Sweet syndrome but bullous or ulcerated lesions, periorbital cellulitis, pyoderma gangrenosum, and tongue swelling are more common in malignancy-associated Sweet syndrome.[20] Anemia and thrombocytopenia are also more common in malignancy-associated Sweet syndrome.

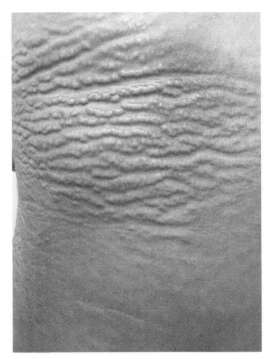

Fig. 4. Skin-colored papules due to scleromyxedema.

SUMMARY

Plasma cell disorders are associated with many different skin syndromes including type I cryoglobulinemia, necrobiotic xanthogranuloma, DNPX, scleromyxedema, and Schnitzler syndrome. PNP is associated with non-Hodgkin lymphoma, and malignancy-associated Sweet syndrome is associated with acute myeloid leukemias. It is important to note that skin biopsy of these cutaneous syndromes generally do not show the malignant cells on histopathology, so knowledge of these patterns is key to establish if there is an associated malignancy.

CLINICS CARE POINTS

- Type 1 cryoglobulinemia is associated with myeloma or leukemia and manifests as a thrombotic vasculopathy.

- Necrobiotic xanthogranuloma is associated with multiple myeloma.

- Extensive erosive stomatitis should prompt workup for PNP associated with lymphoma or leukemia.

- Extensive xanthomas may be associated with lymphoproliferative disease in the absence of any lipid abnormalities.

- Scleromyxedema is a diffuse mucinosis that produces sclerodermoid features and is associated with monoclonal gammopathy.

- Malignancy-associated Sweet syndrome is more likely to have bullae and ulceration and be associated with abnormal laboratory values.

CUTANEOUS METASTASES
Introduction

Metastasis is defined as the spread of cancerous cells from one part of the body to another, either via direct extension, hematogenous, or lymphatic spread.[21] Cutaneous metastases have a highly variable appearance clinically and histologically, which contributes to both diagnostic difficulty and delay in diagnosis. Prompt diagnosis and subsequent treatment has profound implications given that cutaneous metastases can present before, concurrently with, or after diagnosis of primary malignancy (referred to as precocious, synchronous, or metachronous).[22,23] Additionally, spread to the skin may herald recurrence. It is estimated that cutaneous metastasis occurs in 0.6% to 10.4%[22,24,25] of malignancies and 16% to 26% of cutaneous metastases are the presenting sign of cancer.[24] The propensity of a cancer to metastasize to the skin is variable depending on the type of primary cancer. In general, the most common cancers to metastasize to the skin are breast and melanoma followed by lung, gastrointestinal, genitourinary, and oropharyngeal.

Cutaneous metastases generally portend a poor prognosis although this is less true for certain primary cancers than others.[24–26] Below are general principles pertaining to cutaneous metastases as a group but the presentation and prognosis vary according to the primary tumor. Select primary malignancies are listed by site in **Table 2**.

Clinical Variants

Cutaneous metastases will commonly present as a dermal or subcutaneous nodule on the chest, abdomen, or head and neck. They can also present as papules, plaques, or ulcers. As a general principle, cutaneous metastases show a propensity to present within scars from prior surgical sites or needle aspiration biopsies.[27] A patient presenting with cutaneous metastasis is, on average, 62 years old.[26] The historical Sister Mary Joseph nodule is a periumbilical nodular presentation of cutaneous metastasis, usually due to underlying colorectal or gastric cancer but can also be due to others including pancreatic and genitourinary cancers.

Carcinoma erysipeloides (also known as lymphatic carcinomatosis) refers to the clinical presentation of lymphedema and peau d'orange appearance of the skin, which is a consequence of obstruction of dermal lymphatic vessels by neoplastic cells. Although this is classically associated with breast cancer, it has been reported in pancreatic, rectal, ovarian, prostate, parotid, and pulmonary cancers as well. Histopathology demonstrates neoplastic cells obscuring lymphatic vessels.

Mammary Paget disease is the presence of intraductal carcinoma within the epidermis via either lactiferous ducts or direct extension. This clinically presents as unilateral eczematous patches and plaques on the areola or nipple. Histopathologically, pagetoid cells are abundant in the epidermis and stain positively for CK7, carcinoembryonic antigen (CEA), periodic acid-schiff (PAS), and mucin stains, with negative S100 staining[23,25] (**Fig. 5**). The majority of extramammary Paget disease (around 75%) represents de novo primary cutaneous adenocarcinoma derived from Toker cells or adnexal epithelium; however, it is always necessary to distinguish primary from secondary extramammary Paget disease. Secondary extramammary Paget disease represents either direct extension or epidermotropic metastases from an underlying adenocarcinoma—most commonly gastrointestinal or genitourinary. Underlying adenocarcinoma is more likely in the perianal area, as compared with vulvar or scrotal, and with CK20 positivity and gross cystic disease fluid protein 15 (GCFDP-15) negativity. The most common staining pattern for primary extramammary Paget disease is CK7+, cytokeratin 20 (CK20)−, and GCFDP-15+.

Table 2
Clinicopathological and immunohistological characteristics of cutaneous metastases by primary site

Primary	Site Predilection	Histology, IHC Markers	Comments
Colorectal	Abdomen Perineal Head/neck Earlier surgical sites SMJ nodule	"Dirty" neutrophilic debris Karyorrhexis CK20 CEA CDX2 + /CK7−	May mimic hidradenitis suppurativa when presents perineally
Gastric	Abdomen Scars SMJ nodule	CK7 CK20 CDX2 CEA, EMA HIK1083[a]	Occasionally eczematous or inflammatory presentation
Hepatocellular carcinoma	Head/neck Trunk	Trabecular, pseudoglandular patterns Polyclonal CEA: characteristic canalicular pattern AFP A1AT Hepatocyte paraffin 1 monoclonal antibody Arginase-1 (highly sensitive and specific)	Rare May mimic pyogenic granuloma
Gallbladder	Abdominal wall Within scars	None specific	Very rare
Cholangiocarcinoma	Trunk Scars Head/neck	Angulated glands with poorly preserved architecture Desmoplastic stroma CK7+/20+ CDK2−	Very rare, <30 cases (per Alcaraz)
Pancreatic	Umbilicus	Poorly formed glands CA19.9 (highly sensitive, low specificity)	Usually exocrine > neuroendocrine
Esophageal/Oral	Trunk Head/neck	SCC: CK5/6, AE1/3, EMA, Adenocarcinoma: CEA/EMA and CK20	Primary cutaneous SCC vs metastatic oral SCC can be indistinguishable especially in the setting of in actinic damaged skin

Origin	Site	Markers	Notes
Ovarian	Abdomen	CK7 + CK20−[b] CA125 PAX8[c]	Spreads intraperitoneally (HAB 85–89)
Endometrial	Abdomen	CK7 + /CK20− PAX8	Usually adenocarcinoma, presenting late in the disease course
Prostate	Penile Abdomen Groin	PSA NKX3.1 (homeobox protein Nkx-3.1) CD57 Ber-EP4[d]	Usually adenocarcinoma
Testicular	Lower abdomen	Biphasic: syncytiotrophoblastic and cytotrophoblastic Cytokeratin β-Hcg	Usually choriocarcinoma Usually younger men
Thyroid	Seeding after FNA	Papillary: psammoma bodies in 25%, decapitation secretion, TTF and thyroglobulin+ Follicular: follicles containing colloid, Thyroglobulin+ Anaplastic: Thyroglobulin− Medullary: Calcitonin+ PAX8+ in all except medullary	Most common is papillary, followed by follicular, anaplastic, and then medullary
Lung	Scars (thoracotomy, needle aspiration tract) Trunk Upper lip Upper extremities "Clown nose" sign (nasal tip)	Small cell TTF-1 CAM5.2[38] (24, 30, 31 sources in Habermehl) SCC and mesothelioma CK5/6 CK7, Adenocarcinoma BerEp-4[d] CEA	Usually adenocarcinoma NSCLC

(continued on next page)

Table 2
(continued)

Primary	Site Predilection	Histology, IHC Markers	Comments
Carcinoid	Trunk	Trabecular Dense core granules on electron microscopy Neuroendocrine markers: chromogranin, synaptophysin, and NSE CDX2 (intestinal) TTF-1 (pulmonary)	Most commonly bronchial May present with pellagra
Renal	Scalp Genitalia	Prominent vascularity and hemorrhage CK7–/CK20– MNF116 CD31, CD10^e RCC (specific) Adipophilin PAX8	Usually clear cell Clinically can mimic vascular tumor, pyogenic granuloma
Bladder, urothelial, transitional cell	Trunk Upper extremities Groin	HMWK, CK7+ CK20 + /– GATA-3 (50%) Uroplakin III CK14	Variants include squamous differentiation, signet ring cell
Leiomyosarcoma	Variable	Haphazard spindle cells in dermis, SMA Desmin	Important to differentiate from primary cutaneous
Angiosarcoma	Variable	Degree of differentiation highly variable Endothelial markers: Factor VIII-related antigen Ulex europaeus lectin Podoplanin CD31/CD34 MYC is a marker of postradiation angiosarcoma	Breast can extend to overlying skin Hemorrhagic mass, blueish discoloration Epithelioid variant

| Chondrosarcoma | Amputation stumps | GADD45b
+ CD99 (membranous),
Podoplanin
YKL-40
SMA, Desmin
CAM 5.2 |

[a] Monoclonal antibody for gastric o-glycan that is more specific than CK20. Will stain negative in primary sweat gland adenocarcinomas.[38]
[b] May be positive in mucinous carcinomas.
[c] Helpful when differentiating from breast, although will be positive in renal cell, endometrial, and certain thyroid cancers.
[d] Diagnostic pitfall as can be mistaken for BCC.
[e] Can differentiate from nonsebaceous adnexal tumors.

Abbreviations: AFP, Alpha-fetoprotein; BCC, basal cell carcinoma; beta-Hcg, beta-human chorionic gonadotropin; NSE, Neuron specific enolase; SMA, smooth muscle actin; SMJ, Sister-Mary Joseph; TTF, Thyroid transcription factor.

Data from Habermehl and Ko,[38] Alcaraz, Cerroni, Rütten, Kutzner and Requena,[22] and Patterson, Hosler, and Prenshaw.[23]

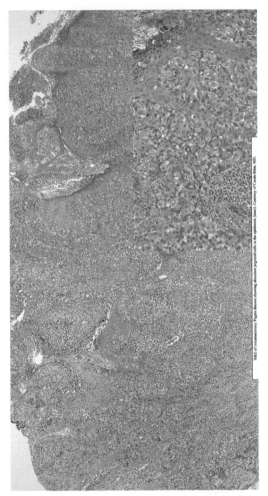

Fig. 5. H&E of extramammary Paget disease showing abundant pagetoid cells in the epidermis (*inset*). (*Courtesy of* Carole Bitar, MD.)

Alopecia neoplastica presents as scarring alopecic plaques due to neoplastic cells obliterating hair follicles, with the majority of cases due to breast cancer (84%). This can easily be misdiagnosed because it can resemble other types of alopecia. Carcinoma en cuirasse, also known as scirrhous carcinoma, presents as thickened plaques on the trunk due to fibrosis of infiltrating tumor cells. This is also more likely associated with breast cancer, and presents as indurated plaques on the chest wall with a peau d'orange appearance. The less common associations are gastric and ovarian cancers.[28,29]

Highly vascular cutaneous metastases can present as friable papulonodules, mimicking pyogenic granuloma. This has been reported in metastatic renal cell, hepatocellular, breast, and colon carcinoma.[30]

General Histologic Characteristics of Cutaneous Metastases

The typical histologic presentation of cutaneous metastasis is a broad-based or inverted wedge-shaped dermal or subcutaneous infiltrate of cytologically atypical cells that characteristically spares the epidermis. The neoplastic cells can exhibit a nodular, infiltrative, diffuse or sheet-like, or intravascular/intralymphatic pattern. Immunohistochemistry is essential to differentiate metastasis from primary cutaneous lesions. The p63 positivity generally supports a primary cutaneous tumor over metastases.[31] p63 will be positive in adnexal malignancies and primary cutaneous squamous cell carcinoma. CK15 and D2-40 (podoplanin) positivity favors primary cutaneous adenocarcinoma over metastatic adenocarcinoma (98% and 96% specificity, respectively). Pathologists should always consider metastasis in the differential when presented with a case that has the aforementioned characteristics without information regarding malignancy history.[32,33]

Although rare, a pure dermal-based nodular melanoma or primary cutaneous squamous cell carcinoma (SCC), which lacks epidermal involvement can occur. There are a few cancers that are highly unlikely to metastasize to the skin. Epidermotropic metastases have rarely been reported in prostate and pancreatic metastases.[34,35]

Breast Cancer

Cutaneous metastasis of breast cancer most commonly presents as painless nodules on the chest or abdomen, with a predilection for surgical scars. The incidence of cutaneous metastasis of breast cancer was 23.9% in a large case series.[25,36] About 3.5% had cutaneous involvement as the presenting sign, and 6.3% had cutaneous manifestation.[37] Carcinoma erysipeloides and Paget disease are commonly thought of in the context of breast cancer, which is likely the function of the higher prevalence. Another variation of cutaneous metastasis is breast carcinoma of the inframammary crease, which is seen underneath pendulous breasts, mimicking squamous cell carcinoma, basal cell carcinoma, or intertrigo.[37] Carcinoma telangiectoides is characterized by pink to violaceous papules, pseudovesicles, and telangiectasias. Histopathologically, neoplastic cells show intravascular invasion. Some have posited a relationship between carcinoma telangiectatoides and estrogen receptor-positive breast cancer. Breast metastases have also been reported to present on the eyelids, either as noduloulcerative lesions or as a "mask like" induration of the periocular skin. This can clinically be mistaken for chalazion or xanthelasma. This presentation is associated with the histiocytoid variant of lobular breast carcinoma and can histologically be misdiagnosed as primary signet ring carcinoma of the eyelid for which p63 and podoplanin negativity favor metastatic over primary cutaneous tumor.[22]

Breast metastases will show dermal or subcutaneous aggregates of neoplastic cells that may intercalate linearly between collagen bundles or form immature glandular structures (**Figs. 6 and 7**). Immunohistochemically, they may stain positive for estrogen (~50% sensitivity) or progesterone receptor, CK7 (~66% sensitivity), mammaglobin (~65-70% sensitivity) GCDFP-15, and GATA-3 transcription factor (GATA-3). The last 2 are nonspecific markers and can stain adnexal or other epithelial neoplasms as well as other carcinomas.[23,38]

Melanoma

Both cutaneous and extracutaneous melanomas can metastasize to the skin. Metastatic lesions tend to be heavily pigmented, and can present as one or few nodular lesions or many smaller pigmented macules or papules, which can be located locoregionally or distant from primary melanoma. Skin metastasis is generally associated with visceral metastasis. Melanocytic origin can be confirmed immunohistochemically with cytoplasmic protein stain (S100), human melanoma black- 45 (HMB-45), transcription factor (SOX10), microphthalmia associated transcription factor (MITF), and/or Melan-A23.[36]

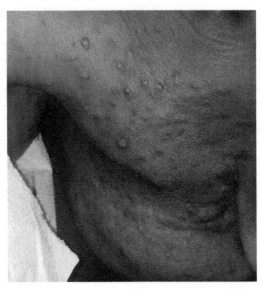

Fig. 6. Breast cancer metastases of the right chest wall. (*Courtesy of* Christopher Haas, MD.)

Specific Metastases by Primary Site

Specific metastases listed by primary site of tumor can be found in **Table 2**. Notably, these are typical staining patterns, as each immunohistochemical stain has its own limitations.

DISCUSSION

Cutaneous metastases remain a diagnostic challenge due to the variability in clinical presentation and limitations of immunohistochemical staining. The clinician should note any suspicion of metastasis on the pathology requisition form but pathologist suspicion should remain high even if a history of cancer is not indicated on the requisition. Most cancers have been reported to have capacity for cutaneous involvement, most commonly breast and lung. No immunohistochemical stains are 100% sensitive and specific; however, considering all stains can help to characterize the likely origin of primary tumor when correlated clinically. **Fig. 8** show a simplified algorithm to interpreting immunohistochemical staining. More specific staining patterns are listed in

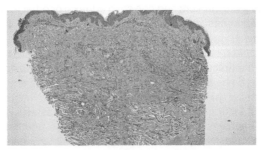

Fig. 7. H&E of metastatic breast carcinoma showing a dermal infiltrate intercalating linearly between collagen bundles (*inset*). (*Courtesy of* Carole Bitar, MD.)

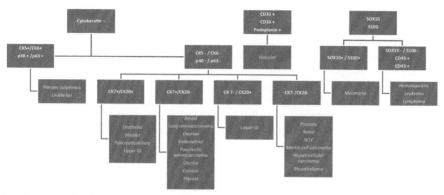

Fig. 8. Algorithm for interpreting immunohistochemical staining in cutaneous metastases. (*Data obtained from* [Habermehl and Ko,[38] Lin and Liu[39]].)

Table 2. Treatment of cutaneous metastases is largely done for palliative or cosmetic reasons as the mainstay of therapy is directed at the underlying cancer.

SUMMARY

Cutaneous metastases are rare and typically portend a poor prognosis. Because they may be a presenting sign of a malignancy or be a harbinger of recurrence, early identification and diagnosis can have profound clinical implications. Clinicians and pathologists should consider cutaneous metastasis in the differential when a patient has a history of cancer, presents with a firm, painless nodule, or an atypical dermal infiltrate is seen on histopathology.

CLINICS CARE POINTS

- Cutaneous metastases most commonly present as a nodule with a predilection for head/neck and trunk.

- Breast cancer commonly has skin manifestations that can range in presentation from eczematous (Paget disease) to inflammatory (carcinoma erysipeloides), and even sclerosing (carcinoma en curiasse) lesions.

- On pathologic condition, cutaneous metastases most commonly exhibit an atypical dermal and/or subcutaneous infiltrate, which can be nodular or infiltrative and requires immunohistochemical staining in combination with clinical correlation to determine primary origin.

DISCLOSURE

Dr A. Murina is a speaker for Abbvie, Amgen, Bristol-Meyers Squibb, and Janssen. She is a consultant for Abbvie, Bristol-Meyers Squibb, Novartis and UCB. Dr A. Allen has no conflicts of interest to disclose.

REFERENCES

1. Valdivielso M, Longo I, Suárez R, et al. Acrokeratosis paraneoplastica: bazex syndrome. J Eur Acad Dermatol Venereol 2005;19(3):340–4.

2. Du G, Patzelt S, van Beek N, et al. Mucous membrane pemphigoid. Autoimmun Rev 2022;21(4):103036.
3. Gasparini G, Cozzani E, Di Zenzo G, et al. Anti-laminin 332 antibody detection using biochip immunofluorescence microscopy in a real-life cohort of Italian patients with mucous membrane pemphigoid. Eur J Dermatol 2022;32(6):756–61.
4. Rongioletti F, Fausti V, Parodi A. Erythema gyratum repens is not an obligate paraneoplastic disease: a systematic review of the literature and personal experience. J Eur Acad Dermatol Venereol 2014;28(1):112–5.
5. Ellis A, Risk JM, Maruthappu T, et al. Tylosis with oesophageal cancer: diagnosis, management and molecular mechanisms. Orphanet J Rare Dis 2015;10:126.
6. Slee PHTJ, van der Waal RIF, Schagen van Leeuwen JH, et al. Paraneoplastic hypertrichosis lanuginosa acquisita: uncommon or overlooked? Br J Dermatol 2007; 157(6):1087–92.
7. Schwartz RA. American academy of D. Sign of leser-trélat. J Am Acad Dermatol 1996;35(1):88–95.
8. Boyce M, Flower C. Tripe palms. N Engl J Med 2022;387(4):355.
9. Tolliver S, Graham J, Kaffenberger BH. A review of cutaneous manifestations within glucagonoma syndrome: necrolytic migratory erythema. Int J Dermatol 2018;57(6):642–5.
10. Tian F, Mazurek KR, Malinak RN, et al. Pseudocellulitis need not be benign: three cases of superficial migratory thrombophlebitis with "negative" venous duplex ultrasonography. J Clin Aesthet Dermatol 2017;10(12):49–51.
11. Terrier B, Karras A, Kahn J-E, et al. The spectrum of type I cryoglobulinemia vasculitis: new insights based on 64 cases. Medicine 2013;92(2):61–8.
12. Nelson CA, Zhong CS, Hashemi DA, et al. A multicenter cross-sectional study and systematic review of necrobiotic xanthogranuloma with proposed diagnostic criteria. JAMA dermatology 2020;156(3):270–9.
13. Wood AJ, Wagner MVU, Abbott JJ, et al. Necrobiotic xanthogranuloma: a review of 17 cases with emphasis on clinical and pathologic correlation. Arch Dermatol 2009;145(3):279–84.
14. Kwatra SG, Boozalis E, Pasieka H, et al. Decreased recognition of paraneoplastic pemphigus in patients previously treated with anti-CD 20 monoclonal antibodies. Br J Dermatol 2019;180(5):1238–9.
15. Svoboda SA, Huang S, Liu X, et al. Paraneoplastic pemphigus: revised diagnostic criteria based on literature analysis. J Cutan Pathol 2021;48(9):1133–8.
16. Cohen YK, Elpern DJ. Diffuse normolipemic plane xanthoma associated with monoclonal gammopathy. Dermatol Pract Concept 2015;5(4):65–7.
17. Dispenzieri A. POEMS Syndrome: 2019 Update on diagnosis, risk-stratification, and management. Am J Hematol 2019;94(7):812–27.
18. Khwaja J, D'Sa S, Minnema MC, et al. IgM monoclonal gammopathies of clinical significance: diagnosis and management. Haematologica 2022;107(9):2037–50.
19. Claveau J-S, Wetter DA, Kumar S. Cutaneous manifestations of monoclonal gammopathy. Blood Cancer J 2022;12(4):58.
20. Raza S, Kirkland RS, Patel AA, et al. Insight into Sweet's syndrome and associated-malignancy: a review of the current literature. Int J Oncol 2013; 42(5):1516–22.
21. Disibio G, French SW. Metastatic patterns of cancers: results from a large autopsy study. Arch Pathol Lab Med 2008;132(6):931–9.
22. Alcaraz I, Cerroni L, Rütten A, et al. Cutaneous metastases from internal malignancies: a clinicopathologic and immunohistochemical review. Am J Dermatopathol 2012;34(4):347–93.

23. Patterson JW, Hosler GA, Prenshaw KL. Weedon's skin pathology. In: Patterson JW, editor. *Skin pathology*. 5th edition. Amsterdam, Netherlands: Elsevier; 2021. p. 1169–80.
24. Choate EA, Nobori A, Worswick S. Cutaneous metastasis of internal tumors. Dermatol Clin 2019;37(4):545–54.
25. American Academy of D, Spangler N, Helm KF. Cutaneous metastases in patients with metastatic carcinoma: a retrospective study of 4020 patients. J Am Acad Dermatol 1993;29(2 Pt 1):228–36.
26. Marcoval J, Moreno A, Peyrí J. Cutaneous infiltration by cancer. J Am Acad Dermatol 2007;57(4):577–80.
27. Strickley JD, Jenson AB, Jung JY. Cutaneous metastasis. Hematol Oncol Clin N Am 2019;33(1):173–97.
28. Rajeshwari M, Sakthivel P, Sikka K, et al. Carcinoma en cuirasse' in the neck: extremely unusual initial presentation of gastric cancer. BMJ Case Rep 2019; 12(4). https://doi.org/10.1136/bcr-2018-228418.
29. Sharma V, Kumar A. Carcinoma en Cuirasse. N Engl J Med 2021;385(27):2562.
30. Verardino GC, Silva RSd, Obadia DL, et al. Rare cutaneous metastasis from a probable basaloid carcinoma of the colon mimicking pyogenic granuloma. Anais Brasileiros De Dermatología 2011;86(3):537–40.
31. Compton LA, Murphy GF, Lian CG. Diagnostic immunohistochemistry in cutaneous neoplasia: an update. Dermatopathology 2015;2(1):15–42.
32. Saeed S, Keehn CA, Morgan MB. Cutaneous metastasis: a clinical, pathological, and immunohistochemical appraisal. J Cutan Pathol 2004;31(6):419–30.
33. Sariya D, Ruth K, Adams-McDonnell R, et al. Clinicopathologic correlation of cutaneous metastases: experience from a cancer center. Arch Dermatol 2007; 143(5):613–20.
34. Manteaux A, Cohen PR, Rapini RP. Zosteriform and epidermotropic metastasis. Report of two cases. J Dermatol Surg Oncol 1992;18(2):97–100.
35. Weidner N, Foucar E. Epidermotropic metastatic squamous cell carcinoma. Report of two cases showing histologic continuity between epidermis and metastasis. Arch Dermatol 1985;121(8):1041–3.
36. De Giorgi V, Grazzini M, Alfaioli B, et al. Cutaneous manifestations of breast carcinoma. Dermatol Ther 2010;23(6):581–9.
37. American Academy of D. Cutaneous metastatic disease. J Am Acad Dermatol 1995;33(2 Pt 1):161–82, quiz 183.
38. Habermehl G, Ko J. Cutaneous metastases: a review and diagnostic approach to tumors of unknown origin. Arch Pathol Lab Med 2019;143(8):943–57.
39. Lin F, Liu H. Immunohistochemistry in undifferentiated neoplasm/tumor of uncertain origin. Arch Pathol Lab Med 2014;138(12):1583–610.

Cosmetic Dermatology Concerns in Older Adults

Sheetal K. Sethupathi, MD[a], Mackenzie Poole, MBA[b],
Kavita Darji, MD[a], Jennifer Fehlman, MD[c],*

KEYWORDS

- Aging skin • Rhytids • Dyspigmentation • Androgenetic alopecia
- Male pattern hair loss • Female pattern hair loss • Cosmetic dermatology
- Cosmetic treatments

KEY POINTS

- Fine rhytids, skin texture, and dyspigmentation are best addressed by a multimodal treatment approach that combines an efficacious topical skin care regimen with resurfacing treatments including chemical peels, microneedling, or laser treatment.
- Dynamic rhytids and volume loss are commonly treated with neuromodulator injections and soft tissue filler injections.
- Hair loss, most commonly in the form of androgenetic alopecia (AGA), is a chronic, progressive process affecting most patients over 65 that can negatively impact self-esteem.
- An abundance of oral and topical medications, nutraceuticals, and minimally invasive treatments are available for AGA. Clinical trials have been largely heterogenous, and efficacy data are mixed.
- An individualized approach is essential in order to meet the specific goals and expectations of each patient when designing a treatment plan for cosmetic concerns.

INTRODUCTION

It is important to understand that each layer of facial tissue, from the underlying facial skeleton to the overlying skin, undergoes significant changes during the aging process. Bony support is lost along the mandible and maxilla and the orbital aperture widens.[1] Superficial and deep fat pads undergo volume loss and migration and the overlying skin begins to reveal signs of both intrinsic aging with skin laxity and fine rhytids as well as extrinsic aging in the form of coarse, deeper rhytids and dyspigmentation.[2,3] In a survey conducted of 610 dermatology patients aged 65 and older regarding

[a] Department of Dermatology, Saint Louis University, 1008 S Spring Avenue, Saint Louis, MO 63110, USA; [b] Saint Louis University School of Medicine, 1008 S Spring Avenue, Saint Louis, MO 63110, USA; [c] Saint Louis University SLU Care Physician Group -SSM Health, 2315 Dougherty Ferry Road, Suite 200C, Saint Louis, MO 63122, USA
* Corresponding author.
E-mail address: jennifer.a.fehlman@health.slu.edu

Clin Geriatr Med 40 (2024) 197–210
https://doi.org/10.1016/j.cger.2023.09.009
0749-0690/24/© 2023 Elsevier Inc. All rights reserved.

geriatric.theclinics.com

dermatologic concerns, one of the main concerns expressed by the patients was "aging/cosmetic."[4] Multiple treatments are available to target these concerns in the aging population including those of dyspigmentation, static and dynamic rhytids, skin laxity, skin texture, volume loss, and hair thinning. This article will focus on these common cosmetic concerns and the available treatment modalities used to address them.

SKIN CONCERNS
Topical Treatments

Approximately 80% of the photoaging of the face can be attributed to ultraviolet (UV) exposure.[5] UV radiation leads to the formation of reactive oxygen species within cells, and this oxidative stress in both the intracellular and extracellular environment is responsible for the findings seen in photoaging, including wrinkling and uneven pigmentation.[6] Therefore, sunscreen is an essential part of a skincare routine as it protects the skin from damaging UV radiation.[7] UVA radiation is responsible for photoaging and wrinkling of the skin, whereas UVB radiation is responsible for sunburns and many types of skin cancer. Broad-spectrum sunscreens protect against both UVA and UVB radiation.[8] Notably, sunscreens can be divided into chemical and physical categories. Chemical sunscreens, such as octinoxate, octisalate, oxybenzone, and avobenzone, contain aromatic compounds that absorb high-energy UV radiation and convert it into lower energy radiation, thus decreasing photo-induced damage to the skin. Comparatively, physical sunscreens, such as zinc oxide and titanium dioxide, reflect UV radiation away from the skin. High-quality evidence has shown that regular use of sunscreen minimizes signs of photoaging, including wrinkling, hyperpigmentation, and telangiectasias, while also decreasing incidence of actinic keratoses, squamous cell carcinoma, and melanoma.[9] The American Academy of Dermatology recommends daily broad-spectrum sun protection factor $\geq$30 sunscreen use with reapplication every 2 hours when outside.[10]

Topical retinoids are another important topical treatment in the prevention and treatment of skin aging. Vitamin A and its related natural and synthetic compounds are referred to as retinoids.[11] Retinoids work via binding to a nuclear receptor with subsequent alteration of gene expression. These compounds prevent and reduce signs of aging both clinically and histologically. Multiple studies have shown that the use of topical tretinoin can prevent and reduce signs of aging, including reducing fine and deep wrinkles, improving skin texture and pigmentation, and decreasing photoaging. Topical tretinoin has also been shown to increase epidermal thickness, increase collagen, and correct keratinocyte and melanocyte atypia.[5] Tretinoin is the most commonly used retinoid and has the most clinical evidence for efficacy in the prevention and treatment of photoaging; however, tazarotene and over-the-counter adapalene can be used as alternatives to tretinoin in the treatment of photoaging.[12] It is essential to educate patients regarding the most common side effects of topical retinoid use, including redness, irritation, dryness, burning, and photosensitization. Consistent use for 3 months is necessary prior to seeing results and patients should practice sun-protective behaviors while using topical retinoids.[5,11] Cosmeceutical alternatives to prescription tretinoin include retinols, which have also been shown to increase epidermal thickness and collagen synthesis. Retinols are often less irritating compared to tretinoin; however, these over-the-counter products are 20 times less potent than tretinoin, highly unstable, and lack robust clinical evidence in the treatment of photoaging.[5,12]

As previously discussed, one of the main factors driving photoaging is the production of free oxygen radicals induced by UV radiation. Vitamin C is an ingredient used in many cosmeceutical products, and it can reduce UV-induced free radical production and damage via its antioxidant properties.[13] Vitamin C is available in many formulations; however, L-ascorbic acid is the most common form and the most well studied. Vitamin C exerts its potent antiaging effects via antioxidant properties, collagen biosynthesis, antipigmentation, and replenishment of vitamin E.[14] Clinical studies have demonstrated efficacy of topical vitamin C in increasing collagen production, increasing thickness of the papillary dermis, and improving wound healing and skin hydration.[13,14] Moreover, studies have also demonstrated synergistic effects of topical vitamin C and vitamin E in cutaneous protection against oxidative stress, protecting against photoaging and tumorigenesis.[15,16] However, it is important to note that in order for vitamin C to have significant clinical effects, it must be in its active form in a concentration of 8% to 20%.[5]

Chemical Peels

Chemical peels are a treatment technique used to induce controlled injury to the layers of the skin with subsequent improvement in cosmesis and signs of UV-induced photoaging.[17] This procedure involves applying a caustic, toxic, or metabolically active substance to the skin by a trained professional with subsequent controlled destruction and exfoliation of layers of the skin and induction of a regenerative response in the epidermis and dermis. Peels can be divided into superficial, medium-depth, and deep peels, and the depth of the peel is determined by the substance used and its concentration.[18,19] Superficial peels exfoliate the epidermis and do not extend beyond the basal layer. Medium-depth peels exfoliate the epidermis and the papillary dermis. Deep peels exfoliate the epidermis and extend down to the lower portion of the dermis, the reticular dermis.[18] Each type of peel has different clinical applications and endpoints and the specific choice of a peel should depend on the patient's main cosmetic concerns.[19] The depth of a peel correlates with improvement in clinical outcomes but also an increased number of complications.[17]

Superficial chemical peels are suited for treatment of abnormal growths of the epidermis, including thin actinic keratoses, uneven epidermal pigmentation, including epidermal melasma and solar lentigines, and acne. Patients will typically experience postoperative peeling and erythema for 3 to 4 days.[19,20] The most commonly used superficial peel is glycolic acid, an alpha-hydroxy acid (AHA).[18] AHAs are weak acids that lead to discohesion of corneocytes in the epidermis with subsequent superficial exfoliation.[21] Glycolic acid has the lowest molecular weight of the AHAs, allowing for increased cutaneous penetration. Clinical studies have repeatedly documented the efficacy of glycolic acid in improving skin texture, reducing pore size, brightening skin, improving dyschromia, and decreasing fine wrinkles and photodamage.[20] Other commonly used superficial chemical peels include pyruvic acid, trichloroacetic acid (TCA) 10% to 30%, salicylic acid, tretinoin, and Jessner's solution. Of these superficial peels, glycolic acid and pyruvic acid are the only substances that require neutralization after application to prevent excess acidification of the skin.[17]

Medium-depth chemical peels are suitable for fine rhytids, skin laxity, and dermal melasma. Since these peels extend down to the papillary dermis, postoperative erythema and peeling last for approximately 7 days, and there is associated higher risk of scarring and post-inflammatory pigment alteration.[19] The classic medium-depth chemical peel is TCA 50%; however, it is rarely used given its unpredictable clinical results and high risk of scarring and dyspigmentation.[22] Instead, clinicians often use TCA 35% in combination with another agent that allows for depth of penetration down to the papillary dermis without the same complications as TCA 50% used alone.[22] Examples include Jessner's solution plus TCA 35%, solid CO_2 plus TCA

35%, and glycolic acid 70% plus TCA 35%.[17,23] The initial agent results in epidermal injury, allowing for deeper penetration of the lower concentration TCA peel with improved treatment outcomes.[22] TCA works via coagulation of membrane proteins and cell necrosis in the epidermis and dermis. After destruction, there is regeneration of new epidermal and dermal cells with synthesis of underlying collagen.[17,18] Complications of medium-depth peels include prolonged postoperative erythema, hyperpigmentation, hypopigmentation, scarring, and bacterial, fungal, and viral infections.[17]

Deep chemical peels are suitable for deep rhytids and scars, and postoperative erythema and peeling last for at least 10 to 12 days. Although these peels are associated with a significant risk for scarring and hypopigmentation, especially in darker Fitzpatrick skin types, they are highly efficacious, predictable, and can provide long-lasting results. Prior to the availability of resurfacing lasers, deep phenol-croton oil peels were the gold standard for facial rejuvenation.[19] However, they have fallen slightly out of favor given their association with significant complications and availability of fractional ablative laser resurfacing.[23] The classic deep chemical peel is the Baker-Gordon phenol-croton oil peel, composed of croton oil, phenol, water, and septisol.[24] Phenol works similarly to TCA in that it causes protein denaturation and coagulation. However, caution should be exercised when working with phenol-based peels due to the significant associated risk of cardiac arrhythmias, hepatic and renal toxicity, and dyspigmentation.[17,19] Intraoperative cardiac monitoring and sufficient hydration with intravenous fluids are imperative when using phenol-based peels. Other risks to note include scarring, usually more prominent along the lower face, acneiform dermatitis, and bacterial, viral, and fungal infections. Given the likelihood of comorbidities when caring for a geriatric patient, these peels may not be the safest treatment option.

Microneedling

Microneedling, or percutaneous collagen induction therapy, is a minimally invasive, less abrasive, and more cost-effective treatment modality for facial rejuvenation and treatment of aging skin. In contrast to resurfacing lasers and deep chemical peels which inflict ablative cutaneous trauma and induce a robust inflammatory response with propensity for scar formation, hypopigmentation, and hyperpigmentation, microneedling results in controlled cutaneous injury, promoting cutaneous regeneration rather than cicatrization.[25] In this therapeutic modality, the skin is repetitively punctured with sterile microneedles, creating minute openings in the epidermis and disrupting thickened papillary dermal collagen. This controlled cutaneous micro-injury stimulates a wound-healing response with the release of growth factors along with the synthesis of new collagen and elastic fibers.[26] The nonablative nature of microneedling nearly eliminates a risk of postoperative dyschromia, making it a safe treatment modality in patients with darker Fitzpatrick skin types.[27]

Histologic studies have shown that microneedling leads to increased epidermal thickness, dermal elastic fiber deposition, and expression of dermal collagens I and III.[28] Additionally, studies have shown that collagen bundles increase in number and thickness and become more loosely woven throughout the dermis.[25] Microneedling has multiple applications and has been used in the treatment of rhytids, skin rejuvenation, acne and postsurgical scarring, dyschromia, and melasma. Microneedling is most well studied in the treatment of acne scars; however, multiple clinical studies have demonstrated efficacy of microneedling in improving the appearance of tissue laxity and rhytids.[29] Needle length can be varied based on desired depth and anatomic area to be treated. Longer needles are usually used for thicker and more sebaceous skin, whereas shorter needles are used for thinner skin.[27]

Microneedling is considered a relatively safe esthetic procedure and is associated with relatively mild side effects and low rates of adverse effects. Common side effects of microneedling include redness, swelling, flaking, and pain of the skin which usually resolve after 2 to 3 days.[26,29] Although rare, microneedling can result in tram tracking.[25] The introduction of certain topical products via micro-conduits in the skin can lead to hypersensitivity reactions and, rarely, granulomatous reactions.[28,29] Therefore, it is important for the clinician to effectively counsel patients on postoperative skin and wound care. Microneedling does not carry the same risk of dyspigmentation as resurfacing lasers and chemical peels and is associated with decreased downtime compared to the aforementioned treatment modalities.[26]

Lasers

Lasers are considered the most effective therapeutic option for skin rejuvenation and the treatment of signs of aging.[25] Various different lasers exist that can be tailored for the treatment of various signs of aging, including benign vascular neoplasms, dyspigmentation, solar lentigines, skin textural changes, tissue laxity, and rhytids.[30]

Vascular lesions constitute one of the most common indications for laser treatment.[31] Cherry angiomas are common benign vascular neoplasms that increase in incidence with age, and telangiectasias are a common feature of facial photoaging.[32,33] The pulsed-dye laser (PDL) is the treatment of choice for many vascular lesions consisting of small vessels, including cherry angiomas and facial telangiectasias.[30] PDL utilizes selective photothermolysis to damage small cutaneous blood vessels and uses a wavelength of 585 to 595 nm to target oxyhemoglobin.[30,34] Side effects of PDL can include redness, swelling, hemorrhagic crusting, temporary or permanent dyspigmentation, and scarring.[34]

Photoaging caused by chronic UV exposure can lead to pigmentary alterations, including lentigines, ephelides, and uneven pigmentation.[35] Lasers for the treatment of pigmented lesions work via targeting the chromophore melanin.[36] When selecting a laser to target pigmented lesions, it is important to consider the patient's Fitzpatrick skin type, type of melanin content (pheomelanin versus eumelanin), and location of melanin in the skin—epidermal versus dermal.[31,36] A Wood's lamp can be used to assist in determining the depth of melanin within a lesion.[31] The main lasers used in the treatment of solar lentigines, which usually contain epidermal eumelanin, include the Q-switched (QS) 532 nm neodymium-doped yttrium aluminum garnet laser(-Nd:YAG), QS 694 nm ruby, and QS 755 alexandrite.[36] Ephelides can also be treated with laser, but response is less predictable compared to the treatment of solar lentigines.[31] Ephelides usually contain epidermal pheomelanin and are best targeted with QS 532 nm Nd:YAG.[31,36] The most common complication associated with laser therapy for pigmented lesions is dyschromia, with hyperpigmentation being more common than hypopigmentation. Of note, patients with darker Fitzpatrick skin type are at an increased risk of posttreatment dyschromia. Therefore, it is important for clinicians to effectively counsel patients prior to treatment. Scarring can rarely occur after treatment with these lasers.[31]

Laser resurfacing has largely replaced the use of chemical peels in the treatment of facial rejuvenation to target tissue laxity, rhytids, and uneven skin texture seen in aging.[37] Resurfacing lasers can be divided into ablative versus nonablative lasers and fractionated versus nonfractionated lasers.[38] Ablative lasers vaporize target tissues, whereas nonablative lasers heat the dermis and subcutaneous tissue, stimulating dermal collagen production and leaving target tissues intact.[38,39] Nonfractionated lasers treat the entire surface area of the target tissue, whereas fractionated lasers treat an evenly distributed percentage of the surface area of the target tissue.[38]

The mainstay ablative lasers include the 10,600 nm CO2 and 2940 nm erbium-doped yttrium aluminum garnet laser (Er:YAG). These ablative lasers target and heat water molecules, which, when turned into gas, lead to vaporization and removal of the epidermal layers. This results in collagen production as well as tightening of the epidermis and dermis.[38] Although highly effective, these ablative lasers are associated with significant adverse effects, including erythema, edema, scarring, dyspigmentation, prolonged postoperative downtime, and risk of bacterial, viral, and fungal infections.[31] Given the significant adverse effects associated with the use of traditional ablative lasers, fractionated ablative lasers have been developed that improve the side effect profile and shorten downtime while still resurfacing the skin more efficaciously compared to their nonablative counterparts.[37]

Nonablative resurfacing lasers are considered a safer alternative to the use of ablative laser given their more favorable side effect profile and shorter downtime.[40] Nonablative nonfractionated lasers stimulate collagen synthesis and remodeling of the dermis. Commonly used nonablative nonfractionated lasers include the 1319 nm, 1320 nm Nd:YAG, and 1450 nm diode. These lasers are gentler on the skin compared to their ablative counterparts, with minimal risk for complications and shorter downtime. However, clinical results are not as impressive and some studies have shown that these lasers produce minimal improvement in rhytids. Despite this, these lasers can be helpful in the treatment of acne and improving skin texture.[38]

Nonablative fractional lasers are gentle but more efficacious compared to nonablative nonfractionated lasers. Nonablative fractional lasers work via fractional photothermolysis—these lasers create microscopic thermal zones of injury in the target tissue that are surrounded by normal, untreated skin. Reepithelialization occurs over the first 24 hours, and there is transepidermal elimination of damaged collagen and dermal contents. Nonablative fractional lasers can be used in the treatment of acne and postsurgical scars, rhytids, dyschromia, and skin laxity.[41] Treatment with this class of lasers requires a moderate amount of downtime; however, they are safer in patients with darker Fitzpatrick skin types. Commonly used nonablative fractional lasers include the 1410 nm, 1440 nm Nd:YAG, 1540 nm, 1550 Er:YAG, and 1927 nm thulium fiber.[38] Nonablative fractional lasers have very low risk of complications, including dyschromia and scarring. However, they are less clinically efficacious than their ablative counterparts and often require multiple treatments.[37]

INJECTABLE TREATMENTS
Volume Loss

As skin ages, subcutaneous fat pad atrophy and volume loss lead to skin laxity, which is further exacerbated by photodamage over the years.[42] Volume loss is a major contributor to facial aging. Over the years, contour alterations lead to skin laxity, prominent nasolabial folds, hollow cheeks, jowling, and deep circles under the eyes. Volume restoration to support the nasojugal fold, malar and buccal fat pads, lateral lip commissures, perioral region, and pre-jowl sulcus can be helpful to create a more youthful appearance.[43] As a result, restoring facial volume by adding curves and contours with dermal fillers has been an important treatment approach in cosmetic dermatology.[44,45]

Various types of fillers exist to replete this facial volume loss. Most commonly used hyaluronic acid fillers consist of hyaluronic acid, an abundant polysaccharide of the extracellular matrix. Crosslinking techniques are used to connect hyaluronic acid polymer chains together, creating a gel.[45] A study of 61 patients with mean age of 57.4 years showed that midface volumization using low volumes of hyaluronic acid filler is effective and well tolerated, with patient-graded Global Aesthetic Improvement Scale scores showing that 73% to 89% of patients were very much to moderately improved.[46]

Non-hyaluronic acid fillers include calcium hydroxylapatite, poly-L-lactic acid, poly-methylmethacrylate, and autologous fat.[47] Calcium hydroxylapatite filler is composed of calcium hydroxylapatite microspheres suspended in an aqueous carrier gel. It is indicated in the United States to correct moderate to deep nasolabial folds as well as lipoatrophy in patients with human immunodeficiency virus.[48] Poly-L-lactic acid is a synthetic, biocompatible, biodegradable polymer that allows for long-lasting restoration of facial volume along with a stimulatory action on collagen formation.[49,50] Nonbiodegradable fillers, including polymethylmethacrylate and silicone, can incite a foreign body reaction that triggers a fibroblastic deposition of collagen around nonabsorbable microspheres.[51]

The use of dermal fillers should be tailored accordingly to each patient and performed by trained professionals to optimize safety and efficacy. Benefits and side effects should be weighed prior to use. Potential side effects of dermal fillers include bruising, edema, erythema, hyperpigmentation, infection, nodules, foreign body granulomas, paresthesia, arterial occlusion, and tissue necrosis.[51]

Muscle Tone & Neuromodulators

Over time, repetitive muscle contraction and muscle tone changes result in the appearance of superficial and deep dynamic rhytids. As a result, lines of facial expression become more apparent both at rest and with activity, contributing to hyperdynamic expressions.[42,52]

Neuromodulators can be used to treat certain facial lines of concern. Botulinum toxin (BTX) is the most common esthetic procedure, and it works to reduce the static and dynamic rhytides associated with the muscles of facial expression.[42] Serotypes A (BTX-A) and B (BTX-B) are commercially available, of which BTX-A is most commonly used to treat rhytids.[42] Currently, several BTXs are commercially available and hold Food and Drug Administration approvals for the treatment of moderate to severe forehead lines, lateral canthal lines, and glabellar lines. However, these products are often used off-label in additional anatomic areas as well. A study including subjects 18 to 75 years old treated with BTX showed progressive improvement in glabellar lines at rest, with the likelihood of significant response noted in older women greater than 55 years old with mild resting lines at baseline.[53] Another study evaluated 2 randomized, controlled phase 3 studies consisting of 1362 patients and concluded that BTX was effective and well-tolerated for lateral canthal line treatment, with injection pattern tailored according to the patient's lateral canthal line pattern.[54] Patient satisfaction has been reported after use of BTX treatment for facial rhytids. In a study of 60 females with mean age 42 ± 8.7 years, approximately 45% to 60% of patients reported looking younger by a mean of 3.5 to 5.8 years.[55]

BTX has been combined with other cosmetic treatment options for improved results. A prospective, randomized study evaluating 10 female patients showed that pretreatment of hyperdynamic facial lines with BTX before laser resurfacing led to improved results.[56] Moreover, in a study of 40 patients, it was shown that using BTX prior to cutaneous CO_2 laser resurfacing led to prolonged correction of movement-associated facial lines.[57] A study of 20 female subjects noted that hyaluronic acid filler and neurotoxin injections combined with a topical skin treatment regimen contributed to improved skin quality, optimized patient appearance, and increased patient satisfaction.[58]

Side effects of cosmetic use of BTX include pain, hematoma, swelling, localized bruising, headaches, injection site discomfort, excessive muscle weakness, and unintended paresis of adjacent muscles.[59] It is important to have knowledge of the target structures to allow for optimal dose and technique when injecting BTX.[60]

There are limited safety and efficacy data on the use of BTX in the elderly. It is important to develop a risk-benefit assessment prior to using BTX in the elderly patient in the setting of concomitant diseases and medications.[61]

HAIR LOSS
Background & Pathophysiology

In order to gain a holistic understanding of one's age-related cosmetic concerns, providers must consider the contribution of thinning hair on the perceived efficacy of facial rejuvenation treatments.[62]

Hair loss usually begins in the third or fourth decade and is a progressive process that impacts both men and women.[63,64] The most common cause of age-related hair loss is androgenetic alopecia(AGA) which leads to male pattern hair loss (MPHL) and female pattern hair loss (FPHL), respectively.[63,64] Peaking during the fifth decade, it is estimated that by age 65, up to 80% of Caucasian males and 75% of Caucasian females will be impacted by this condition.[62–64] Although less prevalent in patients of African, Latino, and Asian descent, AGA is a common source of concern for older adults of all backgrounds in both primary care and dermatology practices.[65,66] In a society that associates hair with physical beauty and youthfulness, the losing of one's hair represents a core loss of identity for many individuals and can lead to emotional distress.[64,66] Investigational studies of patients seeking care for AGA suggest that these patients experience decreased self-esteem, lower quality of life, and higher signs of anxiety and depression than patients without this concern.[62,66,67] It has been noted that the emotional impact of hair loss is more likely to negatively affect women, although both genders report facing increased stigmatization.[66–68] There are many current treatments on the market for hair loss, but these products do little to address the bearing that AGA has on one's self-image and relationships.[67]

It is widely accepted that dihydrotestosterone (DHT), the precursor molecule to testosterone, plays a large role in the pathogenesis of AGA.[63–65,67] DHT acts on androgen receptors in the hair follicle to result in the classic follicular miniaturization that is the hallmark of the condition. The net effect of this interaction is alteration in the hair cycle such that anagen is shortened, telogen is prolonged, and dermal papilla cells are lost into the dermal sheath with each cycle.[65,67] Terminal hairs are gradually converted into vellus hairs with decreased diameter in a typical pattern of distribution.[63,66,68] Cumulative exposure to extrinsic factors such as UV radiation, smoking, and pollution negatively impact the hair's strength and can accelerate hair aging.[62]

Clinical Presentation

Hair loss in AGA is of gradual onset characterized by increased hair shedding in a traditional pattern of distribution.[63] It must be considered that the threshold to perceive hair loss varies; a patient's self-perception of his/her hair loss and the impact it has on his/her quality of life does not always correlate with objective observations of hair loss by clinicians.[62,66] In MPHL, there is bitemporal thinning and recession of frontal hairline followed by thinning and eventual balding at the vertex.[63,68] FPHL often accelerates after menopause and features diffuse thinning between the frontal scalp and vertex, creating a more visible scalp with preserved frontal and temporal hairlines.[63,68] Various scales have attempted to quantify the extent of AGA, although the classification of severity plays little impact on treatment strategy in the clinical setting.[69]

AGA is diagnosed clinically based on the patient's age and pattern of hair loss. Rarely, diffuse alopecia areata may be mistaken for AGA in middle-aged patients.[63] Nevertheless, it may be worthwhile to rule-out underlying or comorbid telogen effluvium (TE), anagen effluvium, or alopecia secondary to a medical condition, specifically in older patients.[63,67] In older women presenting with hair loss and hirsutism, dehydroepiandrosterone sulfate and testosterone levels may be obtained to rule out a virilizing condition along the hypothalamic-pituitary-ovarian axis.[63,67] Thyroid studies may also be considered.[63,67] Iron studies and/or levels of B vitamins may prove useful if concomitant TE is suspected.[63,67] Finally, the patient's prescription medications and supplements should be reviewed, as these can contribute to or accelerate hair thinning.[63]

Topical and Oral Medications

In general, the goal of therapy is to restore and maintain hair density by reversing follicular miniaturization and promoting anagen.[65] Many topical, oral, and minimally invasive treatments for hair loss are commercially available and range extensively in level of proven efficacy, cost, and regulatory approval status. Although multiple therapies have shown benefit for increasing hair count, there has been a paucity of head-to-head trials between agents.[68]

Minoxidil, a vasodilating agent originally marketed for hypertension, has been the mainstay of treatment for AGA for decades in both men and women because of its ability to increase hair density and delay further progression. Topically, it is often prescribed as a 5% solution or foam applied once to twice daily.[62,64] Patients should be informed that they may experience increased hair shedding at the beginning of treatment.[64] Although oral minoxidil is often prescribed off-label, as only topical formulations are approved for AGA in any country, multiple reviews of studies assessing the use of oral minoxidil have found this to be a safe and convenient treatment with 61% to 100% of patients reporting objective clinical improvement.[64,70–72] Daily starting doses of 2.5 to 5 mg for men and 0.5 to 2.5 mg for women with uptitration at 3-month intervals as clinically indicated are recommended.[72] Hypertrichosis can be experienced as a side effect in patients taking oral minoxidil, and although these doses are well below the 10 to 40 mg doses used to treat hypertension, there is a risk of orthostatic hypotension, tachycardia, fluid retention, and renal injury.[64,71,72] This is an important consideration in geriatric patients who may be predisposed to developing hypotension or have existing chronic kidney disease. Patients should understand that oral minoxidil is being prescribed for an off-label indication.[72]

Finasteride, a 5-alpha reductase inhibitor that decreases DHT production, can be used for males with MPHL. It is typically prescribed as a once-daily 1-mg or 5-mg oral dose.[64,65] Patients should be warned about the risk of sexual dysfunction, which sometimes persists past treatment discontinuation, as well as gynecomastia and depression in predisposed individuals.[64,65,68] Patients with an increased risk of prostate cancer should also understand that finasteride may falsely lower prostate specific antigen levels.[64] Evidence suggests that combination therapy with finasteride and topical minoxidil may be more efficacious than either agent used alone.[64,68] For both forms of minoxidil and finasteride, satisfaction with treatment should be re-evaluated after 6 months before deciding whether additional therapy is needed.[64,68]

Nutraceuticals

Given that adequate vitamins and minerals are needed to support the process of hair growth, natural ingredients are often targeted as a hair loss solution. As many as 81% of patients with alopecia report the use of supplements, mostly biotin, vitamin B12, or vitamin D, although no studies have supported their use as monotherapy in alopecia.[73]

While these interventions are generally viewed as harmless, it must be noted that that they can become quite expensive over time and interact with common medications.[68,73] Though many natural products have demonstrated positive results, perhaps the best studied is saw palmetto (Serenoa repens), a 5a-reductase inhibitor.[68,73]

Two multi-ingredient nutraceutical products have gained popularity with patients and providers. Nutrafol (Nutraceutical Wellness) contains a 21-ingredient Synergen complex with antioxidant, anti-DHT, and anti-inflammatory properties; it is taken 4 times daily.[68,73,74] Viviscal (Lifes2good Inc), taken 2 times daily, contains an AminoMar C marine protein complex with extracellular matrix components of sharks and mollusks among other vitamins and minerals.[68,73,74] Both products are sold in multiple formulations and strengths.[73,74] They have been shown to improve the subjective appearance of hair in multiple randomized, double-blind, placebo-controlled clinical trials, although these studies contain relatively few subjects that were selected on the basis of perceived hair thinning alone.[73,74] Patients should be reminded that these supplements are not subject to the same safety and efficacy standards as other medications.[68,73,74]

Adjunctive and Emerging Therapies

Although clinical trials have been limited, several adjunctive therapies exist. Low-level light therapy is a noninvasive option that can be used alone or in combination with topical or oral therapies to promote hair growth through increased vasodilation in the scalp.[64,65,68] Multiple devices are available without a prescription and require patients to wear caps for a specific amount of time each week.[65,68] Platelet-rich plasma (PRP) injections are another investigational therapy performed in the outpatient setting.[64,65,68] Although techniques have not been standardized across clinical trials, treatment is generally performed monthly for several sessions followed by less frequent maintenance therapy.[65,68] Microneedling, especially when used as an adjunct to topical medications or PRP, may promote neovascularization and increase hair counts according to a limited number of studies.[65,68] Finally, hair transplantation can be considered for refractory cases. Graft survival rates are around 90%, and combination therapy with finasteride or minoxidil before and after therapy may limit postoperative progression.[64,68]

Practical Considerations of Therapy

Given the condition's chronicity, treatments require lifelong maintenance in order to be efficacious.[64,65,68] Patients should understand that compliance is paramount in achieving desirable results, and the feasibility of a given treatment strategy should be taken into consideration when tailoring a regimen to an individual patient.[68] While oral medications may be easier from a compliance perspective, they are also associated with an increased risk of adverse effects.[68] The costs associated with lifelong treatment should also be discussed. In medically complex adults, potential side effects and drug/supplement interactions need to be considered to mitigate the risks of polypharmacy. It should also be noted that the median age in most clinical trials of medications and nutraceuticals is between 40 to 50 years of age such that safety profiles from these studies may not be representative of the geriatric population.[64,71,73,74] Given the abundance of possible therapies, it is important for primary care providers to have a basic understanding of the risks, benefits, practicality, and costs of the various options available.[68] Even basic measures such as wearing a hat to decrease UV light and pollutant exposure, ensuring adequate dietary exposure to key vitamins and minerals, and smoking cessation can help slow hair loss.[62,65,67,74] Assessing the patient's chief concerns and esthetic goals in order to ensure that expectations of therapy are realistic can allow providers to understand when referral to a dermatologist or hair loss specialist is necessary.[62,68]

SUMMARY

Cosmetic concerns are common and important to our older patient population. Each patient would benefit from an individualized treatment plan that may include some of the common interventions described earlier, with special consideration to select the modality with a favorable side effect profile given any underlying comorbidities. It is also always critical to set up realistic expectations of results prior to treatment.

DISCLOSURE

The authors have no relevant disclosures.

REFERENCES

1. Mendelson B, Wong CH. Changes in the facial skeleton with aging: implications and clinical applications in facial rejuvenation. Aesthetic Plast Surg 2012;36(4): 753–60.
2. Sunder S. Relevant topical skin care products for prevention and treatment of aging skin. Facial Plast Surg Clin North Am 2019;27(3):413–8.
3. Sadick NS, Dorizas AS, Krueger N, et al. The facial adipose system: its role in facial aging and approaches to volume restoration. Dermatol Surg 2015;41: S333–9.
4. Dabade TS, Shaw RT, Benlagha I, et al. Dermatologic concerns and provider preferences of adults aged ≥65 years: results of a national survey. J Am Acad Dermatol 2022;86(5):1151–4. Epub 20210424.
5. Berry K, Hallock K, Lam C. Photoaging and topical rejuvenation. Facial Plast Surg Clin North Am 2022;30(3):291–300.
6. Masaki H. Role of antioxidants in the skin: anti-aging effects. J Dermatol Sci 2010; 58(2):85–90. Epub 20100317.
7. Bennett SL, Khachemoune A. Dispelling myths about sunscreen. J Dermatolog Treat 2022;33(2):666–70. Epub 20200707.
8. Guan LL, Lim HW, Mohammad TF. Sunscreens and photoaging: a review of current literature. Am J Clin Dermatol 2021;22(6):819–28.
9. Sander M, Sander M, Burbidge T, et al. The efficacy and safety of sunscreen use for the prevention of skin cancer. CMAJ (Can Med Assoc J) 2020;192(50): E1802–8.
10. Dermatology AAo. Sunscreen FAQs: AAD; 2023 23 March 2023. Available at: https://www.aad.org/media/stats-sunscreen.
11. Mukherjee S, Date A, Patravale V, et al. Retinoids in the treatment of skin aging: an overview of clinical efficacy and safety. Clin Interv Aging 2006;1(4):327–48.
12. Milosheska D, Roskar R. Use of retinoids in topical antiaging treatments: a focused review of clinical evidence for conventional and nanoformulations. Adv Ther 2022;39(12):5351–75.
13. Mumtaz S, Ali S, Tahir HM, et al. Aging and its treatment with vitamin C: a comprehensive mechanistic review. Mol Biol Rep 2021;48(12):8141–53. Epub 20211015.
14. Al-Niaimi F, Chiang NYZ. Topical vitamin C and the skin: mechanisms of action and clinical applications. J Clin Aesthet Dermatol 2017;10(7):14–7. Epub 20170701. PubMed PMID: 29104718; PubMed Central PMCID: PMC5605218.

15. Lin FH, Lin JY, Gupta RD, et al. Ferulic acid stabilizes a solution of vitamins C and E and doubles its photoprotection of skin. J Invest Dermatol 2005;125(4):826–32.

16. Lin JY, Selim MA, Shea CR, et al. UV photoprotection by combination topical antioxidants vitamin C and vitamin E. J Am Acad Dermatol 2003;48(6):866–74.

17. Lee KC, Wambier CG, Soon SL, et al, International Peeling Society. Basic chemical peeling: superficial and medium-depth peels. J Am Acad Dermatol 2019; 81(2):313–24. Epub 20181211.

18. Fischer TC, Perosino E, Poli F, et al, Cosmetic Dermatology European Expert Group. Cosmetic Dermatology European Expert G. Chemical peels in aesthetic dermatology: an update 2009. J Eur Acad Dermatol Venereol 2010;24(3): 281–92. Epub 20090908.

19. Obagi S, Dover JS. In: *Chemical peels: procedures in cosmetic dermatology.* 3rd Edition. St. Louis, MO: Elsevier; 2021. p. 1–194.

20. Sharad J. Glycolic acid peel therapy - a current review. Clin Cosmet Investig Dermatol 2013;6:281–8.

21. Moghimipour E. Hydroxy acids, the most widely used anti-aging agents. Jundishapur J Nat Pharm Prod 2012;7(1):9–10. Epub 20120104. PubMed PMID: 24624144; PubMed Central PMCID: PMC3941867.

22. Williams JD, Elston DM, Treat JR, et al. Andrews' diseases of the skin. 13th edition. Philadelphia, PA: Elsevier Inc; 2020.

23. Starkman SJ, Mangat DS. Chemical peel (deep, medium, light). Facial Plast Surg Clin North Am 2020;28(1):45–57.

24. Wambier CG, Lee KC, Soon SL, et al, International Peeling Society. Advanced chemical peels: phenol-croton oil peel. J Am Acad Dermatol 2019;81(2): 327–36. Epub 20181211.

25. Atiyeh BS, Abou Ghanem O, Chahine F. Microneedling: percutaneous collagen induction (PCI) therapy for management of scars and photoaged skin-scientific evidence and review of the literature. Aesthetic Plast Surg 2021;45(1):296–308. Epub 20200901.

26. Sitohang IBS, Sirait SAP, Suryanegara J. Microneedling in the treatment of atrophic scars: a systematic review of randomised controlled trials. Int Wound J 2021;18(5):577–85.

27. Alessa D, Bloom JD. Microneedling options for skin rejuvenation, including non-temperature-controlled fractional microneedle radiofrequency treatments. Facial Plast Surg Clin North Am 2020;28(1):1–7.

28. Juhasz MLW, Cohen JL. Microneedling for the treatment of scars: an update for clinicians. Clin Cosmet Investig Dermatol 2020;13:997–1003.

29. Alster TS, Graham PM. Microneedling: a review and practical guide. Dermatol Surg 2018;44(3):397–404.

30. Fowler GC. Pfenninger & fowler's procedures for primary care. 4th edition. Canada: Elsevier; 2020.

31. Tanzi EL, Dover JS. Procedures in cosmetic dermatology: lasers, lights, and energy devices. 5th edition. Philadelphia, PA: Elsevier; 2023.

32. Buslach N, Foulad DP, Saedi N, et al. Treatment modalities for cherry angiomas: a systematic review. Dermatol Surg 2020;46(12):1691–7.

33. Mekic S, Hamer MA, Wigmann C, et al. Epidemiology and determinants of facial telangiectasia: a cross-sectional study. J Eur Acad Dermatol Venereol 2020; 34(4):821–6. Epub 20191125.

34. Nischwitz SP, Lumenta DB, Spendel S, et al. Minimally invasive technologies for treatment of HTS and keloids: pulsed-dye laser. In: Teot L, Mustoe TA,

Middelkoop E, et al, editors. Textbook on scar management: state of the art management and emerging technologies. Cham: CH; 2020. p. 263–9.

35. Han A, Chien AL, Kang S. Photoaging. Dermatol Clin. 2014;32(3):291–9. https://doi.org/10.1016/j.det.2014.03.015. PubMed PMID: 24891052.

36. Passeron T. Lasers. Ann Dermatol Venereol. 2012;139(Suppl 4):S159–65. https://doi.org/10.1016/S0151-9638(12)70129-1. PubMed PMID: 23522632.

37. Pozner JN, DiBernardo BE. Laser resurfacing: full field and fractional. Clin Plast Surg 2016;43(3):515–25. Epub 20160513.

38. Preissig J, Hamilton K, Markus R. Current laser resurfacing technologies: a review that delves beneath the surface. Semin Plast Surg 2012;26(3):109–16. PubMed PMID: 23904818; PubMed Central PMCID: PMC3580982.

39. Ciocon DH, Doshi D, Goldberg DJ. Non-ablative lasers. Curr Probl Dermatol 2011;42:48–55. Epub 20110816.

40. Akerman L, Mimouni D, Nosrati A, et al. A combination of non-ablative laser and hyaluronic acid injectable for postacne scars: a novel treatment protocol. J Clin Aesthet Dermatol 2022;15(3):53–6.

41. Narurkar VA. Nonablative fractional laser resurfacing. Dermatol Clin 2009;27(4):473–8.

42. Ogden S, Griffiths TW. A review of minimally invasive cosmetic procedures. Br J Dermatol 2008;159(5):1036–50.

43. Carruthers JD, Carruthers A. Facial sculpting and tissue augmentation. Dermatol Surg 2005;31(11 Pt 2):1604–12.

44. Luebberding S, Alexiades-Armenakas M. Facial volume augmentation in 2014: overview of different filler options. J Drugs Dermatol 2013;12(12):1339–44.

45. Wongprasert P, Dreiss CA, Murray G. Evaluating hyaluronic acid dermal fillers: a critique of current characterization methods. Dermatol Ther 2022;35(6):e15453.

46. Wilson MV, Fabi SG, Greene R. Correction of age-related midface volume loss with low-volume hyaluronic acid filler. JAMA Facial Plast Surg 2017;19(2):88–93.

47. Trinh LN, Gupta A. Non-hyaluronic acid fillers for midface augmentation: a systematic review. Facial Plast Surg 2021;37(4):536–42.

48. Graivier MH, Bass LS, Busso M, et al. Calcium hydroxylapatite (Radiesse) for correction of the mid- and lower face: consensus recommendations. Plast Reconstr Surg 2007;120(6 Suppl):55S–66S.

49. Fitzgerald R, Bass LM, Goldberg DJ, et al. Physiochemical characteristics of poly-L-lactic acid (PLLA). Aesthetic Surg J 2018;38(suppl_1):S13–7.

50. Ezzat WH, Keller GS. The use of poly-L-lactic acid filler in facial aesthetics. Facial Plast Surg 2011;27(6):503–9.

51. Funt D, Pavicic T. Dermal fillers in aesthetics: an overview of adverse events and treatment approaches. Clin Cosmet Investig Dermatol 2013;6:295–316.

52. Swift A, Liew S, Weinkle S, et al. The facial aging process from the "inside out". Aesthetic Surg J 2021;41(10):1107–19.

53. Carruthers A, Carruthers J, Fagien S, et al. Repeated OnabotulinumtoxinA treatment of glabellar lines at rest over three treatment cycles. Dermatol Surg 2016;42(9):1094–101.

54. Carruthers A, Bruce S, Cox SE, et al. OnabotulinumtoxinA for treatment of moderate to severe crow's feet lines: a review. Aesthetic Surg J 2016;36(5):591–7.

55. Carruthers A, Carruthers J. A single-center dose-comparison study of botulinum neurotoxin type A in females with upper facial rhytids: assessing patients' perception of treatment outcomes. J Drugs Dermatol 2009;8(10):924–9.

56. Zimbler MS, Holds JB, Kokoska MS, et al. Effect of botulinum toxin pretreatment on laser resurfacing results: a prospective, randomized, blinded trial. Arch Facial Plast Surg 2001;3(3):165–9.

57. West TB, Alster TS. Effect of botulinum toxin type A on movement-associated rhytides following CO2 laser resurfacing. Dermatol Surg 1999;25(4):259–61.

58. Dayan SH, Ho TVT, Bacos JT, et al. A randomized study to assess the efficacy of skin rejuvenation therapy in combination with neurotoxin and full facial filler treatments. J Drugs Dermatol 2018;17(1):48–54.

59. Dorizas A, Krueger N, Sadick NS. Aesthetic uses of the botulinum toxin. Dermatol Clin 2014;32(1):23–36.

60. Wollina U, Konrad H. Managing adverse events associated with botulinum toxin type A: a focus on cosmetic procedures. Am J Clin Dermatol 2005;6(3):141–50.

61. Cheng CM. Cosmetic use of botulinum toxin type A in the elderly. Clin Interv Aging 2007;2(1):81–3.

62. Ahluwalia J, Fabi SG. The psychological and aesthetic impact of age-related hair changes in females. J Cosmet Dermatol 2019;jocd:12960.

63. Feinstein R, Khardori R, Butler D, Chan E, Sperling L. Androgenetic Alopecia. Medscape.

64. Kanti V, Messenger A, Dobos G, et al. Evidence-based (S3) guideline for the treatment of androgenetic alopecia in women and in men – short version. J Eur Acad Dermatol Venereol 2018;32(1):11–22.

65. Wall D, Meah N, Fagan N, et al. Advances in hair growth. Fac Rev 2022;11. https://doi.org/10.12703/r/11-1.

66. Huang CH, Fu Y, Chi CC. Health-related quality of life, depression, and self-esteem in patients with androgenetic alopecia. JAMA Dermatol 2021;157(8):963.

67. Chen S, Xie X, Zhang G, et al. Comorbidities in androgenetic alopecia: a comprehensive review. Dermatol Ther 2022;12(10):2233–47.

68. Nestor MS, Ablon G, Gade A, et al. Treatment options for androgenetic alopecia: efficacy, side effects, compliance, financial considerations, and ethics. J Cosmet Dermatol 2021;20(12):3759–81.

69. Gupta M, Mysore V. Classifications of patterned hair loss: a review. J Cutan Aesthet Surg 2016;9(1):3.

70. Gupta AK, Venkataraman M, Talukder M, et al. Relative efficacy of minoxidil and the 5-α reductase inhibitors in androgenetic alopecia treatment of male patients. JAMA Dermatol 2022;158(3):266.

71. Sharma AN, Michelle L, Juhasz M, et al. Low-dose oral minoxidil as treatment for non-scarring alopecia: a systematic review. Int J Dermatol 2020;59(8):1013–9.

72. Vañó-Galván S, Pirmez R, Hermosa-Gelbard A, et al. Safety of low-dose oral minoxidil for hair loss: a multicenter study of 1404 patients. J Am Acad Dermatol 2021;84(6):1644–51.

73. Drake L, Reyes-Hadsall S, Martinez J, et al. Evaluation of the safety and effectiveness of nutritional supplements for treating hair loss. JAMA Dermatol 2023; 159(1):79.

74. Ring C, Heitmiller K, Correia E, et al. Nutraceuticals for androgenetic alopecia. Journal of Clinical and Aesthetic Dermatology 2022;15(3):26–9.

Moving?

Make sure your subscription moves with you!

To notify us of your new address, find your **Clinics Account Number** (located on your mailing label above your name), and contact customer service at:

Email: journalscustomerservice-usa@elsevier.com

800-654-2452 (subscribers in the U.S. & Canada)
314-447-8871 (subscribers outside of the U.S. & Canada)

Fax number: 314-447-8029

Elsevier Health Sciences Division
Subscription Customer Service
3251 Riverport Lane
Maryland Heights, MO 63043

*To ensure uninterrupted delivery of your subscription, please notify us at least 4 weeks in advance of move.

Printed and bound by CPI Group (UK) Ltd, Croydon, CR0 4YY

03/10/2024

01040473-0004